Navigation Assisted Robotics in Spine and Trauma Surgery

Wei Tian
Editor

Navigation Assisted Robotics in Spine and Trauma Surgery

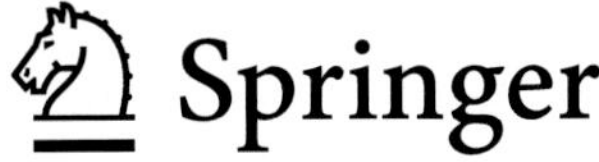
Springer

Editor
Wei Tian
Department of Spine Surgery
Beijing Jishuitan Hospital
Fourth Clinical Hospital of
Peking University
Beijing
China

ISBN 978-981-15-1848-5 ISBN 978-981-15-1846-1 (eBook)
https://doi.org/10.1007/978-981-15-1846-1

This Springer imprint is published by the registered company Springer Nature Singapore Pte Ltd.
The registered company address is: 152 Beach Road, #21-01/04 Gateway East, Singapore 189721, Singapore

Foreword

Computer-assisted orthopedic surgery is undergoing rapid developments in recent years. Professor Tian and his orthopedic team from Beijing Jishuitan Hospital are in the forefront of advancing this field in China by performing a remarkable number of computer-assisted orthopedic cases. Their center have contributed to the international advancement of the field by training computer-assisted surgical techniques to professionals from different countries.

I first met Professor Tian in the spring of 2016 while I was invited to the Jishuitan Forum in Beijing, China. From very first meeting, I noticed his passion for robot-assisted surgery. Later, I continued to collaborate with Beijing medical robotics innovation development center. The first summit of the center in 2018 was organized and managed by Professor Tian. As a colleague, I am proud to see the immense contributions of Professor Tian to the field through his live demonstrations and lectures aiming at improving and popularizing robot-assisted orthopedic surgery in China.

In the recent years, Professor Tian and his team has focused on robotic technique and 5G remote orthopedic surgery capitalizing on the world-wide expansion of 5G communications. Professor Tian performed the world's first robot-assisted upper cervical surgery using Tianji robotic system in 2015. On June 27 2019, the world's first multi-center 5G remote robot-assisted orthopaedic surgery was performed by Prof. Tian's team.

This book compiles a large number of new cases involving robot-assisted minimally-invasive surgical techniques. The book may serve as a great reference for orthopedic surgeons who are interested in performing robot-assisted surgery as it documents the authors' prior valuable experiences. Furthermore, the book nicely represents the contribution of researchers in china to the global progress of robot-assisted orthopaedic surgery. I commend Professor Tian and have the highest appreciation for his continued and tireless efforts to internationally advance and promote collaboration in this exciting field.

Mehran Armand, Ph.D.
Director, Biomechanical- and Image-Guided Surgical Systems Laboratory
Co-director, Laboratory for Neuroplastic Surgery Research
Research Professor, Department of Mechanical Engineering
Associate Professor, Department of Orthopaedic Surgery
Johns Hopkins University, Baltimore, Maryland, USA

Preface

Since the beginning of the twenty-first century, the technological revolution has brought tremendous changes into everyday life. Patients have higher demands for medical service and, thus, minimal invasion has become the primary request for surgical treatment. Conversely, with the explosive development of, both, hardware and software, surgeons have more advanced equipment and techniques to fulfill the patient's need.

The limitations of the human hand and eye have always been an insurmountable obstacle in the development of spine and pelvic surgery. As the spine and pelvis are closely surrounded by vital neural and vascular structures, surgeons must operate with extremely high accuracy to avoid fatal consequences. Furthermore, accurate manipulation is essential for stable fixation and sufficient decompression. To overcome this obstacle, a revolutionary technique known as computer-assisted orthopedic surgery (CAOS) has undergone rapid development in recent years. With the help of navigation and robotic systems, the persistent limitation that followed freehand and intraoperative fluoroscopy techniques could easily be resolved. Minimally invasive spine surgery (MISS) is safer and easier for surgeons to operate using computer-assisted techniques. The huge innovation of CAOS has been of great benefit as a minimally invasive treatment for patients.

Research and development of robot-assisted orthopedic technology in China was initiated nearly 20 years ago. As one of the precursors, I deeply observe the rapid progress in my professional field raised by orthopedic robot technology. As a significant part of CAOS, the importance of orthopedic robotic techniques has been recognized worldwide. Nowadays, more than 30 different types of orthopedic robots have been released, but no more than 10 types have been applied in clinical practice. From 2002, Beijing Jishuitan Hospital started to build a team with Beihang University, Beijing Tinavi Medical Technology Company, and the Shenzhen Institute of Advanced Technology of the Chinese Academy of Science. The Tianji (Tinavi®) orthopedic robotic system, the first Chinese orthopedic robotic system, was developed by this team, which is a collaboration of clinical, industrial, scientific, and commercial power. The invention of the Tianji orthopedic robotic system expands our conception of computer-assisted minimally invasive spine surgery (CAMISS). It is a new milestone in intelligent orthopedics.

In recent years, the sales and application of orthopedic robots have been increasing. However, in China, we found that robotic equipment was often left unused in their hospitals. This was because many surgeons still find this new technique too complex to handle. Contrary to the original intention, the accuracy and safety of the operation can be even worse if the surgeon does not follow the standard procedures of the robotic system. To create a standard operation tutorial for navigation assisted orthopedic robotic surgery, we have edited this book to systemically introduce navigation-assisted robotic surgery in spine and trauma surgery, from equipment to facilities, surgical procedures to postoperative complications, and staff training to perioperative cooperation, we can share our experience in robotic surgery for spine and trauma diseases, especially in minimally invasive surgery. This book was organized into two parts. The first part relates to spine surgery, including pedicle screw fixation on the cervical, thoracic, and lumbar spine; dens and Magerl screw fixations; PVP; PKP; and MED. The second part relates to trauma surgery, which covers screw fixation in pelvic and acetabulum fractures and fibular grafting in femoral head osteonecrosis. We hope this book can serve as an ideal reference for everyone involved in orthopedic robotic surgery, whether they are trainees, senior surgeons, nurses, or technical staff.

I thank all my Jishuitan hospital colleagues, whose precious clinical experience is the absolute core of this book. Special thanks go to Springer and editors, Mrs. Sasirekka Nijanthan and Mr. James Hu, who have contributed to bringing this book to fruition. Without them and all the contributing authors of each chapter, this book could not be published so soon. A sincere thank you to all of you.

Beijing, China
March, 2020

Wei Tian

Contents

List of Contributors

Editor

Wei Tian Department of Spine Surgery, Beijing Jishuitan Hospital, Fourth Clinical Hospital of Peking University, Beijing, China

Beijing Key Laboratory of Robotic Orthopaedics, Beijing, China

Deputy Editor

Xinbao Wu Trauma Orthopedic, Beijing Jishuitan Hospital, Fourth Clinical Hospital of Peking University, Beijing, China

Bo Liu Department of Spine Surgery, Beijing Jishuitan Hospital, Fourth Clinical Hospital of Peking University, Beijing, China

Yajun Liu Department of Spine Surgery, Beijing Jishuitan Hospital, Fourth Clinical Hospital of Peking University, Beijing, China

Junqiang Wang Trauma Orthopedic, Beijing Jishuitan Hospital, Fourth Clinical Hospital of Peking University, Beijing, China

Edit Secretary

Yajun Liu Department of Spine Surgery, Beijing Jishuitan Hospital, Fourth Clinical Hospital of Peking University, Beijing, China

Cheng Zeng Department of Spine Surgery, Beijing Jishuitan Hospital, Fourth Clinical Hospital of Peking University, Beijing, China

Contributors

Yan An Department of Spine Surgery, Beijing Jishuitan Hospital, Fourth Clinical Hospital of Peking University, Beijing, China

Shanlin Chen Department of Hand Surgery, Beijing Jishuitan Hospital, Fourth Clinical Hospital of Peking University, Beijing, China

Guanyu Cui Department of Spine Surgery, Beijing Jishuitan Hospital, Fourth Clinical Hospital of Peking University, Beijing, China

Mingxing Fan Department of Spine Surgery, Beijing Jishuitan Hospital, Fourth Clinical Hospital of Peking University, Beijing, China

Shuo Feng Department of Spine Surgery, Beijing Jishuitan Hospital, Fourth Clinical Hospital of Peking University, Beijing, China

Wei Han Trauma Orthopedic, Beijing Jishuitan Hospital, Fourth Clinical Hospital of Peking University, Beijing, China

Xiao Han Department of Spine Surgery, Beijing Jishuitan Hospital, Fourth Clinical Hospital of Peking University, Beijing, China

Xiaoguang Han Department of Spine Surgery, Beijing Jishuitan Hospital, Fourth Clinical Hospital of Peking University, Beijing, China

Da He Department of Spine Surgery, Beijing Jishuitan Hospital, Fourth Clinical Hospital of Peking University, Beijing, China

Meng He Trauma Orthopedic, Beijing Jishuitan Hospital, Fourth Clinical Hospital of Peking University, Beijing, China

Lin Hu Department of Spine Surgery, Beijing Jishuitan Hospital, Fourth Clinical Hospital of Peking University, Beijing, China

Jile Jiang Department of Spine Surgery, Beijing Jishuitan Hospital, Fourth Clinical Hospital of Peking University, Beijing, China

Peihao Jin Department of Spine Surgery, Beijing Jishuitan Hospital, Fourth Clinical Hospital of Peking University, Beijing, China

Zhao Lang Department of Spine Surgery, Beijing Jishuitan Hospital, Fourth Clinical Hospital of Peking University, Beijing, China

Nan Li Department of Spine Surgery, Beijing Jishuitan Hospital, Fourth Clinical Hospital of Peking University, Beijing, China

Zhiyu Li Department of Spine Surgery, Beijing Jishuitan Hospital, Fourth Clinical Hospital of Peking University, Beijing, China

Bo Liu Department of Spine Surgery, Beijing Jishuitan Hospital, Fourth Clinical Hospital of Peking University, Beijing, China

Wenyong Liu School of Biological Science and Medical Engineering, Beihang University, Beijing, China

Yajun Liu Department of Spine Surgery, Beijing Jishuitan Hospital, Fourth Clinical Hospital of Peking University, Beijing, China

Sai Ma Department of Spine Surgery, Beijing Jishuitan Hospital, Fourth Clinical Hospital of Peking University, Beijing, China

Jianping Mao Department of Spine Surgery, Beijing Jishuitan Hospital, Fourth Clinical Hospital of Peking University, Beijing, China

Yonggang Su Trauma Orthopedic, Beijing Jishuitan Hospital, Fourth Clinical Hospital of Peking University, Beijing, China

Xiaohui Tao Department of Spine Surgery, Beijing Jishuitan Hospital, Fourth Clinical Hospital of Peking University, Beijing, China

Wei Tian Department of Spine Surgery, Beijing Jishuitan Hospital, Fourth Clinical Hospital of Peking University, Beijing, China

Beijing Key Laboratory of Robotic Orthopaedics, Beijing, China

Han Wang Department of Spine Surgery, Beijing Jishuitan Hospital, Fourth Clinical Hospital of Peking University, Beijing, China

Huadong Wang Department of Spine Surgery, Beijing Jishuitan Hospital, Fourth Clinical Hospital of Peking University, Beijing, China

Junqiang Wang Trauma Orthopedic, Beijing Jishuitan Hospital, Fourth Clinical Hospital of Peking University, Beijing, China

Yongqing Wang Department of Spine Surgery, Beijing Jishuitan Hospital, Fourth Clinical Hospital of Peking University, Beijing, China

Yu Wang School of Biological Science and Medical Engineering, Beihang University, Beijing, China

Yi Wei Department of Spine Surgery, Beijing Jishuitan Hospital, Fourth Clinical Hospital of Peking University, Beijing, China

Jingye Wu Department of Spine Surgery, Beijing Jishuitan Hospital, Fourth Clinical Hospital of Peking University, Beijing, China

Xinbao Wu Trauma Orthopedic, Beijing Jishuitan Hospital, Fourth Clinical Hospital of Peking University, Beijing, China

Xinfeng Wu Department of Spine Surgery, Beijing Jishuitan Hospital, Fourth Clinical Hospital of Peking University, Beijing, China

Bin Xiao Department of Spine Surgery, Beijing Jishuitan Hospital, Fourth Clinical Hospital of Peking University, Beijing, China

Yonggang Xing Department of Spine Surgery, Beijing Jishuitan Hospital, Fourth Clinical Hospital of Peking University, Beijing, China

Yunfeng Xu Department of Spine Surgery, Beijing Jishuitan Hospital, Fourth Clinical Hospital of Peking University, Beijing, China

Kai Yan Department of Spine Surgery, Beijing Jishuitan Hospital, Fourth Clinical Hospital of Peking University, Beijing, China

Jie Yu Department of Spine Surgery, Beijing Jishuitan Hospital, Fourth Clinical Hospital of Peking University, Beijing, China

Ning Yuan Department of Spine Surgery, Beijing Jishuitan Hospital, Fourth Clinical Hospital of Peking University, Beijing, China

Qiang Yuan Department of Spine Surgery, Beijing Jishuitan Hospital, Fourth Clinical Hospital of Peking University, Beijing, China

Cheng Zeng Department of Spine Surgery, Beijing Jishuitan Hospital, Fourth Clinical Hospital of Peking University, Beijing, China

Ning Zhang Department of Spine Surgery, Beijing Jishuitan Hospital, Fourth Clinical Hospital of Peking University, Beijing, China

Teng Zhang Trauma Orthopedic, Beijing Jishuitan Hospital, Fourth Clinical Hospital of Peking University, Beijing, China

Chunpeng Zhao Trauma Orthopedic, Beijing Jishuitan Hospital, Fourth Clinical Hospital of Peking University, Beijing, China

Jingwei Zhao Department of Spine Surgery, Beijing Jishuitan Hospital, Fourth Clinical Hospital of Peking University, Beijing, China

Shan Zheng Department of Spine Surgery, Beijing Jishuitan Hospital, Fourth Clinical Hospital of Peking University, Beijing, China

Li Zhou Trauma Orthopedic, Beijing Jishuitan Hospital, Fourth Clinical Hospital of Peking University, Beijing, China

Gang Zhu School of Biological Science and Medical Engineering, Beihang University, Beijing, China

The History and Development of Robot-Assisted Orthopedic Surgery

1

Wei Tian, Yi Wei, and Xiaoguang Han

Abstract

Orthopedic surgical robot is the core intelligent equipment to promote the development of precision, minimally invasive orthopedics surgery, which has become the focus of international researches. This chapter introduces the development of orthopedic surgical robots and the typical products of orthopedic robots.

Keywords

Robot · Robot-assisted orthopedic surgery

Several definitions of "robot" exist. According to The Robot Institute of America, the robot is defined as a reprogrammable, multifunctional manipulator designed to mover material, parts, tools, or specialized devices through various programmed motions for the performance of a variety of tasks. Robots entered the orthopedic field in the mid-1990s and have demonstrated excellent clinical performance, such as improved surgical accuracy, reduced surgical damage, and reduced labor intensity. At present, many institutions have developed prototype systems for orthopedic robots. Some systems have been successfully converted into commercial products and are being promoted and applied worldwide.

The orthopedic robot has received extensive and long-term attention since its birth. The main robot products include Caspar (Ortomaquet, Germany), Renaissance (Mazor, Israel), ROSA spine (MedTech, France) for assisted positioning, and robots such as PinTrace (Medical Robotics, Sweden), RoboDoc (Think Surgical, USA), RIO (Mako Surgical, USA), Acrobot Sculptor (Acrobot), for intraoperative smart operation.

The first orthopedic robot developed was a completely autonomous system that was mainly used for joint replacement. In 1986, IBM and UC Davis jointly developed an intelligent system for hip arthroplasty. Based on this, the Integrated Surgical Systems of the United States (USA) introduced RoboDoc, an active orthopedic robotic product in 1992. Studies have shown that RoboDoc had significant improvement in fit, fill, and alignment compared with conventional techniques. However, system failure, long femoral stem treatment time, and high complication rates also represented specific problems, which hindered the widespread use of this system (Schulz et al. 2007; Spencer 1996; Taylor 1993; Cowley 1992).

W. Tian (✉)
Department of Spine Surgery, Beijing Jishuitan Hospital, Fourth Clinical Hospital of Peking University, Beijing, China

Beijing Key Laboratory of Robotic Orthopaedics, Beijing, China
e-mail: tianweijst@vip.163.com

Y. Wei · X. Han
Department of Spine Surgery, Beijing Jishuitan Hospital, Fourth Clinical Hospital of Peking University, Beijing, China

W. Tian (ed.), *Navigation Assisted Robotics in Spine and Trauma Surgery*,
https://doi.org/10.1007/978-981-15-1846-1_1

In order to improve the safety of robotic surgery, doctors are becoming an integral part of the closed loop of robot operation control. During the automatic operation of the robot, the doctor can directly "modify" the movement of the robot under certain conditions by taking the initiative to intervene. Precise and safe surgery can be performed under the cooperation of man and machine; therefore, such systems are also known as "handheld" robots. The CASPAR robot that emerged in 1997 is a RoboDoc-like system that can be used for bone treatment in artificial total knee and total hip arthroplasty and bone tunnel drilling of implants during cruciate ligament reconstruction. It shows that CASPAR has obvious advantages over traditional technology (Paul 1999). The Acrobot robot (the latest version is Acrobot Sculptor), which appeared in 2001, is the first orthopedic robot to use the concept of active constraint. During procedures, it is necessary to fix the reference tracker to the femur and tibia to achieve optimal coordination. It is mainly used for total knee replacement and minimally invasive knee joint replacement (Davies et al. 2006).

Later, with the advancement of research, a more specialized robot ontology form appeared. The Robotic Arm Interactive Orthopedic System (RIO) (MAKO Surgical Corp., Fort Lauderdale, Florida) is an example of a commercially available, tactile robotic system that requires active participation of the surgeon to complete a unicompartmental knee replacement (UKR). Up to 2015, the global installed capacity is about 200 units, and the total number of surgical operations have exceeded 50,000. Previous studies have found that RIO robot-assisted joint replacement surgery has smaller incisions and shorter recovery time, better patellofemoral angle, and functional scores, compared with traditional surgery (Lonner 2009). The Acrobat system (The Acrobot Company, London, United Kingdom) is a similar device to the RIO system. The mini bone-attached robotic system (MBARS) robot, which was developed at Carnegie Mellon University (Pittsburgh, Pennsylvania, USA), mounts onto the femur and completes the bone resection cuts during total knee replacement (TKR) procedures.

For spine surgery, the SpineAssist/Renaissance robot (Mazor Robotics Inc., Orlando, Florida, USA) is the most reported product. It is a miniature bone-mounted robot with 6° of freedom. A preoperative computed tomography (CT) scan is used to plan trajectories, and intraoperative fluoroscopy is used to register the images. The robot then guides the surgeon to the appropriate trajectory. Several studies have demonstrated advantages of improved surgical accuracy and reduced radiation exposure for both patients and clinical staff (Togawa et al. 2007; Sukovich et al. 2006; Shoham et al. 2003). However, the accuracy of the device varies in relatively highly in the literature, and some studies have even demonstrated a significantly reduced accuracy of robot-assisted surgery (85%) compared with the fluoroscopic-guided technique (93%, $P = 0.019$). The lesser accuracy may be attributed to the reduced working volume of the robot, which makes them less able to withstand reactive forces and leads to movement of the robot arm relative to the patient.

Another spinal robot is the ROSA robot (Medtech, Montpellier, France), which comprises a patient-side cart (bearing the robotic arm with 6° of freedom and a workstation) and an optical navigation camera. Either intraoperative fluoroscopy or intraoperative CT scan can be used for planning. However currently, it is only approved for lumbar screw position by the FDA (Lonjon et al. 2016; Chenin et al. 2016; Lefranc and Peltier 2015).

A major breakthrough for spinal robotic surgery came in 2015. The TiRobot system (TINAVI Medical Technologies Co., Ltd.) was produced. It is a multi-indication orthopedic surgical robot, suitable for use in the spine, pelvic, and limb surgeries using both open and minimally invasive approaches (Tian et al. 2016; Tian 2016). It is also the first orthopedic surgical robot entirely created in China and obtained CFDA(China Food and Drug Administration) approval in 2016. In the TiRobot device, a robotic arm with tracking abilities is combined with an intraoperative 3D navigation system. After preoperative imaging acquisition and planning of the desired screw trajectories, the surgeon manually performs the drilling and screw insertion.

In summary, precision and minimally invasive treatment are the main fields of the development of orthopedic surgery in the twenty-first century and have become the development trend of orthopedic clinical treatment. Orthopedic robotics consist of core intelligent equipment to promote the development and popularization of precision and minimally invasive surgery. It has broad development prospects and an enormous market. After more than 30 years of development, orthopedic surgery robot technology is developing in the direction of comprehensive human–computer interaction, fine graphic images, miniaturization of hardware, non-invasive surgery, and smooth operation of remote operations.

References

Chenin L, Peltier J, Lefranc M. Minimally invasive transforaminal lumbar interbody fusion with the ROSA(TM) Spine robot and intraoperative flat-panel CT guidance. Acta Neurochir. 2016;158:1125–8.

Cowley G. Introducing "Robodoc". A robot finds his calling—in the operating room. Newsweek. 1992;120(21):86.

Davies B, Jakopec M, Harris SJ, et al. Active-constraint robotics for surgery. Proc IEEE. 2006;94(9):1696–704.

Lefranc M, Peltier J. Accuracy of thoracolumbar transpedicular and vertebral body percutaneous screw placement: coupling the Rosa® Spine robot with intraoperative flat-panel CT guidance—a cadaver study. J Robot Surg. 2015;9:331–8.

Lonjon N, Chan-Seng E, Costalat V, Bonnafoux B, Vassal M, Boetto J. Robot-assisted spine surgery: feasibility study through a prospective case-matched analysis. Eur Spine J. 2016;25:947–55.

Lonner JH. Robotic arm—assisted unicompartmental arthroplasty. Semin Arthroplast. 2009;20(2):15–22.

Paul A. Surgical robot in endoprosthetics. How CASPAR assists on the hip. MMW Fortschr Med. 1999;141(33):18.

Schulz AP, Seide K, Queitsch C, et al. Results of total hip replacement using the Robodoc surgical assistant system: clinical outcome and evaluation of complications for 97 procedures. Int J Med Robot. 2007;3(4):301–6.

Shoham M, Burman M, Zehavi E, et al. Bone-mounted miniature robot for surgical procedures: concept and clinical applications. IEEE Trans Robot Autom. 2003;19(5):893–901.

Spencer EH. The ROBODOC clinical trial: a robotic assistant for total hip arthroplasty. Orthop Nurs. 1996;15(1):9–14.

Sukovich W, Brink-Danan S, Hardenbrook M. Miniature robotic guidance for pedicle screw placement in posterior spinal fusion: early clinical experience with the spine assist. Int J Med Robot. 2006;2(2):114–22.

Taylor KS. Robodoc: study tests robot's use in hip surgery. Hospitals. 1993;67(9):46.

Tian W. Robot-assisted posterior C1-2 transarticular screw fixation for atlantoaxial instability: a case report. Spine. 2016;41:1.

Tian W, Wang H, Liu Y. Robot-assisted anterior odontoid screw fixation: a case report. Orthop Surg. 2016;8(3):400.

Togawa D, Kayanja MM, Reinhardt MK, et al. Bone-mounted miniature robotic guidance for pedicle screw and translaminar facet screw placement: part 2-evaluation of system accuracy. Neurosurgery. 2007;60(2):129–39.

Basic Principle of Robot-Assisted Orthopedic Surgery

2

Yajun Liu, Peihao Jin, Wenyong Liu, and Wei Tian

Abstract

The collaboration between robot and medical environment (including medical staff) plays a critical role through the entire procedure of robot-assisted orthopedic surgery. From aspects of surgical informatization and interactivity, this chapter introduces the functional configuration (workflow and basic setup) and the human–robot interaction modes in the orthopedic operating room. Suggestions for improving the performance and the clinical acceptability of the robot system is also briefly discussed.

Although various robot-assisted surgical systems have been widely adopted in clinical orthopedics, the system configuration and operation procedure are dramatically unfamiliar for different orthopedic indications. It is essential to analyze the basic principle of robot-assisted orthopedic surgery for designing or adopting a robot system.

Y. Liu · P. Jin · W. Tian (✉)
Department of Spine Surgery, Beijing Jishuitan Hospital, Fourth Clinical Hospital of Peking University, Beijing, China
e-mail: tianweijst@vip.163.com

W. Liu
School of Biological Science and Medical Engineering, Beihang University, Beijing, China
e-mail: wyliu@buaa.edu.cn

1 Functional Configuration of Robot-Assisted Orthopedic Surgery

The potential benefits of robotics in the clinical orthopedics mainly focuses on two kinds of functional enhancements. One is to expand the operation capacity of surgeon with the assistance of robotic manipulator in the ROM (range of motion). Another is to augment the decision-making capacity of surgeon through enriching the information display in the FOV (field of vision) with the assistance of computer navigation and virtual reality. Motivated by these two kinds of enhancements, several robots (e.g., RoboDoc, SpineAssist, among others) and navigation systems (e.g., Stryker, BrainLab, among others) were set up and quickly applied into orthopedic surgery by the end of 2010. The clinical outcomes had already shown the unique advantages of robot or navigation system in the aspects of positioning accuracy and operation safety.

Since 2010, navigation-guided robot-assisted operation mode was paid more attention in the clinical orthopedics (Fig. 2.1). Integration of computer navigation in the robot system forms a closed-loop tracking control which can monitor positions and poses of environmental components including robot and patient, among others. This operation mode can track any intraoperative changes of environmental components and real time correct the motion deviation of the robot end-effector from the

W. Tian (ed.), *Navigation Assisted Robotics in Spine and Trauma Surgery*,
https://doi.org/10.1007/978-981-15-1846-1_2

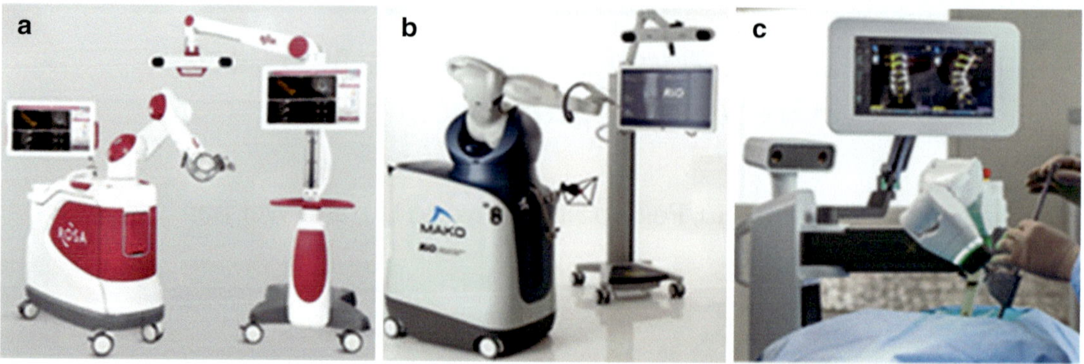

Fig. 2.1 Typical navigation-guided robot-assisted operation systems in orthopedics. (**a**) Rosa. (**b**) Rio. (**c**) MazorX

planned trajectory or region so as to guarantee the operation safety of robot system.

However, it should be noticed that the entire environment of operating room is still characterized with the *unstructured* and *dynamically variable* configuration. This characterization has two kinds of meanings. The first meaning is that the environmental components in an operating room (OR), including medical staff and patient, are individualized and unstructured. In order to achieve the operational automation of surgical procedure, it is necessary to real time digitalize the entire operation environment. The second one is that the environmental configuration in OR is dynamically changing for the different surgical indications. For example, robotic surgeries for the intramedullary nailing of femoral neck and the transpedicular screwing have dramatically different configurations (Fig. 2.2). Take the robotic surgeries in the Beijing Jishuitan Hospital as examples. For the intramedullary nailing, a compact biplanar robot (TINAVI, China) and a C-arm fluoroscope are deployed into OR. For the transpedicular screwing, a TiRobot robot (TINAVI, China), a Polaris tracking sensor (NDI, USA), and an ARCADIS-Orbic 3D C-arm device (Siemens, Canada) are deployed into OR. In order to minimize configuration variation in OR during changing surgical indication, it is necessary to enhance the function generalization (or multifunctions) ability of robot, to standardize the interfaces between different environmental elements in OR and to standardize or regulate the information flow during the procedure.

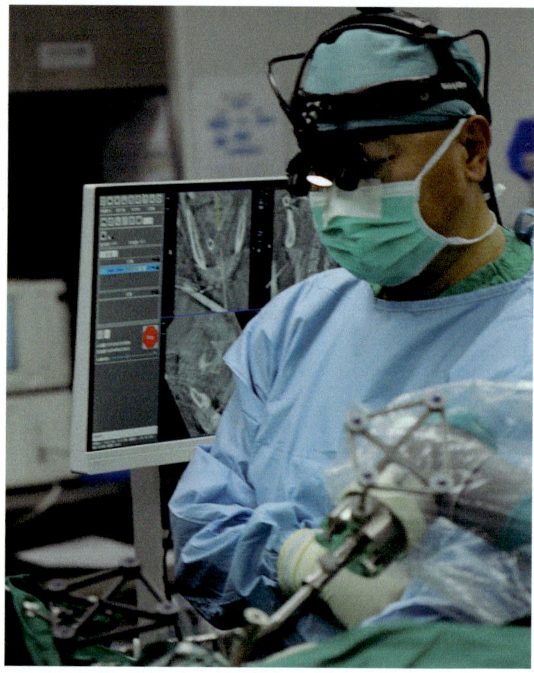

Fig. 2.2 Different OR configuation for different surgical indications in the Beijing Jishuitan Hospital. (**a**) Fluoroscopy-based intraledullary nailing. (**b**) Cone beam CT-based transpedicular screwing

1.1 Workflow of Robotic Operation Procedure

From the viewpoint of information processing, Russell H. Taylor at the John Hopkins University proposed the CIS (computer integrated surgery) concept, the workflow of which divides the operation procedure into several steps including the patient information acquisition (patient-specific information and general information), the surgical planning, the surgical action (with robot or navigation), and the result analysis, among others (Taylor and Stoianovici 2003). All these steps in the CIS form a closed-loop information flow, and the robot itself is just a node in the loop. That is to see, the design of orthopedic robot system is not only a robot design but also an entire information system optimization for surgery.

We know that the CIMS (computer integrated manufacturing system) concept is used for describing the workflow of the modern manufacturing industry. In Fig. 2.3, if we take the patient, the surgeon, and the OR to replace the mechanical material, the operator, and the machining center, respectively, in the CIMS, the CISS (computer integrated surgical system) concept is proposed to depict the workflow of modern surgery. Referencing the workflow modules of CIMS, the CISS workflow can be divided into the surgical CAD (surgical modeling), the surgical CAPP (trajectory or region planning), the surgical CAM (robot execution), and the surgical TQM (outcome evaluation). Current researches mainly focus on first three modules. The last one (TQM) should be paid more and more attention with the further application of the evidence-based statistics analysis in the robotic surgery.

1.2 Basic Setup of Computer-Assisted Orthopedic Surgery System

In the CAOS (computer-assisted orthopedics surgery) field, although robot and navigation are designed and implemented in numerous technical methods, their basic conceptual design is very similar. Different setups of CAOS at least involve three components: a

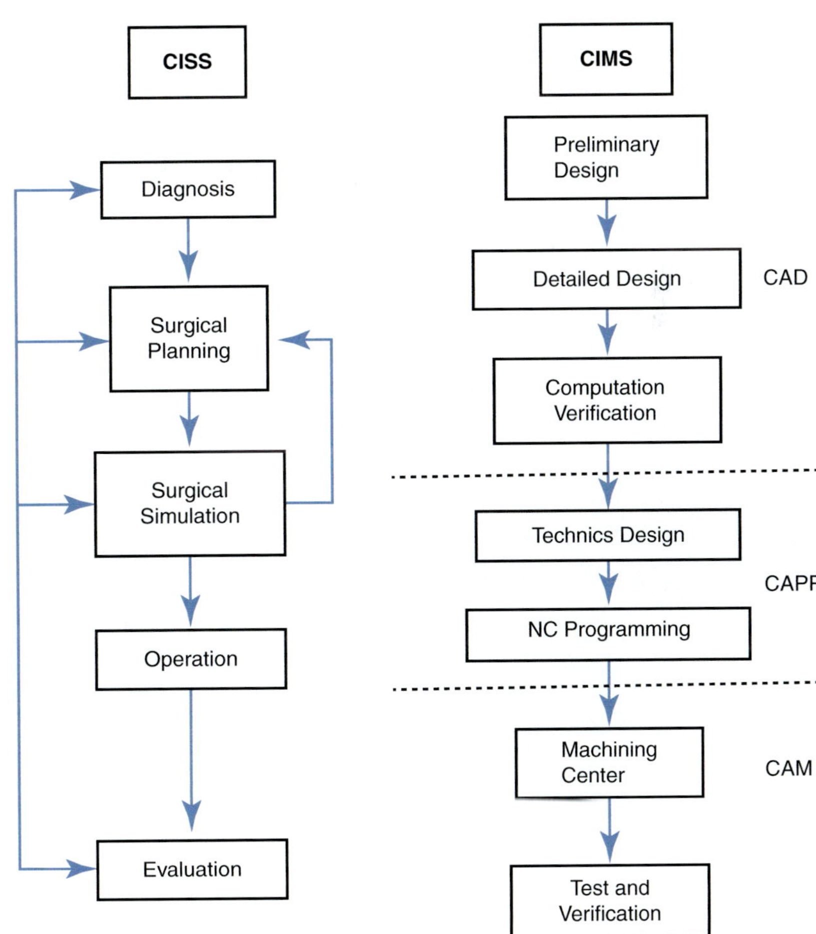

Fig. 2.3 Comparison between concepts of CISS and CIMS (Taylor and Stoianovici 2003) (Redrawn from Russell H. Taylor, Dan Stoianovici. Medical robotics in computer-integrated surgery. IEEE Transactions on Robotics and Automation, 2003, 19(5): 765–781. https://doi.org/10.1109/TRA.2003.817058)

therapeutic object (TO) which is the treatment target of surgery, a virtual object (VO) which is the virtual representation in the planning or navigation software, and a navigator that links both TOs and VOs (Nolte and Beutler 2004; Zheng and Nolte 2015).

The navigator is the core component of a CAOS system and a bridge to enable the transmission of locational information among the end-effectors (EEs), the Vos, and the TO. The navigator can establish a 3D global coordinate system (COS) in which the TO is to be treated and the current position and pose of the adopted EEs are tracked and calculated in real time. EEs are usually a passive surgical instrument, but can also be a semi-active or active instrument. For robotic devices, the robot itself plays the role of the navigator; while for surgical navigation, a position tracking device is adopted (Zheng and Nolte 2015). The coaction of these three entities (TO, VO, and EE) can be used to establish a CAOS system.

A typical CAOS system can be established by three technical steps including calibration, registration, and referencing. First, *calibration* of an EE is used to describe the geometry and shape parameters of the EE in the navigator's COS. it is necessary to establish a local COS on the EE. Second, *registration* among VO, TO, and EE is used to provide a geometrical transformation between these three kinds of entities in order to display the end-effector's position and orientation with respect to the virtual representation, similar to the application of GPS-based navigation system for locating a car in the map. Third, *referencing* for compensating for possible motions of the TO or the EE relative to the navigator during surgery is conducted real time. This step can be done by two approaches: the tracking of DRBs (dynamic reference bases) on TO and the rigid immobilization of TO with respect to the navigator (Zheng and Nolte 2015).

2 Human–Robot Interaction Mode in Orthopedic Operating Room

Human–robot interaction (HRI) capacity and efficiency play an important role in robotic surgery, especially for the dynamically variable and unstructured OR environment in orthopedics. Based on the relative relation among patient, surgeon, and robot, Narendra Nathoo (Nathoo et al. 2005) at the Cleveland Clinic Foundation proposed three kinds of HRI modes which can also be applied to robotic orthopedics.

2.1 Supervisory Control

This kind of HRI mode separates the operation procedure into two stages: surgical planning and robot automatic execution (Fig. 2.4). During the procedure, the robot and surgeon are independent to do different tasks: path planning and path implementation. The general opera-

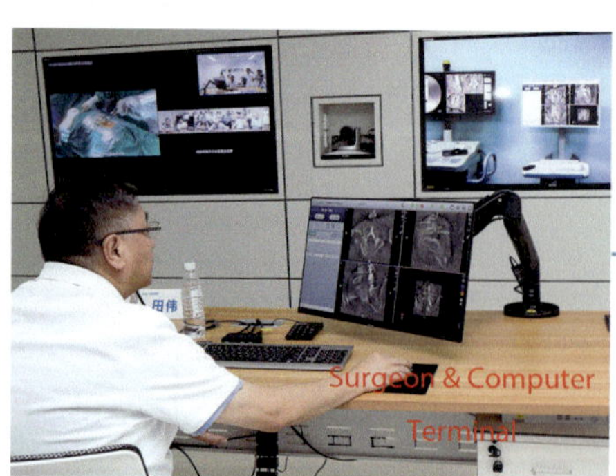

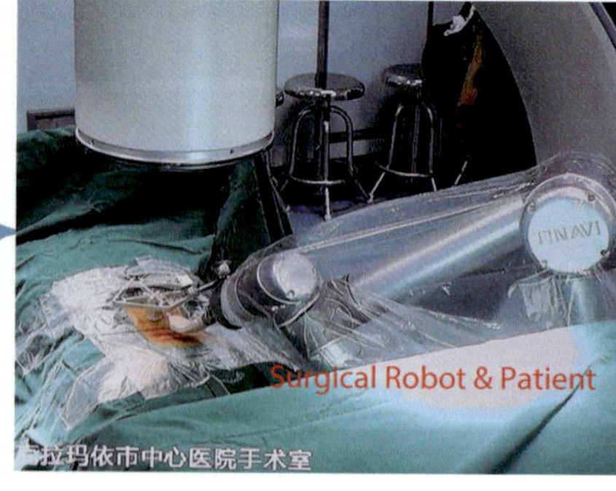

Fig. 2.4 Supervisory control mode

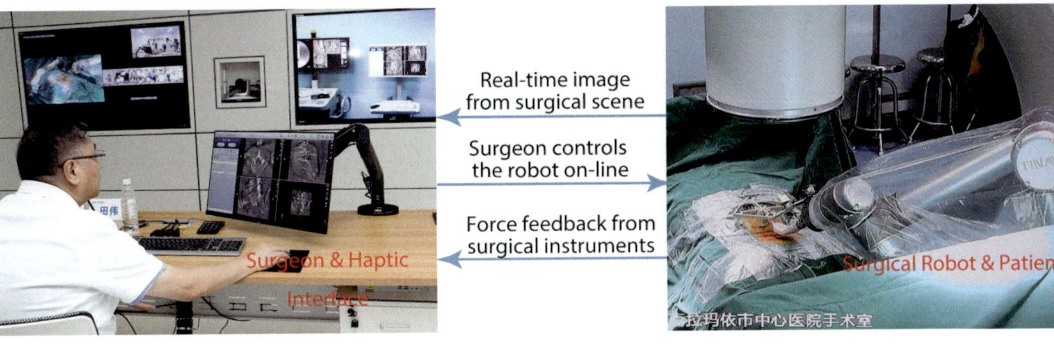

Fig. 2.5 Teleoperation mode

tion steps can be summarized as follows: First, the surgeon conducts the surgical planning pre- or intraoperatively on a computer-generated model of the patient such as CT–MRI scans, 2D–3D fluoroscopy. Second, the surgeon downloads the surgical plans to the surgical robot. Then, the robot downloads the surgical plans while the surgeon monitors the surgical robot's operation.

Supervisory control mode is widely adopted at the early development stage of orthopedic robot system. The robot adopted here must have a fully programmed task written in its control system. The RoboDoc robot (named THINK for the latest version) is a typical supervisory controlled robotic system.

2.2 Teleoperation

This type of HRI mode can geographically separate the surgeon and patient (Fig. 2.5). The general operation steps can be summarized as follows: The surgeon operates the robot in real time through the haptic (haptic device) and the visual (camera) interfaces. The master–slave operation is the mostly adopted option for this mode.

The surgeon site (with a master robot–manipulator) and the patient side (with a slave robot) can be deployed into different ORs at the same or different hospital, even different city of countries. The renowned Operation Lindbergh is a typical robotic telesurgical operation which utilized the Zeus robot at the patient side. The first clinical trial for orthopedic robot teleoperation in China is carried out in 2006. A compact biplanar robot was adopted. The expert surgeon and the patient were separated approximately 1000 km from each other between Beijing city and Yan'an city in China.

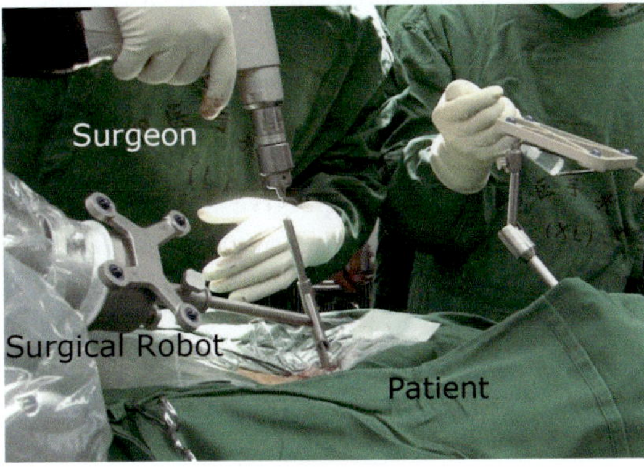

Fig. 2.6 Shared-control mode

2.3 Shared-Control Mode

In this type of HRI mode, the surgeon and robot remain jointly in control. The surgeon remains in the close loop of control while the robot provides steady manipulation of the instrument. This mode not only provides the high accuracy and dexterity but also can guarantee safety during the entire operation, as surgeon can actively control robot's motion when necessary (Fig. 2.6). In orthopedics, Mako is a typical shared control system that has been applied in arthroplasty.

3 Summary

Robotics which is being routinely used in some orthopedic procedures is expected to innovate operation instruments and revolute the traditional orthopedic procedures. Although robotic surgery is still at the beginning of evolution, the newly emerging techniques (the artificial intelligence, the 5G communication, etc.) will constantly be integrated as the development of robotic systems which will allow the surgeon to use any combinations of the above described concepts or modes. The complicated laboratory evaluation platform should be set up as any new techniques, and instruments should be first tested before their clinical acceptance. Besides, more prospective and retrospective studies for scientific evaluation of the outcome of robotic procedures with long follow-up time should be conducted and integrated in the basic principle of robotic-assisted orthopedic surgery.

References

Nathoo N, Cavusoglu MC, Vogelbaum MA, et al. In touch with robotics: neurosurgery for the future. Neurosurgery. 2005;56(3):421–33. https://doi.org/10.1227/01.NEU.0000153929.68024.CF.

Nolte LP, Beutler T. Basic principles of CAOS. Injury. 2004;35(S):A6–A16. https://doi.org/10.1016/j.injury.2004.05.005.

Taylor RH, Stoianovici D. Medical robotics in computer-integrated surgery. IEEE Trans Robot Autom. 2003;19(5):765–81. https://doi.org/10.1109/TRA.2003.817058.

Zheng G, Nolte LP. Computer-assisted orthopedic surgery: current state and future perspective. Front Surg. 2015;2:66. https://doi.org/10.3389/fsurg.2015.00066.

Use of Artificial Potential Field Theory to Determine the Spatial Position of a Navigation-Guided Orthopedic Surgical Robot

3

Yu Wang, Gang Zhu, Yajun Liu, Jingwei Zhao, and Wei Tian

Abstract

During the surgery, the surgical robot should neither touch any of the objects or patient on the operation table nor obstruct the operating of the surgeon. This requirement could be described as a trajectory plan problem for the robot manipulator. In this chapter, an artificial potential field theory is introduced to determine the optimal manipulator pose of the surgical robot.

Keywords

Artificial potential field · Redundant Trajectory · Collision avoid

To set up an orthopedic robot-assisted system into a limited space in an operation room (OR), it is important to consider the interactions between the robot and environment. Set up beside the operating table, the robot should neither touch any of the obstacles nor obstruct the activity of the surgeon. This requirement could be described as a trajectory plan problem for the six degrees of freedom (DOF) manipulator. The efficiency of trajectory planning has a significant effect on the ease of use of surgical robots. This chapter introduces a novel trajectory planning method to deal with environment interaction complications.

1 Nonstructured Environment and Redundant Degrees of Freedom Issues

Different from the structured environment in a traditional factory (Flordal et al. 2006; Schou et al. 2018), the environment in the OR is nonstructured (Hagn et al. 2008). This means that for each type of surgical procedure, or even with each patient, the position of the obstacle (such as the C-arm or the operation table) in the OR will differ. Thus, a trajectory planning method would be used continuously as long as the surgical robot is needed (Fig. 3.1).

To build a nonstructured OR environment, the simultaneous localization and mapping (SLAM) technique is used (Izadi et al. 2011). Infrared depth sensors such as Kinect® and RealSense® are used to obtain a quick scan of the OR (Newcombe et al. 2011). Considering the blocking of an infrared ray, the model of the possible obstacles would be scanned in detail before surgery. Through point cloud registration, for example, an iterative closest point (ICP) algorithm (Besl & McKay 1992) is

Y. Wang · G. Zhu
School of Biological Science and Medical Engineering, Beihang University, Beijing, China
e-mail: wangyu@buaa.edu.cn

Y. Liu · J. Zhao · W. Tian (✉)
Department of Spine Surgery, Beijing Jishuitan Hospital, Fourth Clinical Hospital of Peking University, Beijing, China
e-mail: tianweijst@vip.163.com

W. Tian (ed.), *Navigation Assisted Robotics in Spine and Trauma Surgery*,
https://doi.org/10.1007/978-981-15-1846-1_3

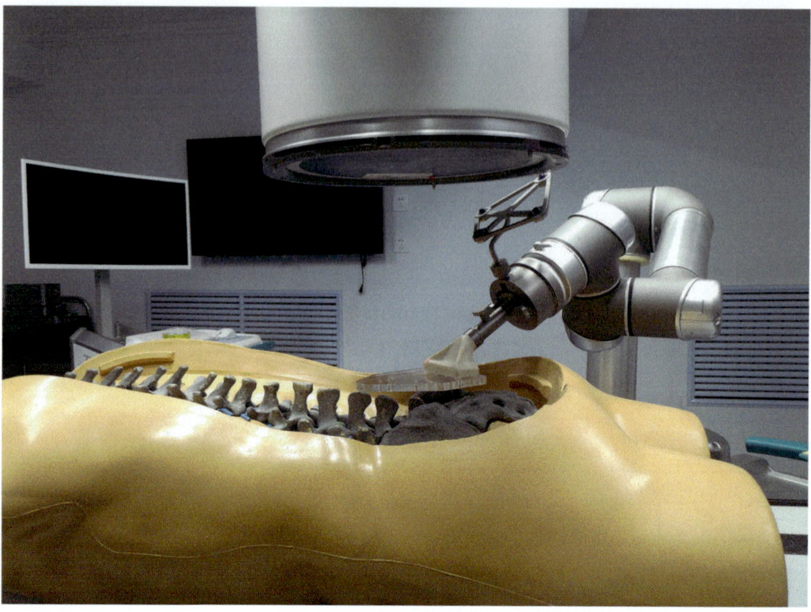

Fig. 3.1 Narrow space for surgical tool insertion

applied to generate and transform the matrix from an obstacle model reference to a robot reference. At this point, the nonstructured environment of the OR has been built.

To provide an optimal positioning of the robot, at least one redundant DOF should be present. For this reason, a collaborative manipulator for industry use would usually consist of seven DOFs. However, there would be little difference for the surgical robot. The main task for surgical navigation robot is to guide a surgical tool into an accurate position, such as a K-wire or a hip reamer. Generally, these surgical tools have a self-spinning axis. Thus, the guide for those tools on the manipulator would rotate along this axis, but this would have no effect on the accuracy of navigation. This means that a normal 6-DOF manipulator would have a redundant DOF for optimization. To date, the redundant DOF has been considered a problem, and many researchers have solved this problem by adding several constraints (Patel et al. 2009). For example, they attribute a minimal motion path which is the manipulator or apply some empirical spatial constraints. Considering the obstacle avoiding requirement, we believe the redundant DOF should be used for trajectory planning.

For example, in pedicle screw fixation surgery, the surgeon is asked to plan an entry point and a stopping point, which determines a spatial line in CT images. Then, the robot will move a surgical tool guide to the accurate spatial position for K-wire guiding. Indeed, if the K-wire guide rotates along the spatial line, there will be no difference in the K-wire guiding result. Ultimately, the trajectory of every possible position for robot navigation would be a spatial circle around the planned spatial line. In order to determine an optimal position for the robot, an environment-related parameter is required to evaluate the distance from the robot to each obstacle. In this context, Artificial Potential Field (APF) theory can be introduced (Fig. 3.2).

2 Artificial Potential Field Algorithm and its Application

The artificial potential field (APF) algorithm was proposed by Khatib (1986). This algorithm was first used for manipulator trajectory but soon was found to be more suitable for a mobile

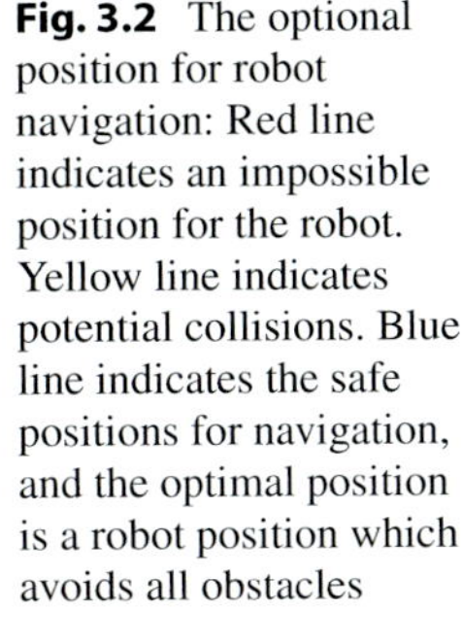

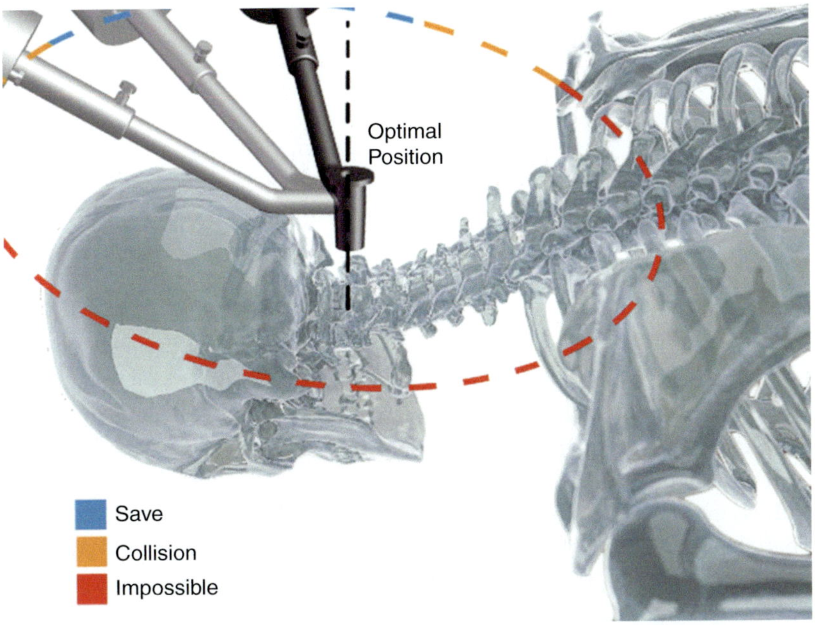

Fig. 3.2 The optional position for robot navigation: Red line indicates an impossible position for the robot. Yellow line indicates potential collisions. Blue line indicates the safe positions for navigation, and the optimal position is a robot position which avoids all obstacles

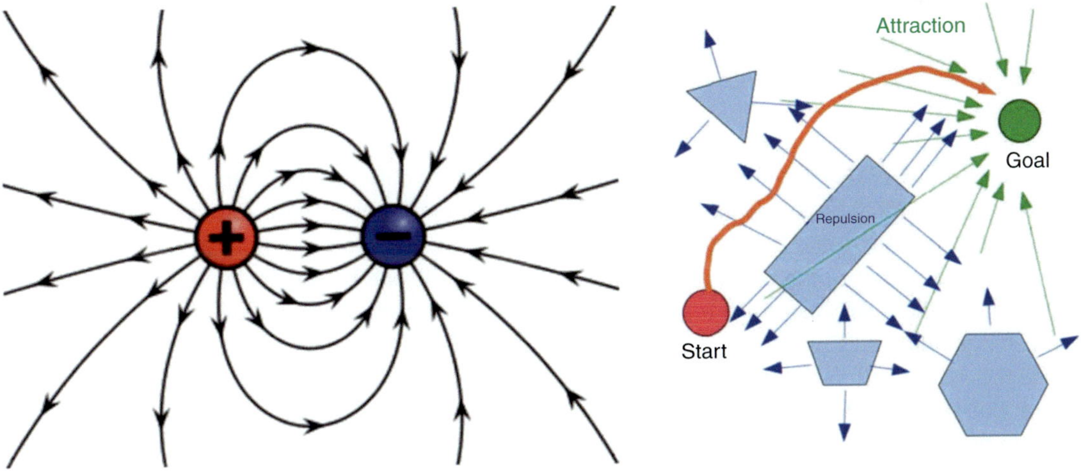

Fig. 3.3 Electrostatic field for avoiding obstacle

robot. The most widely used potential field is an electrostatic field. In this field, the difference the object generates is either an attractive force or a repulsive force to the robot, and the force is correlated with the distance. The attractive force to the robot would lead the robot to move to the assigned target position, and the repulsive force would keep the robot away from obstacles (Koren 1991) (Fig. 3.3).

To determine an optimal position for the robot, a nonstructured environment should be built before surgery. Although the positions of obstacles in OR are uncertain, the shape of the obstacles will not change. The shape of an obstacle such as C-arm was acquired through 3D scanning and is transformed into $1 \times 1 \times 1$ cm^3 voxel model. The artificial potential field value of every voxel near the model is calculated using the repulsive equation below:

$$f(x) = \begin{cases} k * \left(\frac{1}{d_{\min}^{2}} - \frac{1}{d_{\max}^{2}} \right)^{2} & d < d_1 \\ k * \left(\frac{1}{d_i^{2}} - \frac{1}{d_{\max}^{2}} \right)^{2} & d_1 < d < d_0 \\ 0 & d > d_0 \end{cases}$$

$$d_i = \operatorname{argmin}\left(\left| {}_{\text{robot}}^{i}T \cdot P_{\text{robot}} - P_i \right| \right)$$

where $d_{\min}$ is the collision distance, defined as the radius of arm of the robot; $d_{\max}$ is the longest distance for APF, which is five times the radius; and d_i is the shortest distance from any spatial point to the obstacle *i*. Since the APF value is summable, the points on the robot have several APFs for different obstacles referenced, and the ${}_{\text{robot}}^{i}T$ is a matrix used to transform the points on the robot reference to one obstacle reference. These matrices are acquired through the registration algorithms mentioned above (Fig. 3.4).

Once calculated, the APF value for all the points on the robot axis, the value could be widely applied. First of all, it can be applied for collision detection. The APF value is related to the distance from the robot to the obstacle. As long as the radius of the manipulator rod L is measured, the corresponding APF value *f*(*L*) is determined. Since the APF function is a decreasing function, if any points on robot axis APF value is calculated to be larger than the *f*(*L*), this would represent a collision situation. For the safety of the manipulator moving within the OR, a collision position should be excluded before any other calculation (Fig. 3.5).

According to the definition, the APF value decreases when the distance increases. Therefore, a long distance from the robot to all the obstacles is considered a safety index. Thus, if we sum all the APF values on the robot axis and choose the smallest one among the redundant solutions, an optimal target manipulator position is acquired (Fig. 3.6).

The APF function also gives a direction for manipulator trajectory planning. The whole potential field would have the fastest gradient descent direction, which leads the manipulator to move away from the obstacles.

Thus, the trajectory planning step involves: determining the target spinning line, excluding the collision redundant solutions, finding an optimal target position, determining a linear trajectory, collision detection for the trajectory, using the APF fastest gradient descent direction to replan the collision trajectory, and finally, manipulator movement. These steps will only take less than 1 min in the operation. As a comparison, the APF built before surgery would require several hours for each obstacle, but once completed, the APF file will not change any further.

Some modifications can be used to improve the APF algorithm for the operating room. For example, different APF values could have a different weight when being summed. The collision would bring higher danger to the unconscious patient; hence, the weight should be larger than the weight of the C-arm or the operating table. The surgeon is more flexible in the OR; thus, the APF of surgeon should be used during target position optimization but may be ignored during trajectory planning.

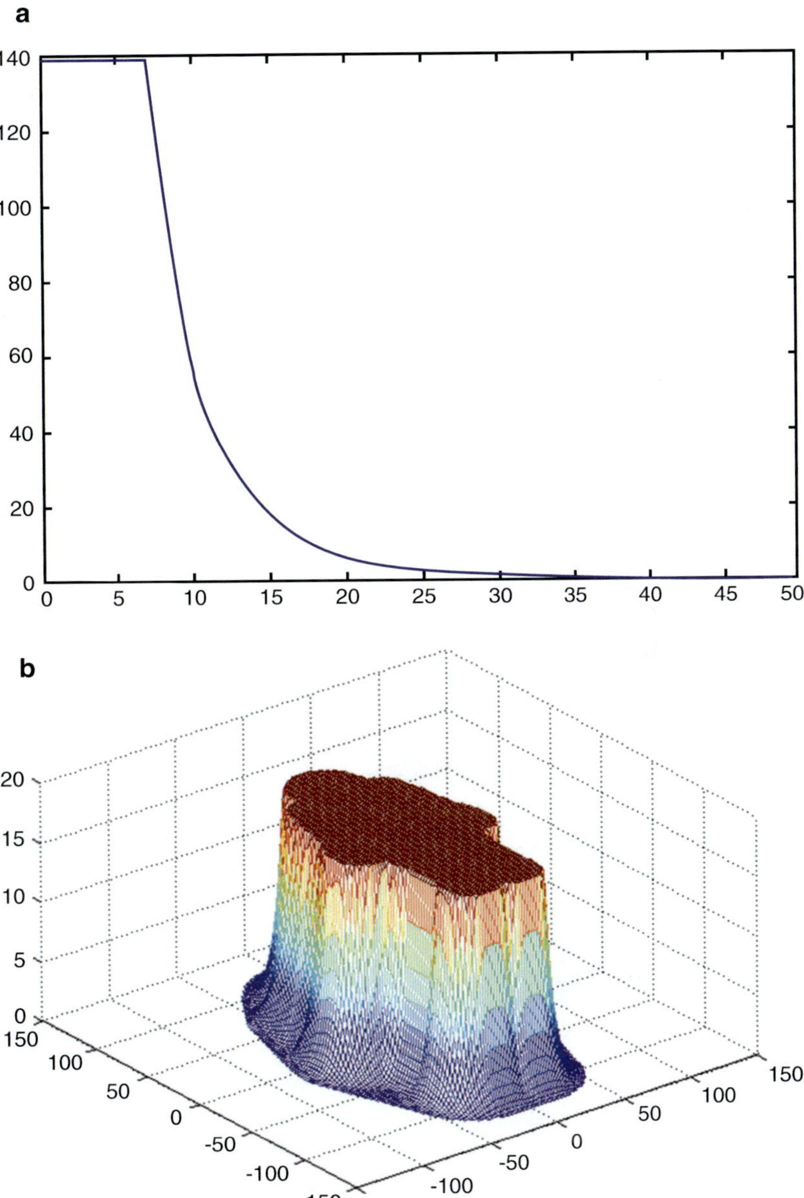

Fig. 3.4 (**a**) Repulsive function image for the artificial potential field (APF). (**b**) APF of the model

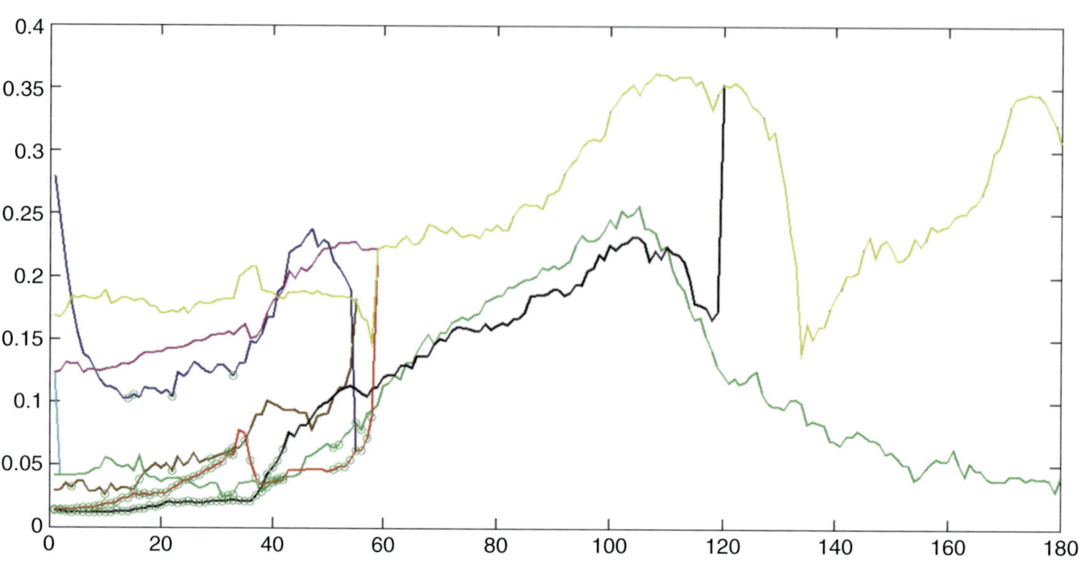

Fig. 3.5 The artificial potential field (APF) value for all the possible robot positions

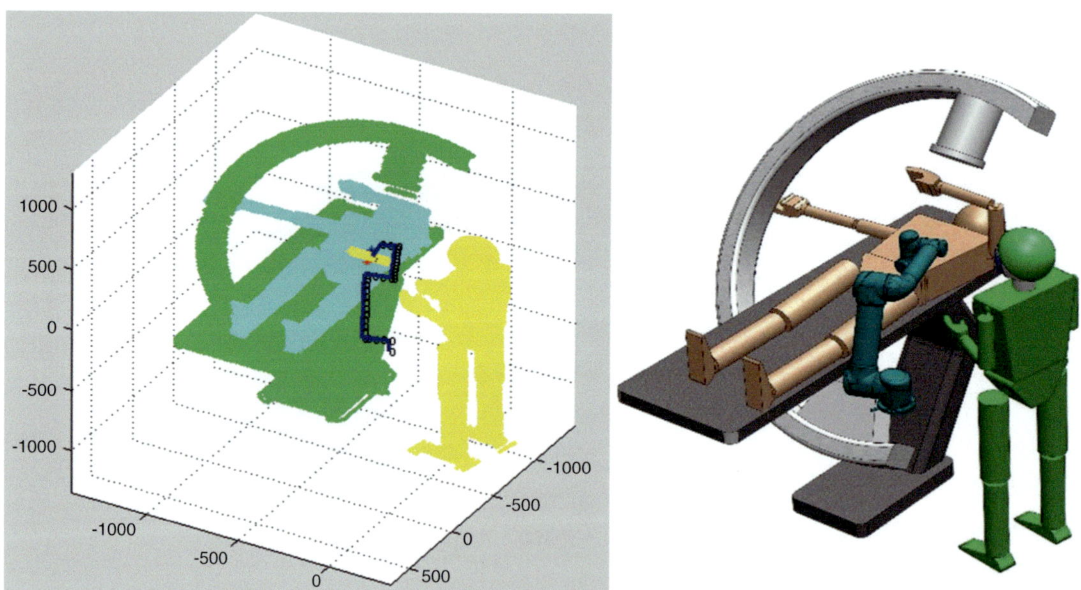

Fig. 3.6 The optimal position for one of the robot navigation surgery

References

Flordal H, Fabian M, Åkesson K, Spensieri D. Automatic model generation and PLC-code implementation for interlocking policies in industrial robot cells[J]. Control Eng Pract. 2006;15(11):1416.

Schou C, Andersen RS, Chrysostomou D, et al. Skill-based instruction of collaborative robots in industrial settings[J]. Robot Comp Int Manuf. 2018; 53(1):72–80.

Hagn U, Nickl M, Jörg S, et al. The DLR MIRO: a versatile lightweight robot for surgical applications[J]. Ind Robot. 2008;35(4):324–36.

Izadi S, Kim D, Hilliges O, Molyneaux D, Newcombe R. Kinectfusion: real-time 3D reconstruction and interaction using a moving depth camera [J]. Proc Uist. 2011:559–68.

Newcombe RA,Davison AJ,Izadi S,Kohli P, Hilliges O,Shotton J,Fitzgibbon A. KinectFusion: Real-time dense surface mapping and tracking[C]. Mixedand augmented reality, IEEE International Symposium on 2011, 127–136.

Besl PJ, McKay ND. A method for registration of 3D shapes. IEEE Trans Pattern Anal Mach Intell. February 1992;14:239–56.

Patel RV, Talebi HA, Jayender J, et al. A robust position and force control strategy for 7-DOF redundant manipulators[J]. IEEE/ASME Trans Mech. 2009;14(5):575–89.

Khatib O. Real-time obstacle avoidance for manipulators and mobile robots[J]. Int J Robot Res. 1986;5(1):90–8.

Koren Y. Potential field methods and their inherent limitations for mobile robot navigation[C]//. IEEE Int Conf Robot Autom. 1991;2:1398–404.

Future Trends and Perspectives

4

Wei Tian, Wenyong Liu, and Mingxing Fan

Abstract

Clinical-oriented robot configuration and data-driven artificial intelligence is evolving robotic orthopedics. This chapter summarizes the harmonious collaboration trend among surgeon–robot–environment interaction in the OR from aspects of the rigid–flexible–soft hybrid mechanical configuration and the environmental structurization, the data-driven trend from aspects of the surgical data science idea, and the artificial intelligence applications in the orthopedics.

Robotics is dramatically changing surgical ideas and operation techniques in orthopedics. More and more technicians and surgeons are involved in the innovation research and development of new robotics. The data-driven design idea and the surgeon–robot collaborative mode have become the future trend of surgical robotics.

W. Tian (✉) · M. Fan
Department of Spine Surgery, Beijing Jishuitan Hospital, Fourth Clinical Hospital of Peking University, Beijing, China
e-mail: tianweijst@vip.163.com

W. Liu
School of Biological Science and Medical Engineering, Beihang University, Beijing, China
e-mail: wyliu@buaa.edu.cn

1 Natural Collaboration Among Surgeon–Robot Environment

Natural collaboration of environmental components in OR may create a harmony workflow which can improve the quality of operation procedure with the minimal interference to the surgeon's habits. To achieve this goal, two trends have emerged and should be paid more attention. First, the collaborative robot (so-called *cobot*) has become the most adopted platform for developing new robotic surgery system. Second, digitalization of the entire OR environment can provide a unified framework for intelligent orthopedic surgery.

1.1 Rigid–Flexible–Soft Hybrid Mechanical Configuration for Collaborative Robot

The rigid–flexible–soft hybrid mechanical configuration is essential for safe and natural interaction among the patient, surgeon, and environment. On the one hand, the surgeon is a key role in the traditional surgical procedure. However, in most surgical robot systems, the surgeon's role is weakened, and more efforts emphasize the technical development and integration. It is very hard to form a stable and robust closed-loop control in robotic system without

W. Tian (ed.), *Navigation Assisted Robotics in Spine and Trauma Surgery*,
https://doi.org/10.1007/978-981-15-1846-1_4

the surgeon. Surgeon–robot–environment interaction in one workflow and control loop is receiving more and more attention. On the other hand, rigid configuration in traditional mechanical design always interferes with the surgeon during surgical operation. As the human body (surgeon and patient) is a kind of nonrigid object, in order to make the surgeon–robot coupling system have more flexible performance, it is better to design a hybrid mechanical configuration with rigid, flexible, and soft properties.

Actuator is a key component for fabrication of the rigid–flexible–soft hybrid mechanical configuration. Several typical actuators were proposed in recent years, such as a novel soft-and-rigid hybrid actuator, a reconfigurable hybrid actuator with rigid and soft components, a compliant Omni-direction bendable hybrid rigid-and-soft Omni-crawler module, a natural orifice soft robot, among others. These actuators have not yet been used in orthopedic robot system. Their integration and testing in orthopedics should be further researched.

1.2 Environmental Structurization and Digitalization in Operating Room

The modern OR is characterized with unstructured, dynamically variable environment. Real-time monitoring of the entire OR environment can guarantee the safety of robotic surgery. Technically, digitalization involves the accurate calibration of intrinsic parameters and the standardized data input–output interface for each component; structurization involves OR space partition based on certain rules such as safety hierarchy. For the accurate calibration of each component, there are many different technologies for a specific device.

For the OR space partition, the optimal partition scheme should be further investigated so as to improve the feasibility of OR structurization. In order to achieve full tracking of the entire OR environment during surgical procedure, the multimode, synchronous tracking technologies should be further designed and integrated into the robot system, so as to realize the unblocked, high accurate tracking of the entire OR environment.

2 Data Driven in Intelligent Orthopedics

Data and their processing methods are fundamentals to implement collaborative operation in the robotic OR. In the concept of CIS, Russel H. Taylor established a closed-loop workflow according to the data flow direction. With the recent development of intelligent orthopedics, the size and type of data produced from each stage of surgical procedure, including the surgical planning, the robot execution, and the environmental sensing are exponentially increasing. The appropriate acquiring, storing, processing, and utilization of these data can dramatically improve clinical efficiency and outcomes of robotic surgery.

2.1 Surgical Data Science in Orthopedics

In 2017, the concept of SDS (surgical/interventional data science) was proposed and was regarded as the main engine to promote the next generation of surgical technology. According to the definition proposed by Lena Maier-Hein et al., SDS involves four components which is used for handling not only biomedical data but also the procedural data (Maier-Hein et al. 2017; Vedula and Hager 2017). SDS is an emerging cross-disciplinary field between medicine and engineering and can be used for efficiently leveraging and scientifically evaluating the methodology, the principle, the techniques, and the medical knowledge during the design and application of intelligent medical devices or instruments (Fig. 4.1).

In the intelligent orthopedics, robotic–navigated surgery is characterized as the dynamic and procedural processes. Thus, SDS in orthopedics includes not only the *measured dynamic* data such as the planned path, the intrinsic parameters of devices the motion data of robot manipulators, among others, but also the *procedural modeling*

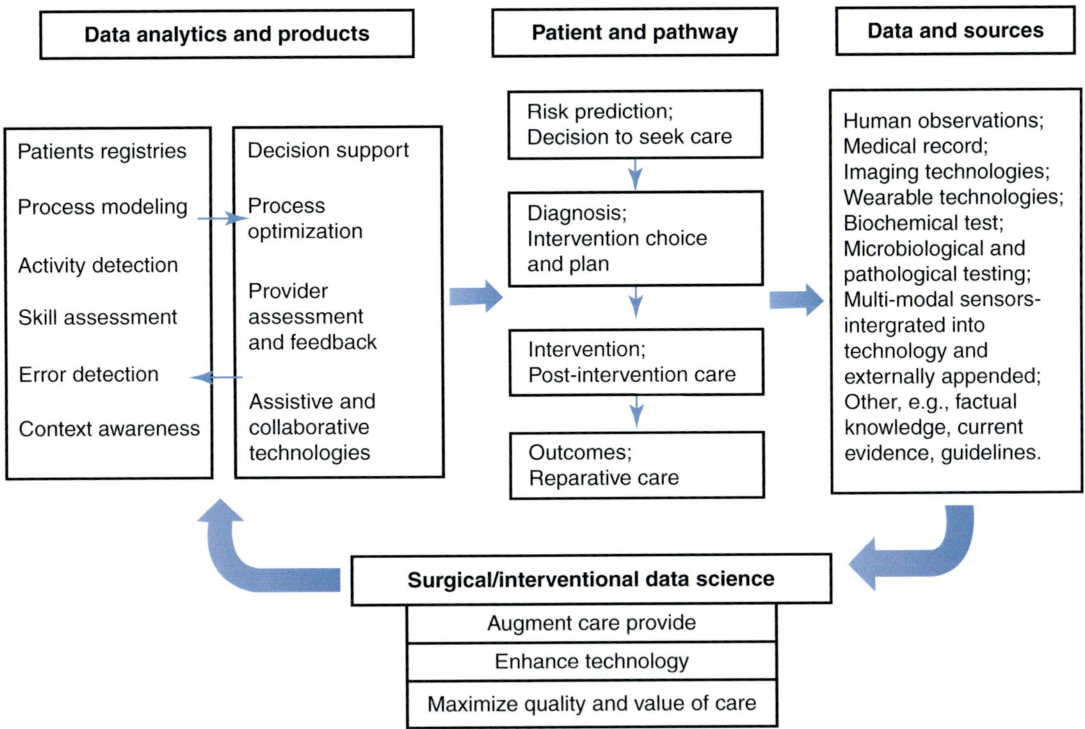

Fig. 4.1 SDS concept and domains (Vedula and Hager 2017) (Redrawn from S. Swaroop Vedula and Gregory D. Hager. Surgical data science: the new knowledge domain. Innov Surg Sci 2017, 2(3): 109–121. https://doi.org/10.1515/iss-2017-0004)

data such as the ergonomic representation of OR environment, the safety levels in different operation space, etc. More attention should be focused on SDS-driven, seamless, efficient integration of robot/navigation with the OR environment.

2.2 Artificial Intelligence in Surgical Interventions

The big data and artificial intelligence (AI) are changing the medical diagnosis and healthcare screening. For the orthopedics application of AI, existed researches mainly focused on the image segmentation and anatomical model reconstruction, which is rarely used for surgical intervention such as the automation of surgical planning. The possible reason is that, compared with the access of diagnosis images in medical checking, the access of intervention images and data (can be modified as some kinds of labels) in surgery is very difficult.

For the automatic localization of 3D vertebral bodies (VB) from medical images, Chu et al. (2015) proposed a unified random forest (RF) regression and classification framework which achieved satisfied accuracies both in localization and segmentation. However, the VBs in the clinical always have some kind of pathological structure with unclear image boundaries, image artifacts, and traces of surgical activities, etc. In order to further automatically segment such pathological VB structures, Bulat Ibragimov et al. (2017) proposed a landmark-assisted deformable model which can be used for efficient segmentation with pathological shape. These segmented shapes can be used for the path planning in robotic or navigated spine surgery. Especially in spine milling procedures such as the decompression of vertebral lamina, the accurate model is very important to precisely plan the boundary of milling region (Fig. 4.2).

Applications of robot in orthopedics are producing high-volume intervention images and

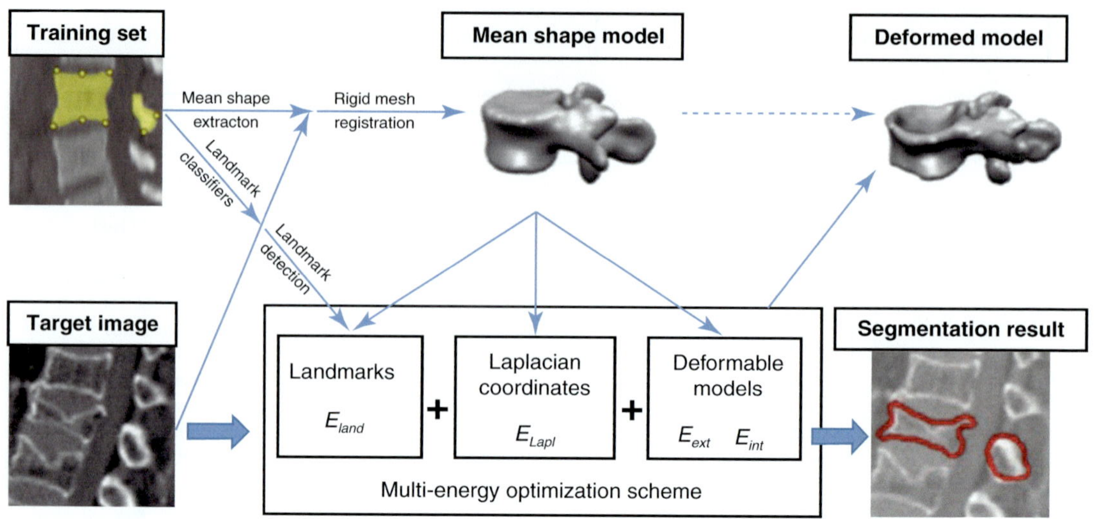

Fig. 4.2 Workflow of the segmentation framework (Ibragimov et al. 2017) (Redrawn from Bulat Ibragimov, Robert Korez, Boštjan Likar, et al. Segmentation of pathological structures by landmark-assisted deformable models. IEEE Transactions on Medical Imaging, 2017, 36(7): 1457–1469. https://doi.org/10.1109/TMI.2017.2667578)

data which form the data base for AI researches in orthopedic interventions. Based on our clinical experiences, the path planning step in robotic surgery is very time-consuming and technical. Thus, the automatic learning of individualized surgical path from the patient's image and the training framework should be further researched. Besides, AI algorithm can also be used for the motion identification of the robot, the risk prediction in OR, and the evidence-based analysis of patient's outcome after robotic surgery.

3 Summary

Innovation of surgical robotics is consistently paving the fast growth of robot application in orthopedics and also proposes a series of challenges in aspects of the collaborative mechanical configuration, the OR structurization, the big data, and AI in orthopedics. For the collaborative configuration, the rigid–flexible–soft hybrid control, the mechanical behavior analysis, and the robot stiffness regulation should be further researched. For the OR structurization, the space partition scheme, and multimode, full tracking of the entire OR environment should be optimized. For the big data and AI in orthopedics, the concrete definition of SDS in orthopedics, the learning-based framework for surgical intervention, and the evidence-based statistical evaluation should be carefully investigated.

References

Chu C, Belavý DL, Armbrecht G, et al. Fully automatic localization and segmentation of 3D vertebral bodies from CT/MR images via a learning-based method. PLoS One. 2015;10(11):e0143327. https://doi.org/10.1371/journal.pone.0143327.

Ibragimov B, Korez R, Likar B, et al. Segmentation of pathological structures by landmark-assisted deformable models. IEEE Trans Med Imaging. 2017;36(7):1457–69. https://doi.org/10.1109/TMI.2017.2667578.

Maier-Hein L, Vedula S, Speidel S, et al. Surgical data science: enabling next-generation surgery. arXiv: 1701.06482. 2017. https://arxiv.org/abs/1701.06482. Accessed 5 Nov 2018.

Vedula SS, Hager GD. Surgical data science: the new knowledge domain. Innov Surg Sci. 2017;2(3):109–21. https://doi.org/10.1515/iss-2017-0004.

Magerl Method of C1–C2 Transarticular Screw Fixation

5

Yongqing Wang, Cheng Zeng, and Wei Tian

1 Introduction

Posterior C1–C2 transarticular screw fixation surgery, also known as the Magerl method, was first suggested by Magerl in 1987 (Jeanneret and Magerl 1992). Two screws are placed from the C2 pars inferior posteriorly to the C1 anterior arch, to obtain a stable fixation of C1 and C2 vertebrae.

1.1 Indication

1. Traumatic atlantoaxial instability (dens fracture, transverse ligament tearing, etc.)
2. Congenital atlantoaxial instability (congenital dens anomalies, etc.)
3. Inflammatory arthropathy (rheumatoid arthritis, etc.)
4. Former C1–C2 fixation failure.

1.2 Contraindication

1. Severe C1–C2 anatomy mutation, i.e., C2 lateral mass collapse.
2. Vertebral artery mutation.
3. Incapable of robot-guided screw placement, such as severe obesity or thoracic kyphosis.

Y. Wang · C. Zeng · W. Tian (✉)
Department of Spine Surgery, Beijing Jishuitan Hospital, Fourth Clinical Hospital of Peking University, Beijing, China
e-mail: wangyongqing@medmail.com.cn; tianweijst@vip.163.com

2 Difficulties of Traditional Methods and Advantages of Robotic Surgery

The Magerl technique of transarticular screw fixation provides a stronger stability compared with other techniques. But screw trajectory through C2 pedicle and C1–C2 joint is restricted because of its anatomy in the medulla oblongata and vertebral artery and other vital structures. Previous reports of surgery complications include fixation failure, C2 occipitalis major nervus injury, O-C1 articular injury, hypoglossal nerve injury, medulla spinalis injury, vertebral artery injury, etc. In particular, vertebral artery injury is always the key concern of surgeons. According to previous studies, 20% of patients cannot have a safe placement of bilateral Magerl screws because of the high incidence of vertebral artery endangering (Madawi et al. 1997).

After passing through the foramina transversaria at the C1, the vertebral artery follows posteriorly medially, and course follows behind the C1 articular mass along the groove in C1 posterior arch. Once the screw breeches this groove, the incidence of artery injury is very high.

Using the computer-assisted navigation technique, the insertion of transarticular screw could be monitored and controlled in real time. Further,

W. Tian (ed.), *Navigation Assisted Robotics in Spine and Trauma Surgery*,
https://doi.org/10.1007/978-981-15-1846-1_5

with the help of a robot system, a stable screw trajectory could be provided to improve the accuracy and safety of the surgery. Moreover, the robot system could be used for preoperative planning and for identifying the most optimal screw trajectory. Thus, the robot system has a great advantage in the Magerl method of C1–C2 transarticular screw fixation, especially for patients with severe abnormal upper cervical anatomy.

3 Imaging and Positioning

A posterior-anterior view plane radiograph with open mouth is required. Patient-controlled flexion-extension plane radiographs may be beneficial if possible.

An MRI scan is required for identification of soft-tissue injury. CT scan with sagittal and coronal reconstruction is required for diagnosis and preoperative planning.

4 Surgical Technique

Copy CT images to the platform of the robot system. Plan preoperative and confirm an optimal screw trajectory. Measure the length and diameter of the screw. The procedures were shown in (Figs. 5.1–5.15).

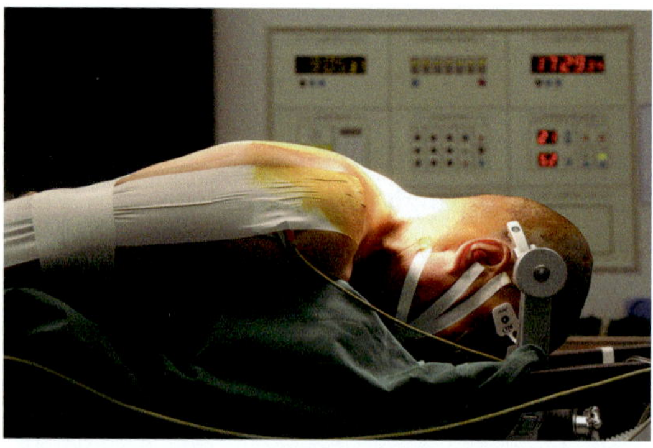

Fig. 5.1 The patient under general anesthesia is placed in the prone position. The head is rigidly held using Mayfield tongs. The shoulders and arms are tucked using tapes at the patient's side. After the patient is positioned, the proper alignment and reduction of C1–C2 joint should be confirmed radiographically

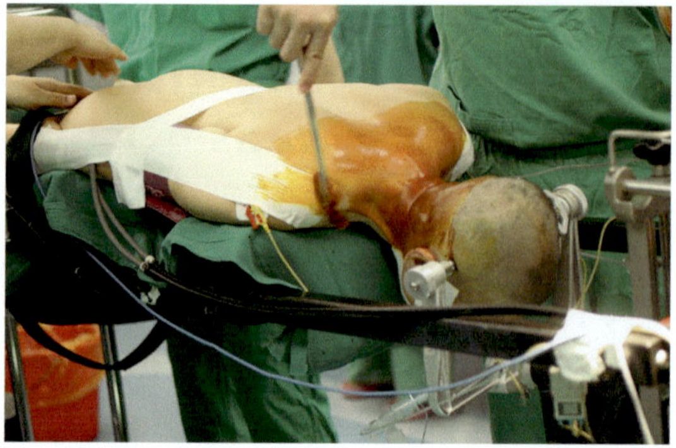

Fig. 5.2 The occiput, posterior neck, and posterior iliac crest should be prepped and draped according to the standard procedure

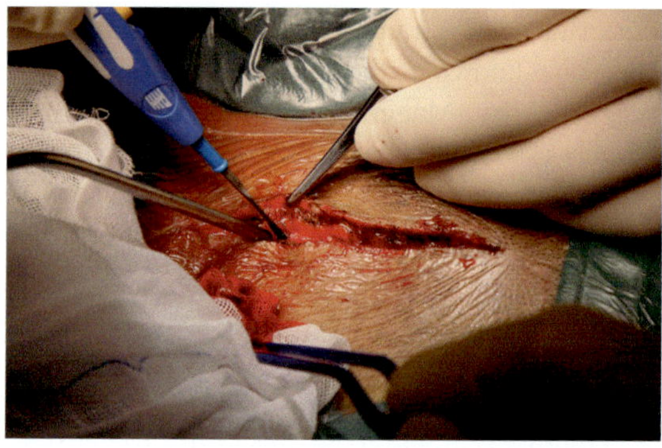

Fig. 5.3 A midline posterior skin and subcutaneous incision is made from occiput to the C2 level

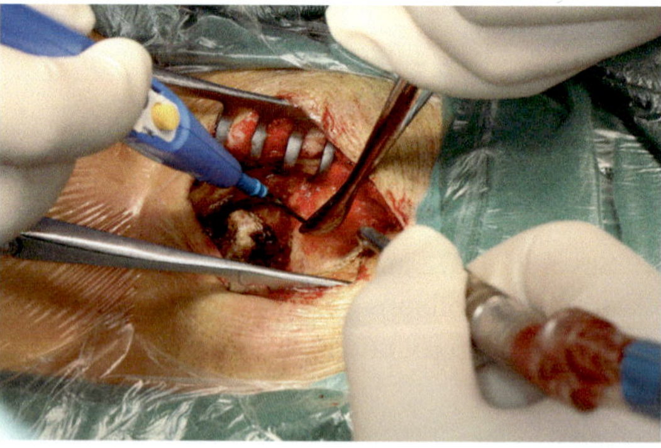

Fig. 5.4 The posterior arch of C1 down to the inferior margin of the lamina of C2 is exposed with meticulous subperiosteal dissection. Exposure is carried out laterally to visualize the superior and medial surfaces of the C2 pars. The C2–3 facet capsule should not be disturbed

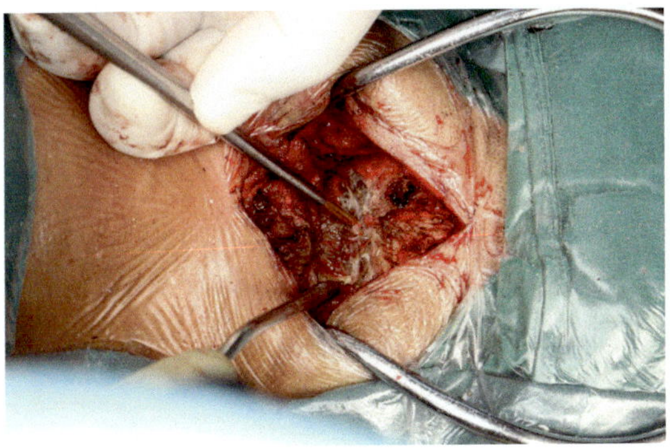

Fig. 5.5 The ligamentum flavum between the C1 and the occiput and between C1 and C2 are sharply divided. Confirm that there are no dural adhesions in the sublaminar space

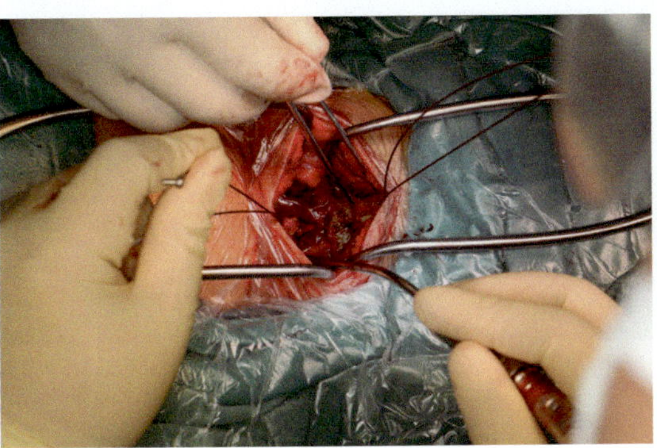

Fig. 5.6 Pairs of titanium cables are passed under each side of the arch of C1 followed by C2

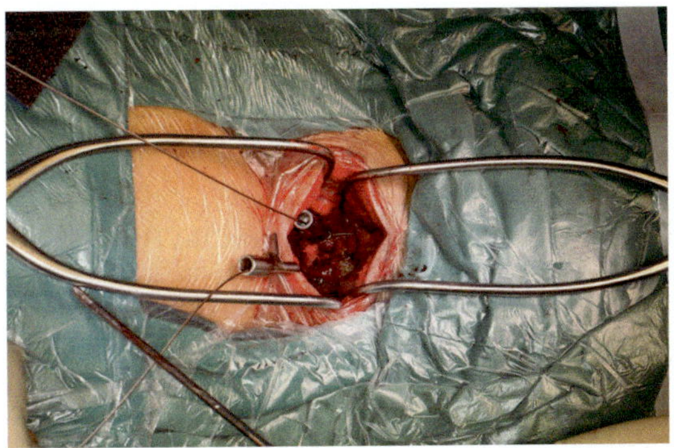

Fig. 5.7 Clips are used to temporally hold the cables

Intraoperative real-time 3D images are obtained by C-arm and transmitted to the robot system. The registration and reconstruction of image series will be completed automatically by the system.

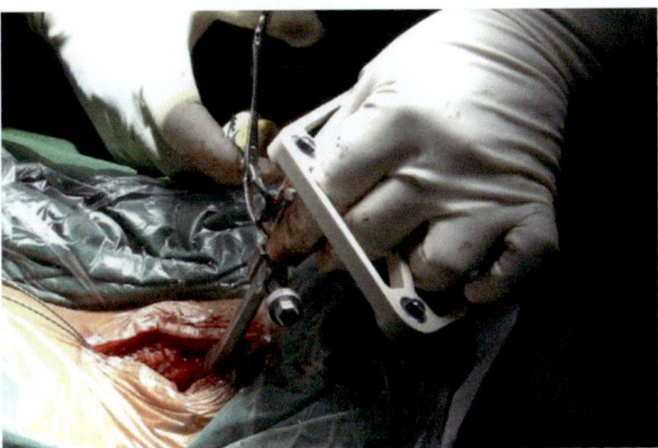

Fig. 5.8 C1–C2 reduction is confirmed with a fluoroscope. Patient tracker of the robot system is settled

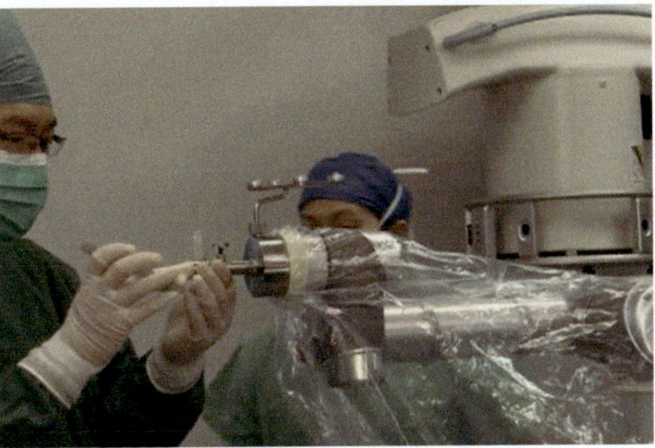

Fig. 5.9 The C-arm is registered and calibrated

5 Tips

1. A bur should be used to make a dip at the entrance point to avoid slipping of the K-wire, which is extremely dangerous.
2. Since the relationship between C1 and C2 obtained on intraoperative fluoroscopy may change during the operation, even with the help of Mayfield tongs, caution should be exercised for gentle manipulation and reduction.
3. The reliability of the real-time images should always be verified before drilling.

6 Typical Cases

A 60-year-old man presented with limb numbness for 1 year and progressive difficulty in walking for 4 weeks. On physical examination,

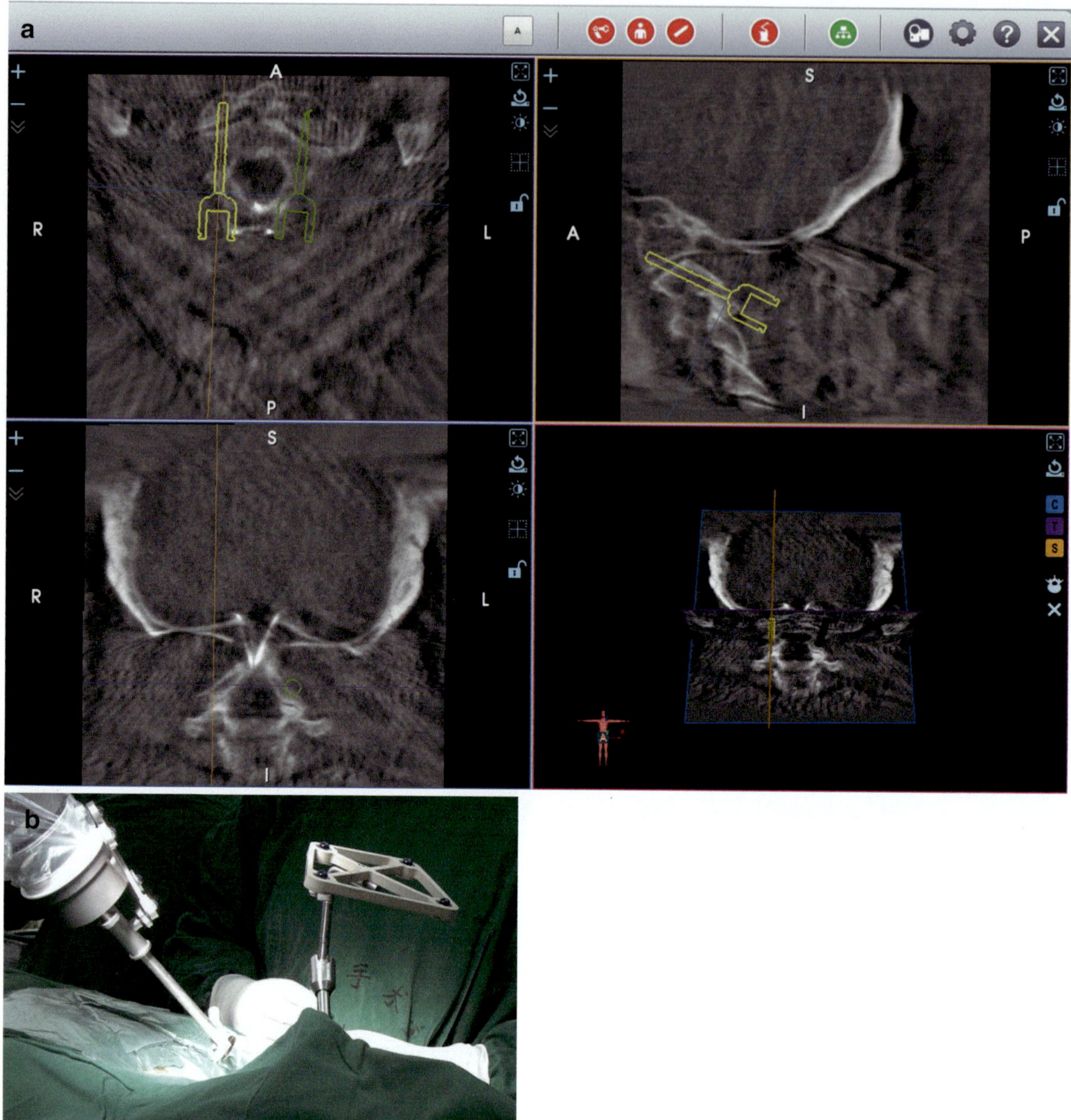

Fig. 5.10 (**a**) The starting point on the C2 pars and direction are confirmed using the robot system. (**b**) The robot arm with a drilling sleeve will be guided to the starting point and stopped automatically according to the intraoperative planning

he had difficulty with fine motor movement of the hands, Hoffmann's sign (+), Romberg's sign (+), Tandem gait (+), Babinski's test (+), hyperreflexia in the legs, and clonus (−). He had difficulty with walking distances more than 200 m. Pre-op images were shown in (Fig. 5.16).

Diagnosis: Os odontoideum, atlantoaxial instability, cervical spinal cord injury.

Robot-assisted Magerl method of C1–C2 transarticular screw fixation and Brooks' method of wire fixation were performed (Fig. 5.17).

Based on the 1-year follow-up, his limb numbness was relieved significantly; independent ambulation distance was more than 5 km. No bone graft nonunion was found according to follow-up images (Fig. 5.18).

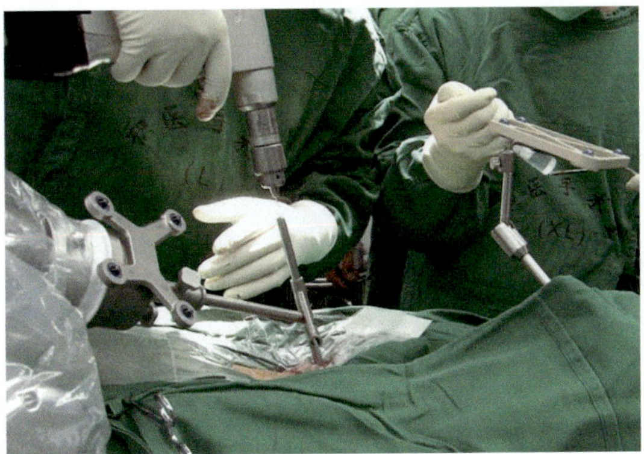

Fig. 5.11 A 1.2 mm K-wire is directly drilled following the drilling sleeve of the robot arm. Repeat the steps and drill another K-wire on the other side

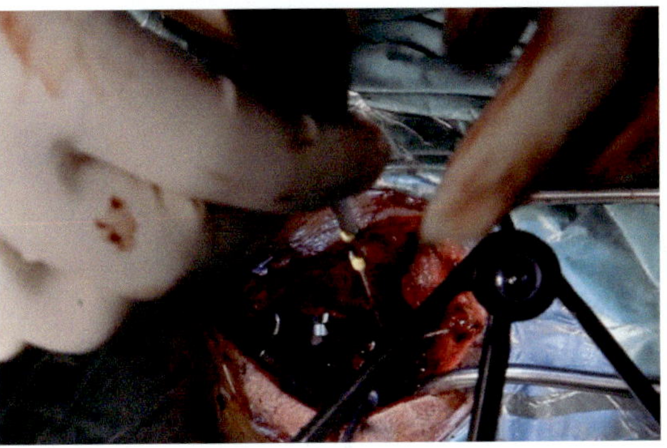

Fig. 5.12 Confirm the localization of the K-wires is satisfied on fluoroscopic images. Two screws are inserted following the K-wires

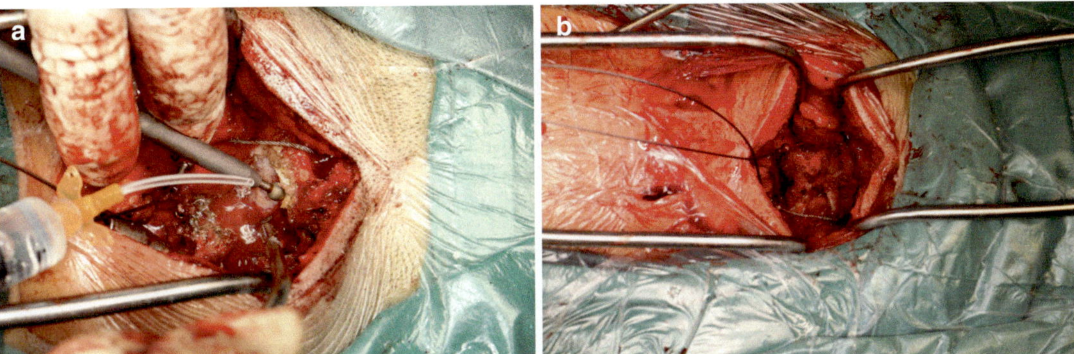

Fig. 5.13 (**a**, **b**) Release the pairs of clips that hold the titanium cables. The posterior arches of C1 and C2 are decorticated

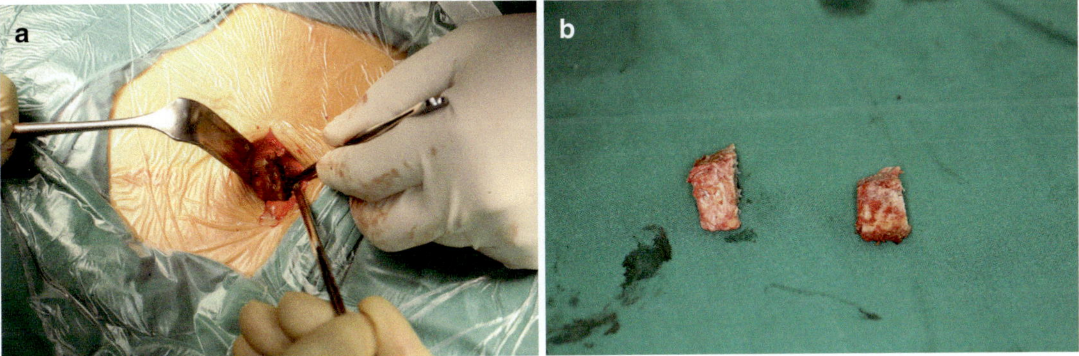

Fig. 5.14 (**a**, **b**) Two full-thickness rectangular bone grafts measuring approximately 1.25 × 3.5 cm are taken from the iliac crest

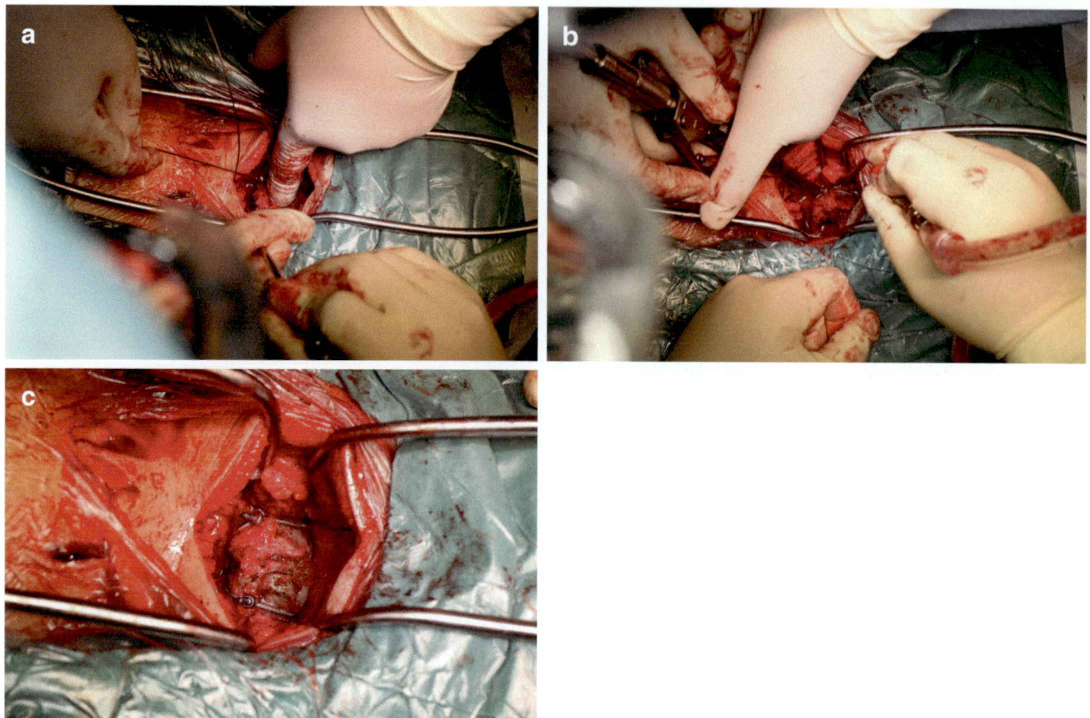

Fig. 5.15 (**a**, **b**, and **c**) The bone grafts are beveled to fit the interval between the C1 and C2 laminae and placed on each side. The bone grafts are then held in place by securing the cables

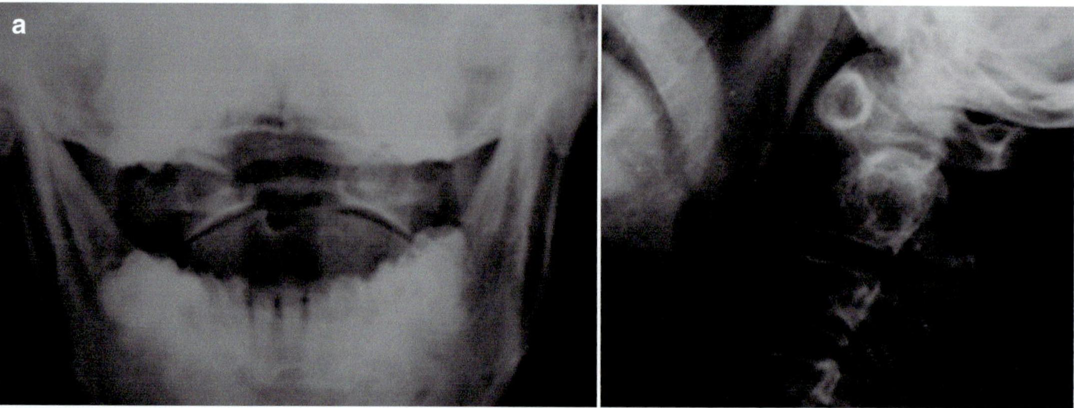

Fig. 5.16 (**a**) The "open mouth" view and lateral view of X-ray; (**b**) the extension-flexion view of X-ray; (**c**) the MRI images

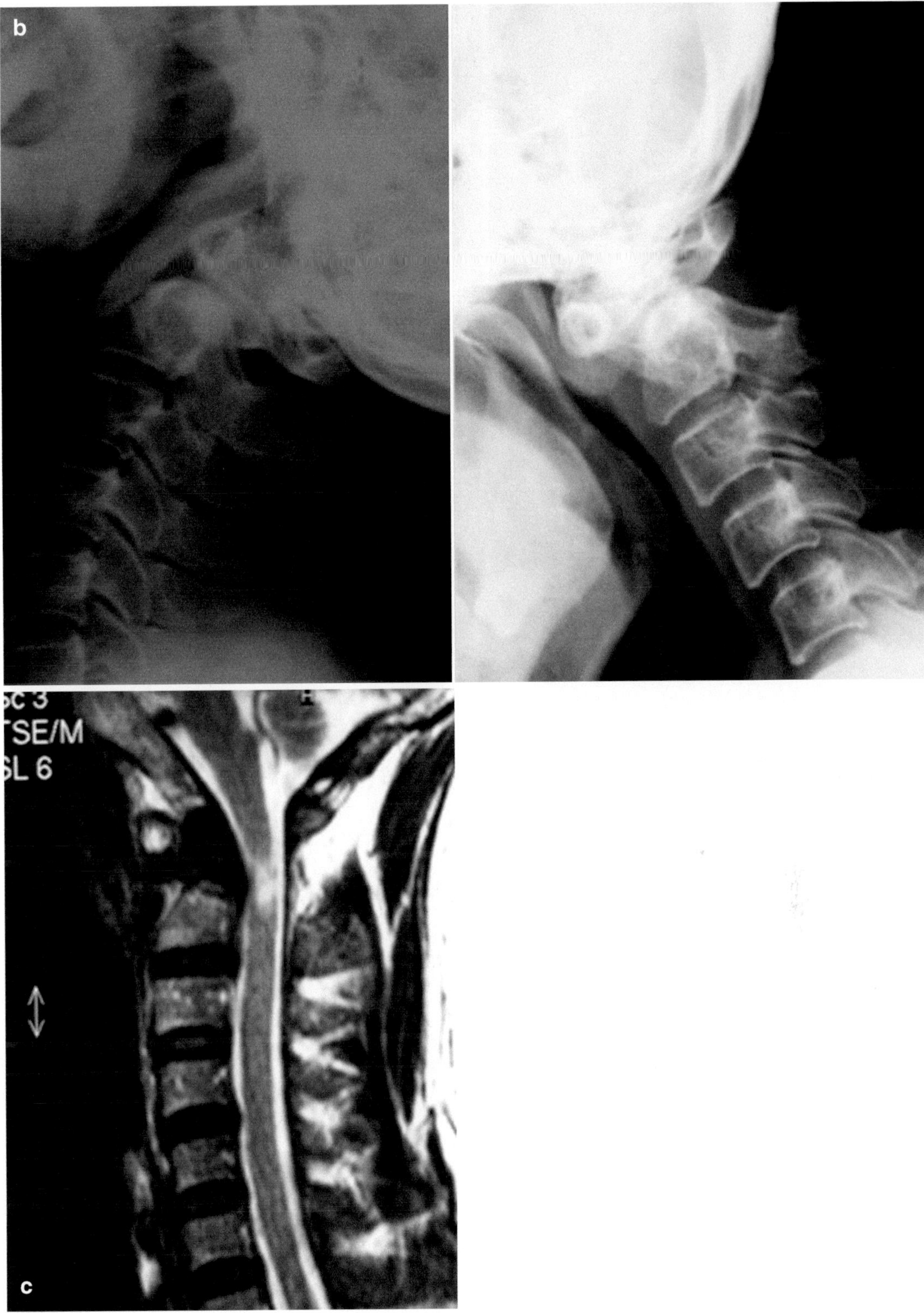

Fig. 5.16 (continued)

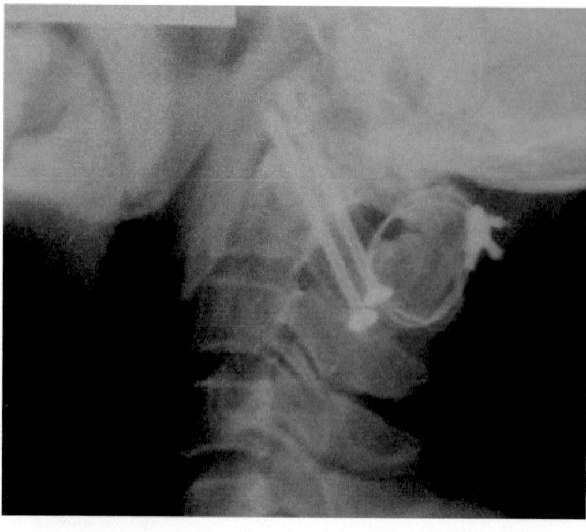
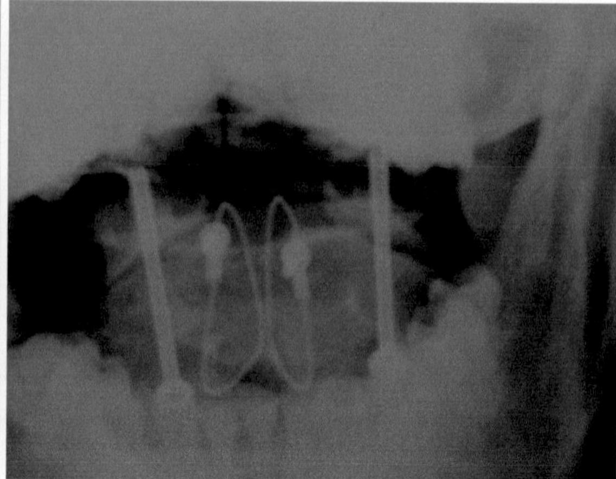

Fig. 5.17 Post-op X-ray images

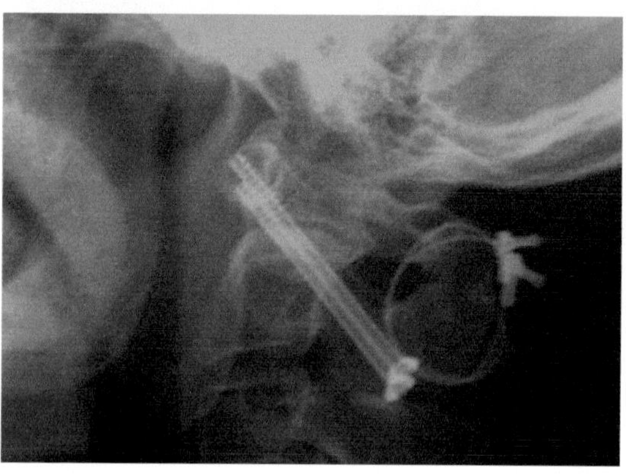

Fig. 5.18 The X-ray image in 1-year follow-up

References

Jeanneret B, Magerl F. Primary posterior fusion of C1/2 in odontoid fractures: indications, techniques, and results of transarticular screw fixation. J Spinal Disord. 1992;5(4):464–75.

Madawi AA, Casey AT, Solanki GA, et al. Radiological and anatomic evaluation of the atlantoaxial transarticular screw fixation technique. J Neurosurg. 1997;86(6):961–8.

Robot-Assisted Posterior C1 and C2 Screw Fixation

6

Lin Hu, Ning Zhang, and Wei Tian

Abstract

The posterior atlantoaxial fixation technique has been widely used for the treatment of upper cervical trauma, atlantoaxial instability, tumors, congenital malformation, and other diseases. However, the design and selection of internal fixation methods have changed greatly due to large anatomical variations in the upper cervical spine. The C1 lateral mass screw and C2 screw fixation system provide more choices for patients with abnormal bone structure and abnormal course of the vertebral artery. Likewise, there is also a reduction in force during the operation. The operation assisted by the surgical robot can effectively improve the accuracy of screw placement, reduce the vertebral artery and nerve injury, and facilitate the development of minimally invasive surgery.

Keywords

Robot-assisted surgery · Harms · C1–C2 posterior fixation · Cervical spine · Robotic surgery procedure

L. Hu · N. Zhang · W. Tian (✉)
Department of Spine Surgery, Beijing Jishuitan Hospital, Fourth Clinical Hospital of Peking University, Beijing, China
e-mail: tianweijst@vip.163.com

1 Introduction

The atlantoaxial lateral mass screw technique was first reported by Goel and Laheri (1994) of Mumbai, India, in 1994 and was fixed using a nail plate system. Harms (2001) and Merlcher (2003) improved and popularized this technology in 2001, using a multi-axis nail rod system. Before this, the C1–C2 joint screw (Magerl operation) was the most effective method to fix the atlantoaxial joint, but due to anatomical variability, a certain percentage of patients had difficulty in undergoing the Magerl procedure (1987). The lateral mass of atlas is relatively large, and the tolerance of placing nails is better than that of the Magerl operation. Likewise, because the nail channel does not pass through the joint of the lateral mass of the atlas and axis, the possibility of vertebral artery injury is reduced. In addition, the nail rod system can exert a reduction in force to a certain extent, thus its widespread use.

Harms first proposed to use the posterior midpoint of the lateral mass under the posterior arch of the atlas as the nail entry point. During the operation, the subperiosteal dissection was suggested to protect the C2 nerve and its surrounding venous plexus. The nail path must be parallel to the C1 rear arch plane (Goel et al. 2002). Some researchers believe that the C2 nerve roots can be cut off directly, but this is not widely accepted. In order to solve this problem, Harms improved the technique by using the posterior arch of the atlas

W. Tian (ed.), *Navigation Assisted Robotics in Spine and Trauma Surgery*,
https://doi.org/10.1007/978-981-15-1846-1_6

as the screw entry point (Tan et al. 2003). Kuroki et al.(2005) measured cadaver specimens and alleged that the average thickness of the posterior arch at the vertebral artery sulcus was 3.95 mm, and only 6.9% of women and 17.4% of men could safely insert 3.5 mm pedicle screws. Initially, the C1 lateral mass was mostly fixed using a double cortex. Recently, its necessity has also been questioned. Literature data show that the strength of the standard atlas pullout strength of a single cortical screw is much greater than the previous requirement for cervical vertebra screw pullout strength (Leconte 1964). Double cortical screws may damage the anterior internal carotid artery and hypoglossal nerve.

Anatomically, the pedicle of the axis is the connecting part between the C2 vertebral body and the posterior structure, presenting a coronal plane. Numerous authors have described the isthmus as the pedicle of the vertebral arch. A French doctor Robert Judet introduced the C2 pedicle screw technique for the first time in 1962 (Joes et al. 1997). Resnick et al. (2002) discovered through the simulated screw channel of the Xavier CT scan that the risk of transpedicular screw is equivalent to that of transpedicular screw. Later, a large number of researchers carried out anatomical studies and established a consensus on the method of setting screws, which actually involves isthmus screws rather than of pedicle screws. Different researchers have suggested different nail feeding points, head and inner inclinations. Subsequently researchers found that due to the greater variation of the axis and the greater potential for directing the nail canal, the standardized nail placement method was inappropriate, and it was necessary to devise an individualized design based on thin-layer CT data before operation (Moftakhar et al. 2008).

2 Indication

1. Instability of atlantoaxial joint caused by various reasons.
2. Transverse ligament fracture, odontoid fracture, and Jefferson fracture caused by trauma.
3. Rheumatoid arthritis.
4. Congenital and developmental malformation.
5. Tumor or infection.
6. Especially suitable for fracture of the odontoid process.

The fracture block is displaced backward. When the anterior odontoid screw fixation needs to adopt the posterior extension position of the cervical vertebra, the fracture reduction is difficult. The posterior-anterior flexion position can be used to reduce the fracture, and Harms operation can be performed to temporarily fix the atlantoaxial, maintain the fracture alignment, and remove the fixation after healing. Harms surgery is a good alternative for cases where the cervical curvature cannot be fixed by the Magerl method.

3 Preoperative Preparation

Preoperative patients should take X-ray positive side and open position films centered on the upper cervical vertebra to observe the deformity and dislocation of the bone joints. If the condition permits, they should assume flexion and extension positions to observe the changes of dislocation. CT and MRI were used to judge the nerve compression. Cervical angiography or CTA examination should be performed when conditions permit or there is a preoperative suspicion of vascular variation, so as to observe the course of the blood vessels in the atlantoaxial region, especially the vertebral artery and internal carotid artery, which is helpful for achieving an intraoperative response.

CT data should be imported into the preoperative design software before surgery. The best nail placement channel should be found in the reconstruction images considering various angles, and the appropriate length of screws should be measured for reference in surgery. For some patients with preoperative CT in the dislocation position, a virtual reduction can be carried out by referring to the position of preoperative dynamic X-ray in the software, and then the method of nailing can be evaluated after reduction (Fig. 6.1). It is important not to wait until the surgery to plan the screws. As some patients with a deformity have too narrow a bone structure, the vertebral body to be operated on may not have a suitable nail passage to pass through, and other surgical methods need to be temporarily replaced.

The position and length of a single screw are of course important for designing a screw channel, and the sequence of the screws is also very important. If the screw position is too asymmetric, this may cause relative rotation between C1 and C2 vertebral bodies (Fig. 6.2).

For patients with atlantoaxial instability, it is necessary to assess whether there are neurological symptoms under hyperextension and flexion before surgery, in order to determine the range of position placement during the operation.

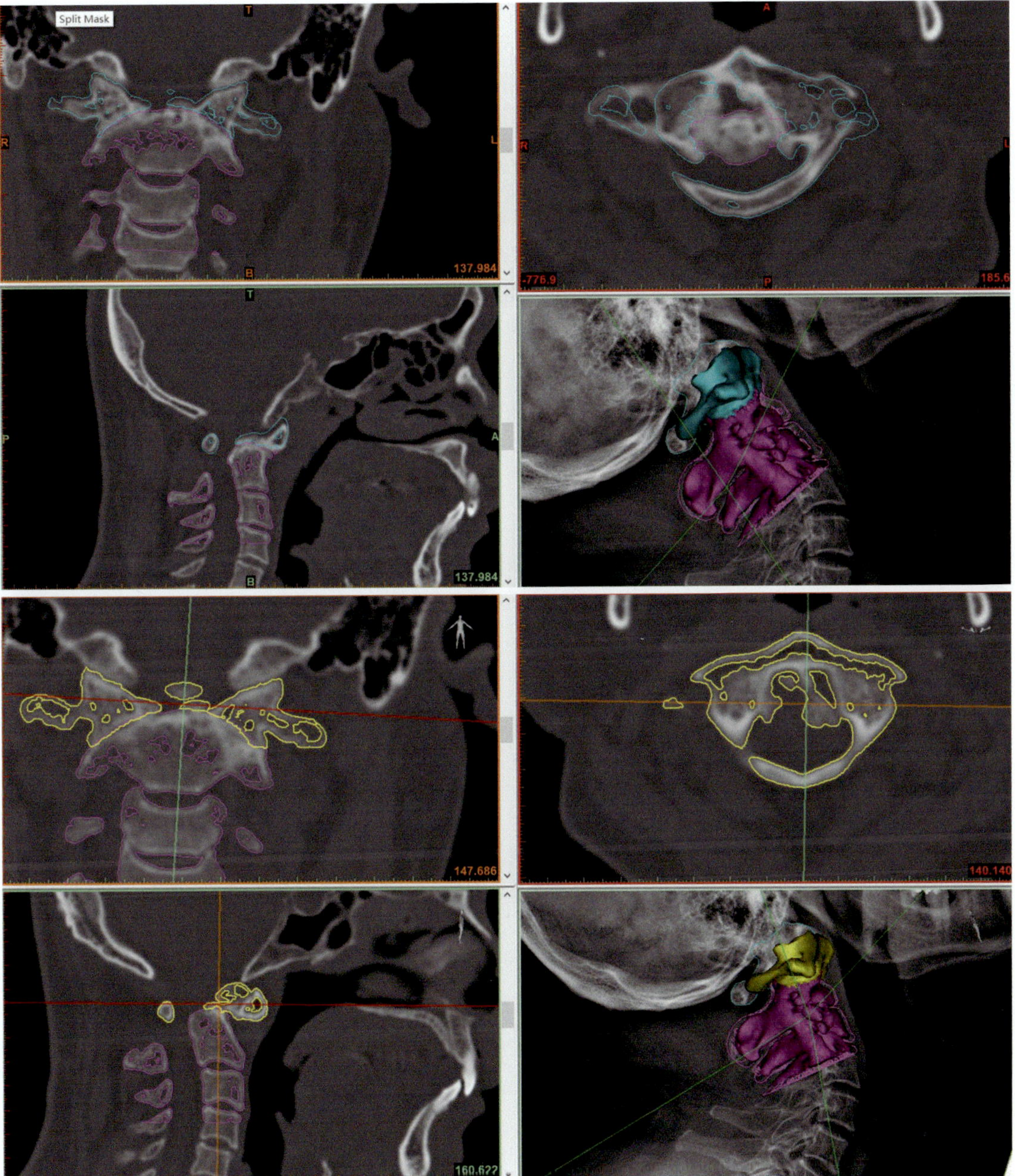

Fig. 6.1 The application of software provides a visualized simulation of reduction

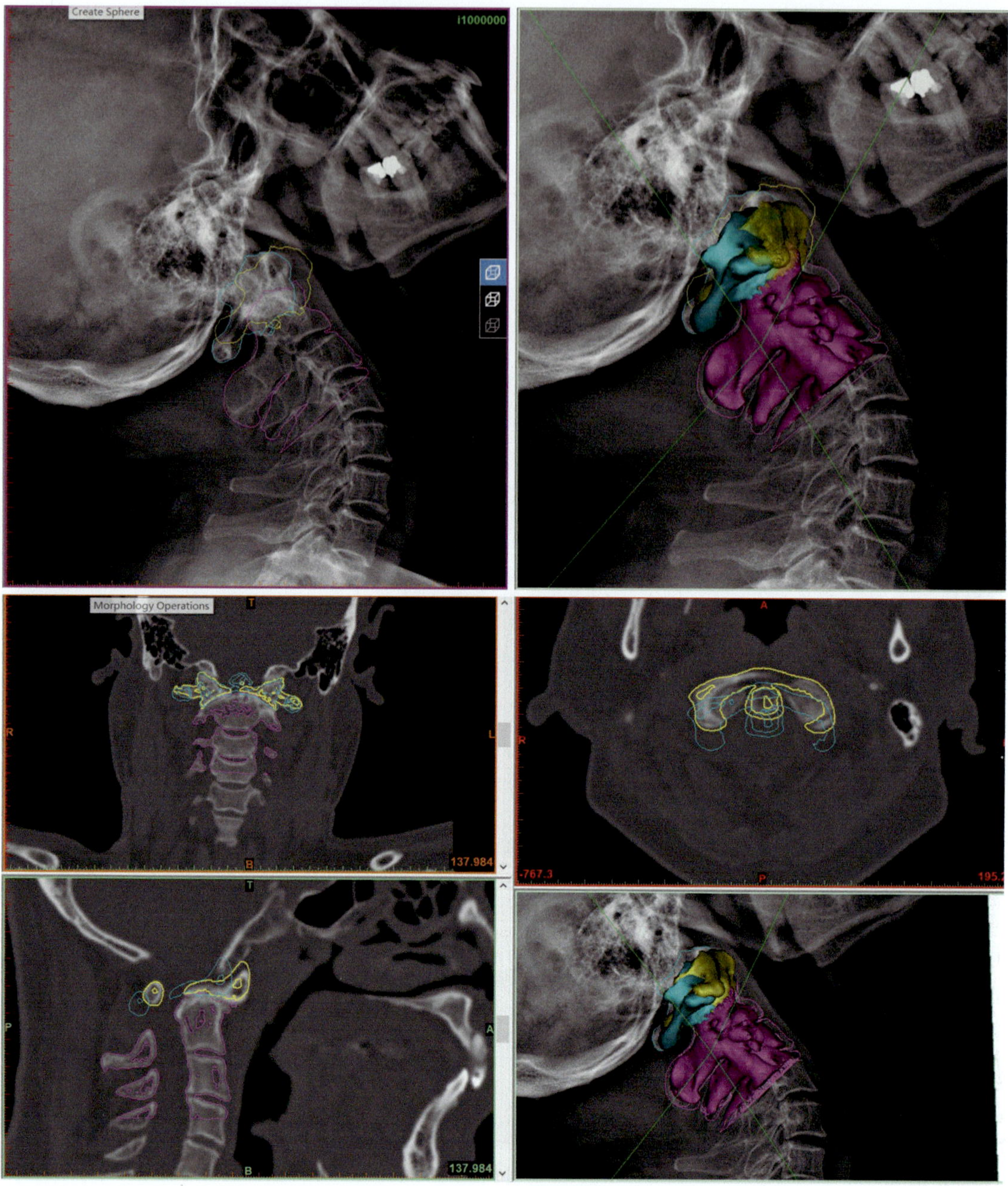

Fig. 6.1 (continued)

4 Procedures

1. The operation was performed under general anesthesia with endotracheal intubation. Place the patient in the prone position and use the Mayfield headrest to secure the head (Fig. 6.3).
2. The headrest is connected with the operating bed to ensure that the operating position is relatively fixed during the operation. The upper limbs of both sides are fixed to the side of the body. According to the operation requirements, adjust the neck flexion and

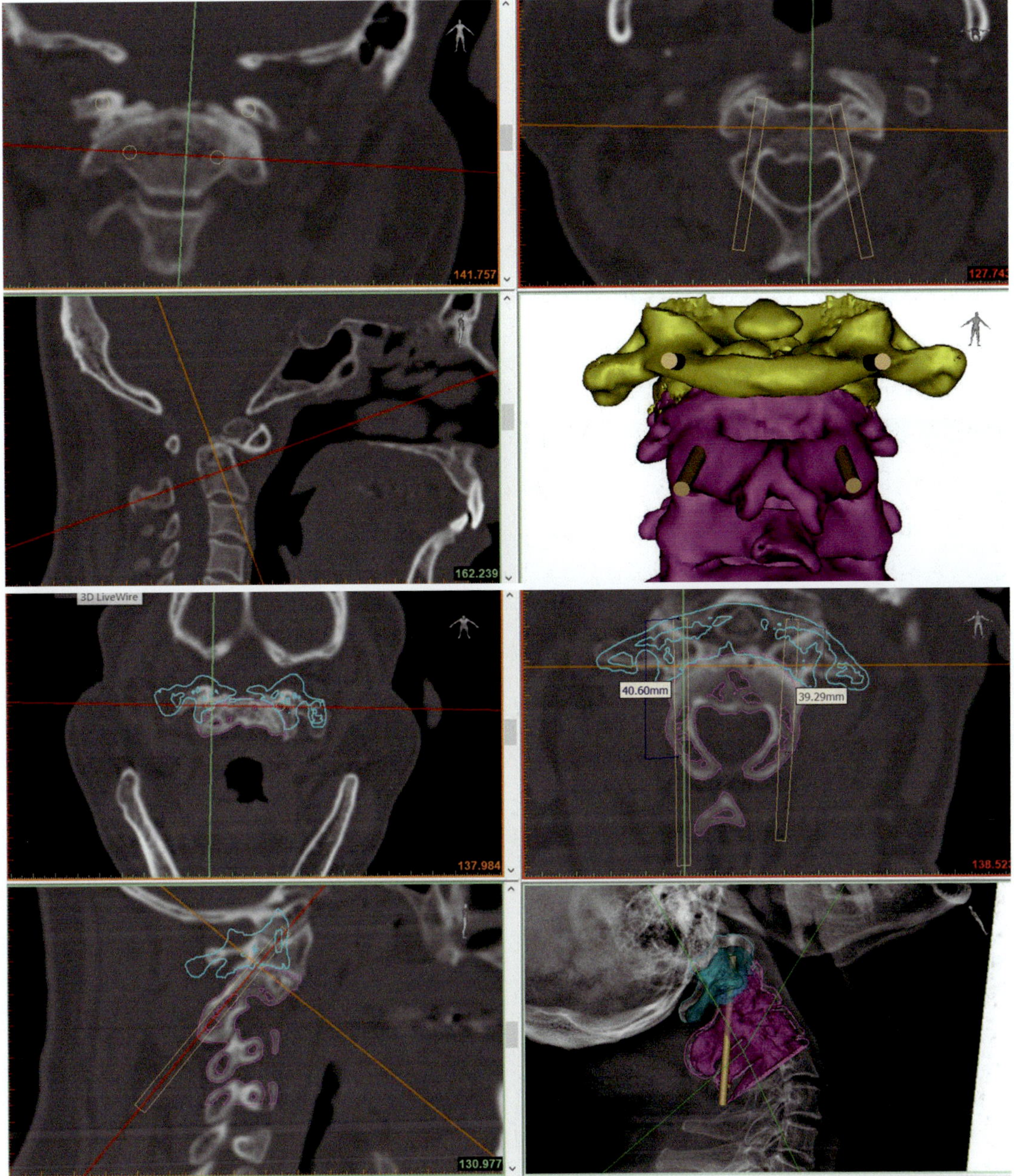

Fig. 6.2 The preoperative design of screw placement in software

extension position to suit the operation. Use the 3-D C-arm to capture the positive side slice (Fig. 6.4).

3. After the routine disinfection, make the skin incision to fully expose the nail point, and protect the peripheral vascular nerves (Fig. 6.5).
4. Next, use the Brooks method to achieve complete reduction (Fig. 6.6).
5. Place the navigation tracer in the head frame and attempt to get as close to the operation field as possible (Fig. 6.7). It can also be exposed and fixed to the C2 spinous process

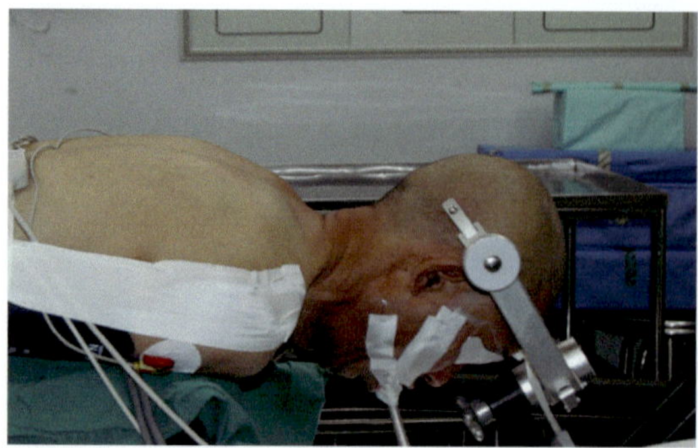

Fig. 6.3 Place the patient in the prone position and use the Mayfield headrest

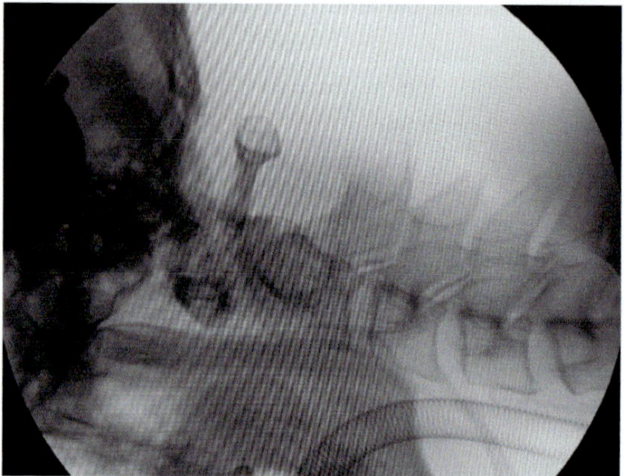

Fig. 6.4 Verify the neck is in a proper traction via fluoroscopy

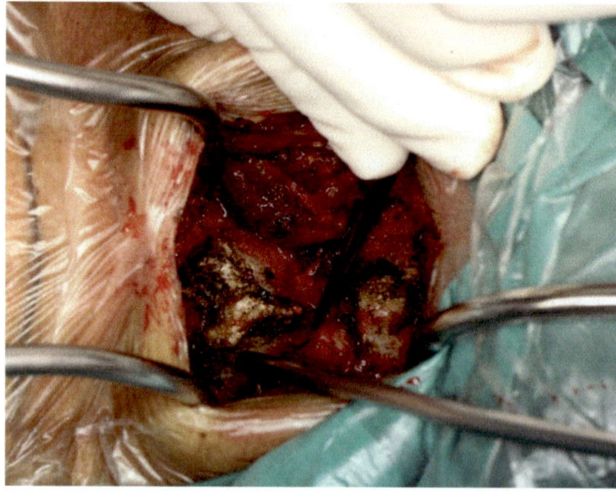

Fig. 6.5 Approach and exposure

based on the situation. Start the robot and enter patient information.

6. Use the 3-D C-arm to scan the surgical field and transmit the data to the robot system. The preoperative design shall be completed by a specialist, including the nail insertion point, screw length, and diameter (Figs. 6.8 and 6.9). After the design is completed, the overall position of the screw can be observed on the three-dimensional image.

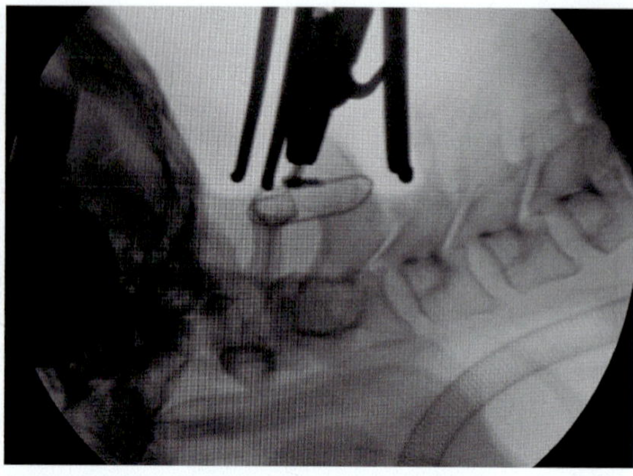

Fig. 6.6 The intraoperative fluoroscopy shows a satisfied reduction of the Brooks method

7. Operate the mechanical arm to move it to the preset nail path, pay attention to the soft tissue tension, and confirm that the error value of the current position is less than 0.5 mm. Place the sleeve to ensure that the tip of the sleeve touches the bone surface. The length of the K-wire tip is preset according to the screw length designed before the operation, and a 1.2 mm K-wire with the preset length is placed along the sleeve. Remove the sleeve and implant the K-wire according to the preoperative plan (Fig. 6.10).
8. The 3-D C-arm scan confirms that the K-wire was in good position (Fig. 6.11).
9. Use a hollow drill for drilling holes along the K-wire, pull out the K-wire, implant a 4.5 mm diameter screw, and install the connecting rod (Figs. 6.12–6.14).

5 Tips

1. When the Kirschner wire is implanted, if the bone cortex is too hard, the Kirschner wire may slip and screw misplacement may occur. The surrounding structures (vertebral artery at

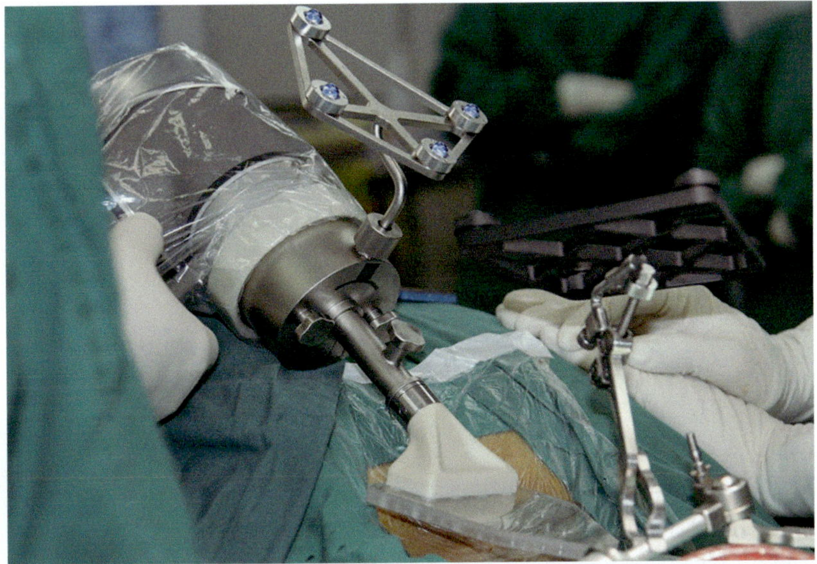

Fig. 6.7 The registration and calibration of the robot system

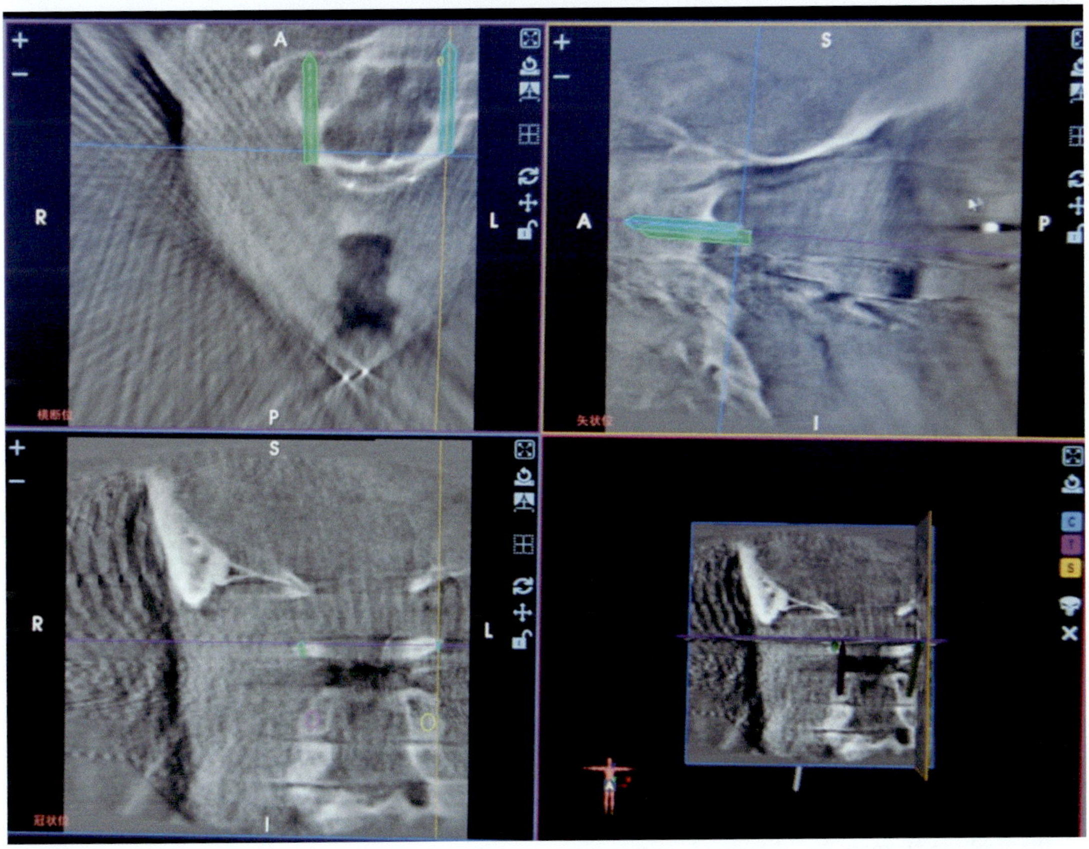

Fig. 6.8 The planning of the superior 2 screws

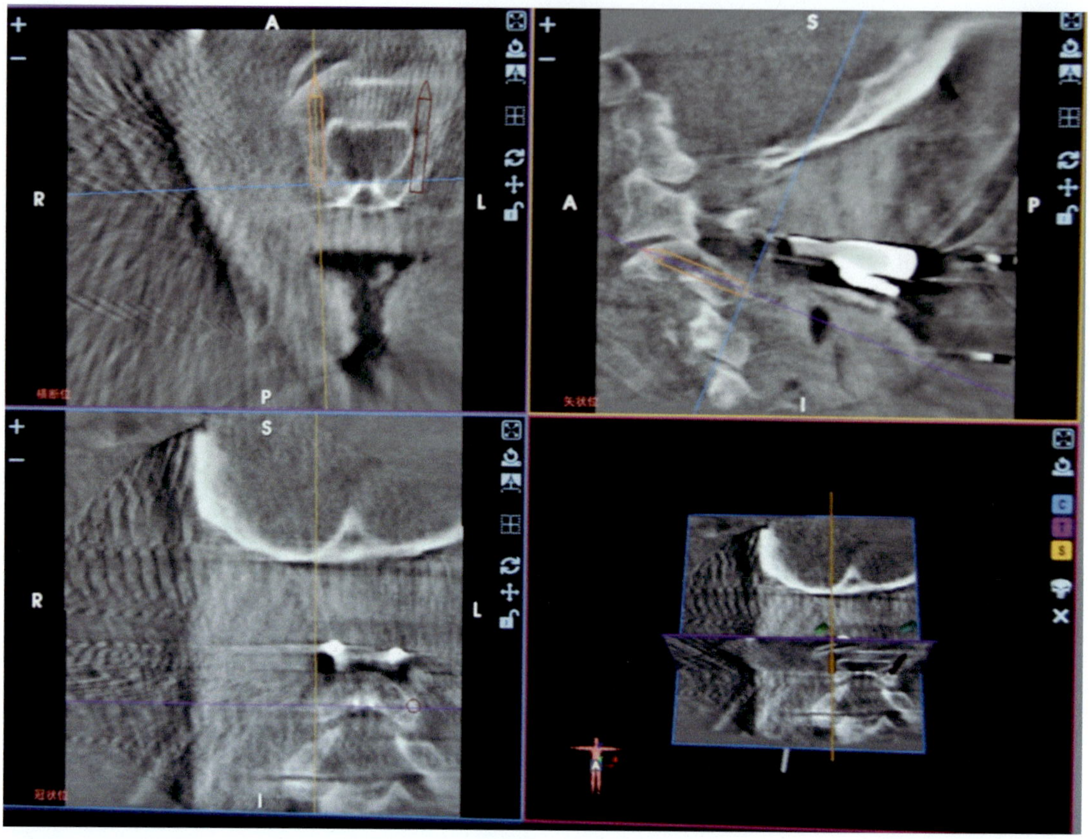

Fig. 6.9 The planning of the inferior 2 screws

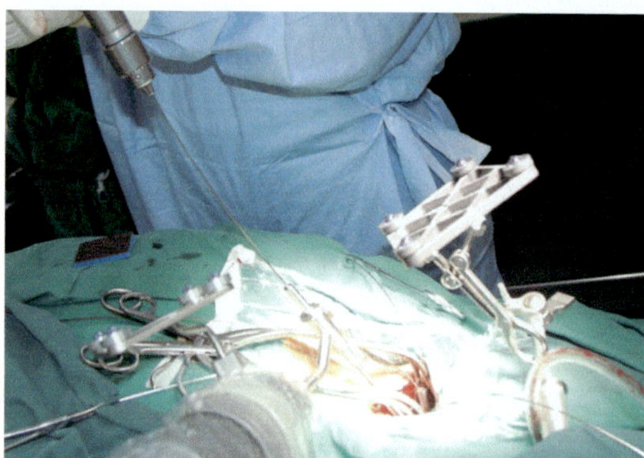

Fig. 6.10 Insert the K-wires followed the pathways that the robot arm automatically provides as planned

the head end and the vascular nerve bundle at the tail end) may be damaged, especially when the C1 side block screws are implanted through the posterior arch. The diameter of the C1 posterior arch is relatively small. Before implanting the Kirschner wire, it is possible to mark the access point, remove the robot slightly, use a small diameter abrasive drill to drill holes at the access point, and then implant the Kirschner wire, which can effectively prevent the phenomenon of Kirschner wire slipping.

2. The Kirschner wire and screw should be implanted to avoid excessive soft tissue tension, which may be indicated by the accuracy of the image for the nail placement. Some patients have thick muscle and soft tissue at the back of the neck. When fixing the C2 vertebral body, if the pedicle screw technique is selected, it may not be possible to complete it due to excessive soft tissue tension. Small incisions are needed to assist in reducing the soft tissue tension on both sides of the inci-

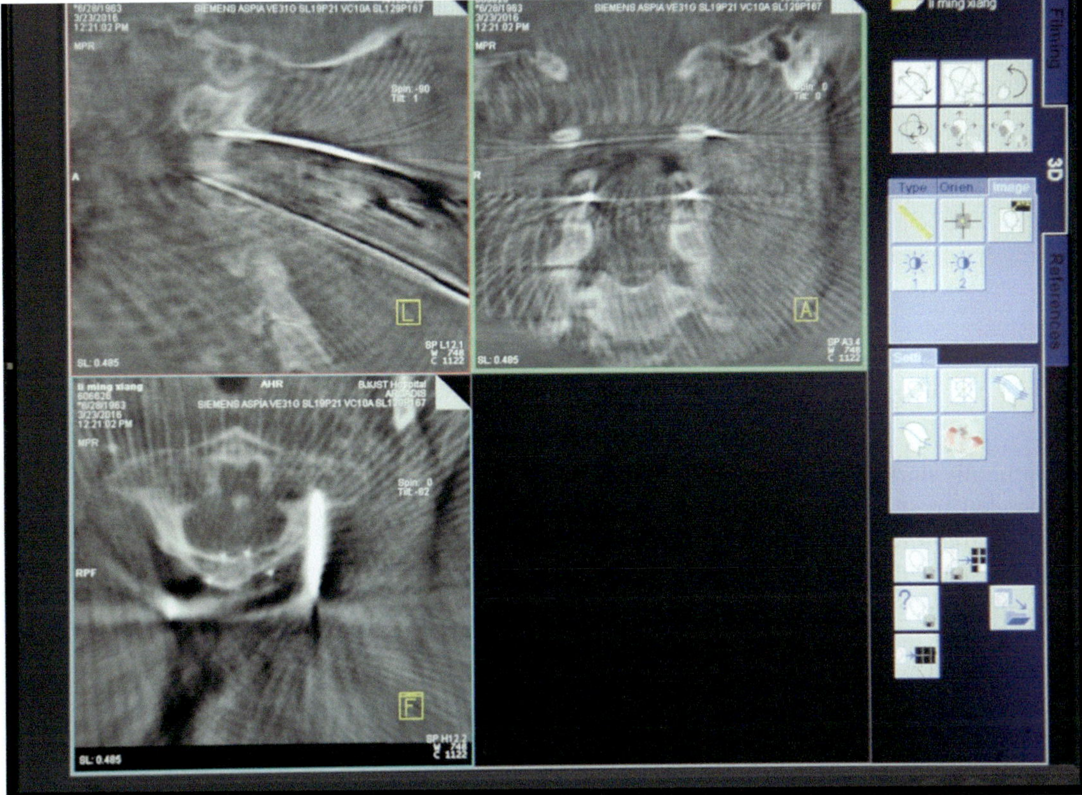

Fig. 6.11 Scan the postions of K-wires using 3D C-arm

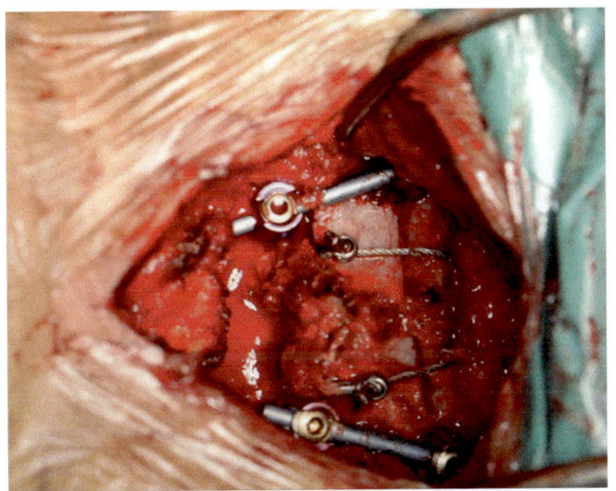

Fig. 6.12 Implant the screws and rods

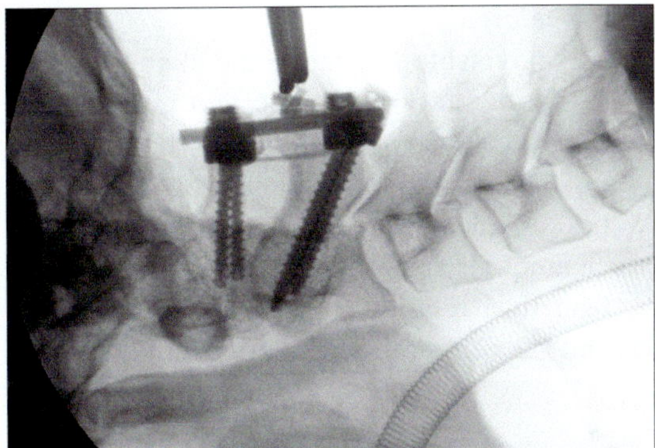

Fig. 6.13 The lateral view of intraoperative fluoroscopy

sion. For odontoid fractures, no bone grafting or fusion is needed, and nails can be placed directly from the bilateral paravertebral approach to reduce the influence of soft tissue tension.

3. Even if the three-dimensional scan shows the Kirschner wire has been positioned

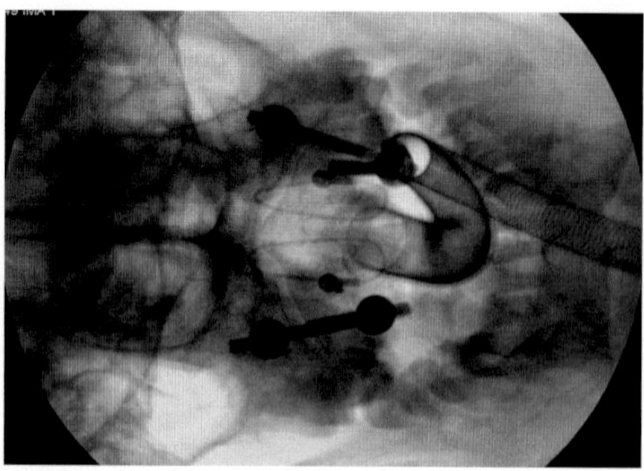

Fig. 6.14 The AP view of the intraoperative fluoroscopy

optimally during the operation, it is recommended to scan the position of the screw again after the nail placement is completed. Because the diameter of the Kirschner wire is small, even if the position is perfect, when the thicker screw is inserted, the direction may shift when it passes through the narrowest part of the bony channel, and cortical damage at the lateral foramen is likely to occur. This situation may be avoided by optimal preoperative planning. If the bony channel is too narrow before surgery, other fixation methods should be considered.

4. It is advisable to change the channel of the C2 vertebral body to a certain range. If the screw rod system is required to be reset during the operation, the screw sequence should be considered before designing the screw channel. If it is too asymmetric, this may lead to a relative rotation between the C1 and C2 vertebral bodies after reduction.

6 Typical Cases

A 45-year-old man was hurt in a traffic accident and presented to the ER. The patient felt severe neck pain but had no neurological symptoms. CT scan showed Type II odontoid fracture (Fig. 6.15).

Screw fixation was performed (Figs. 6.16–6.19).

According to the 1-year follow-up, the fracture had healed (Fig. 6.20).

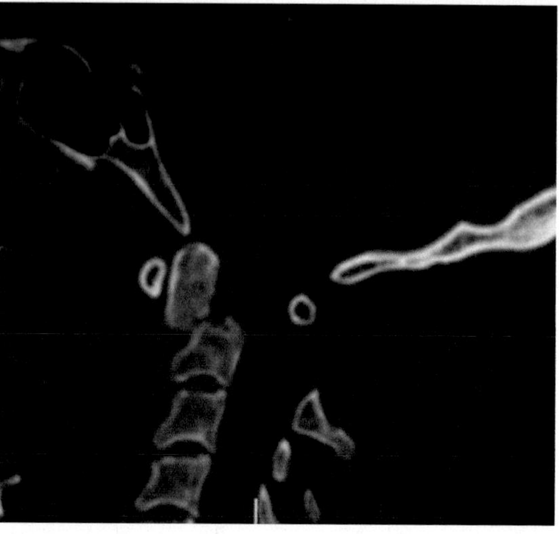

Fig. 6.15 The pre-op CT image

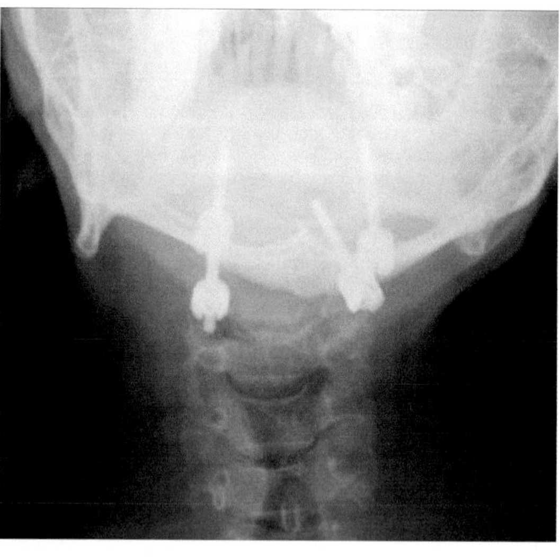

Fig. 6.16 The post-op PA view X-ray image

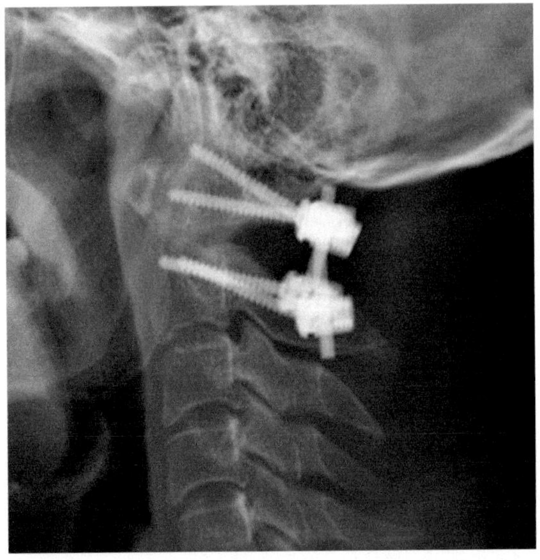

Fig. 6.17 The post-op lateral view X-ray image

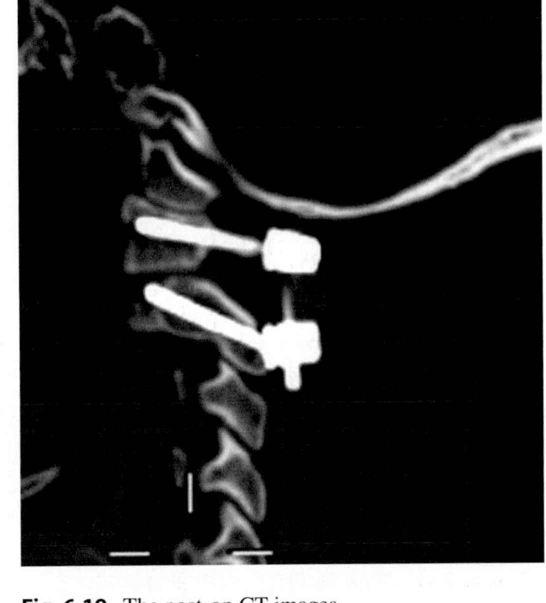

Fig. 6.19 The post-op CT images

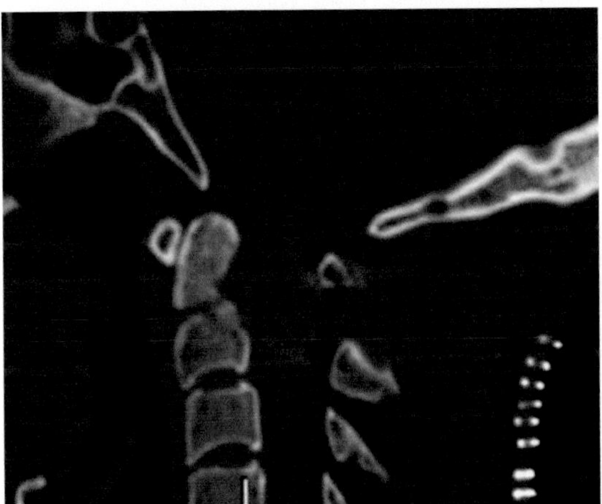

Fig. 6.18 The post-op CT images

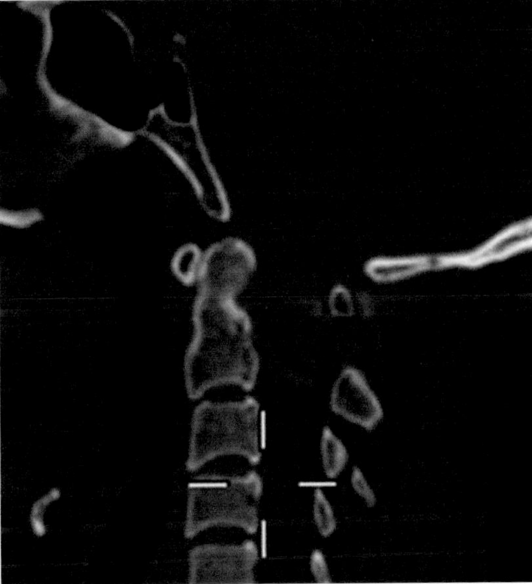

Fig. 6.20 the CT image in 1-year follow-up

References

Goel A, Laheri V. Plate and screw fixation for atlanto-axial subluxation. Acta Neurochir(Wien). 1994;129:47–53.

Harms J, Melcher RP. Posterior C1-C2 fusion with polyaxial screw and rod fixation. Spine. 2001;26:2467–71.

Melcher RP, Harms J. C1-C2 posterior screw-rod fixation. In: Bradford DS, Zdeblick T, editors. Master techniques in orthopaedic surgery: the spine. 2nd ed. Philadelphia: Lippincott, Williams & Wilkins; 2003. p. 129–45.

Margel F, Seemann PS. Stable posterior fusion of the atlas and axis by transarticular screw fixation. In: Kehr P, Weidner A, editors. Cervical spine. Wien: Springer; 1987. p. 322–7.

Goel A, Desai KI, Muzumdar DP. Atlantoaxial fixation using plate and screw method: a report of 160 treated patients. Neurosugery. 2002;51:1351–6. discussion 1356–1357

Tan M, Wang H, Wang Y, et al. Morphometric evaluation of screw fixation in atlas via posterior arch and lateral mass. Spine (Phila Pa 1976). 2003;28:888–95.

Kuroki H, Rengachary SS, Goel VK, et al. Biomechanical comparison of two stabilization techniques of atlantoaxial joints: transarticular screw fixation versus screw and rod fixation. Neurosurgery. 2005;56:151–9. Discussion 151-159

Leconte P. Fracture et luxation des deux premieres vertebres cervicales. In: Judet R, editor. Luxation Congenitale de la Hanche. Fractures du Cou-de-Rachis Cervical. Actualites de Chirurgie Orthopedique de l' Hospital Raymond-Poincare, vol. 3. Paris: Masson et Cie; 1964. p. 14–166.

Joes EL, Heller JG, Silcox DH, et al. Cervical pedicle screws versus lateral mass screws. Anatomical feasibility and biomechanical comparison. Spine(Phila Pa 1976). 1997;22:977–82.

Renick DK, Lapsiwala S, Trost GR. Anatomic suitability of the C1-C2 complex for pedicle screw fixation. Spine(Phila Pa 1976). 2002;27:1494–8.

Moftakhar P, Gonzales NR, Khoo LT, et al. Osseous and vascular anatomical variations within the C1-C2 complex: a radiographical study using computed tomography angiography. Int J Med Robot. 2008;4:158–63.

Robot-Assisted Odontoid Fracture Anterior Screw Fixation

7

Jianping Mao, Yunfeng Xu, and Wei Tian

Abstract

Odontoid anterior screw fixation has been proved to be an effective treatment for type IIB odontoid fracture. However, the traditional anterior screw fixation is technically challenging, due to difficult approach and high risk of screw malposition; even manipulators are exposed to high irradiation doses. With the new robot system (TiRobot), the entry point and trajectory of screw can be designed and sand to TiRobot, and then the robotic arm spontaneously moves accurately to the required position and guide the procedure. The details of TiRobotic procedure and tips are presented, which may help operators to achieve accurate odontoid anterior screw fixation.

Keywords

Robot-assisted surgery · Odontoid fracture · Anterior screw fixation · Cervical spine · Robotic surgery procedure

J. Mao · Y. Xu · W. Tian (✉)
Department of Spine Surgery, Beijing Jishuitan Hospital, Fourth Clinical Hospital of Peking University, Beijing, China
e-mail: tianweijst@vip.163.com

1 Introduction

Fractures of the odontoid process of the axis are common in the upper cervical region and comprise 7.7% of cervical spine fractures in adults (Goldberg et al. 2001). Odontoid fractures occur as a result of trauma to the cervical spine. The odontoid process, or dens, is a superior projecting bony element from the axis, and the atlas rotates around it to provide 50–60% rotation of the cervical spine (White 3rd. 1989). Stability is supported by the apical and paired alar ligaments that tether to the occipital and the transverse ligament that band to encircle the dens. Due to the specificity of the anatomy of the odontoid, surgical procedures for odontoid fractures represent a difficulty in spine surgery.

2 Classification

Anderson and D'Alonzo's classification system (Anderson and D'Alonzo 1974) for odontoid fractures is universally accepted clinically. They divided fractures into three categories (Fig. 7.1):

1. Type I, fracture through the upper part of the odontoid, near the tip of the dens. This injury commonly occurs due to pulling forces from the apical ligament and attachment to the odontoid process, which is rare.

W. Tian (ed.), *Navigation Assisted Robotics in Spine and Trauma Surgery*,
https://doi.org/10.1007/978-981-15-1846-1_7

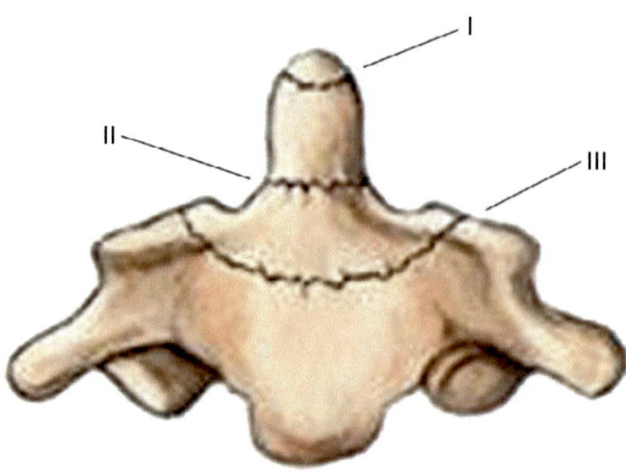

Fig. 7.1 Anderson and D'Alonzo classification of odontoid fracture. (1) Type I fractures involve the upper part of the odontoid. (2) Type II fracture occurs at the junction of the dens and the body of the axis. (3) Type III fracture extends into the body of the axis

2. Type II fracture occurs at the junction of the dens and the body of the axis. This is the most common type, occurring in 65–74% of cases (Anderson and D'Alonzo 1974; Dumonski and Vaccaro 2010; Müller et al. 2003). A common mechanism of injury is the hyperextension of the cervical spine, the anterior arch of the atlas stems backward, and in transmitting this rearward displacement to the odontoid processes causes the odontoid break at its base. This type fracture can also be associated with excessive cervical flexion, and the transverse ligament can transmit excessive anterior forces to the odontoid to cause further facture.
3. Type III, fracture extending into the body of the axis, may involve the atlantoaxial joint. This type of fracture is the second most common type and has a similar mechanics as type II.

While type I and III fractures are stable forms and are generally treated conservatively with rigid immobilization, type II fractures are unstable fractures, and the nonunion rate of conservative management ranges from 16 to 54% (Osman et al. 2017; Platzer et al. 2007; Govender et al. 2000; Koivikko et al. 2004). Grauer et al. (2005) published a subtype classification of type II facture. Type II A, odontoid fracture, has a transverse pattern at the base with no displacement. Type II B displays an oblique fracture line from the anterosuperior to the posteroinferior portion of the dens or transverse fracture with a displacement more than 1 mm. Type IIC is an anteroinferior to posterosuperior oblique fracture or comminuted fracture. Type II A is the stable fracture and can be managed with external fixation. Types IIB and IIC are indications for surgery: type IIB with anterior screw fixation, type IIC with posterior fusion (Grauer et al. 2005).

The factors that have been reported to be associated with nonunion include degree of comminution at the base of the dense, age, rupture of the transverse ligament, delayed start of treatment, and fracture displacement (Govender et al. 2000; Koivikko et al. 2004; Hanigan et al. 1993; Lennarson et al. 2000; Joaquim and Patel 2010a, b).

3 Anterior Odontoid Screw Fixation

Anterior odontoid screw fixation was first described by Bohler (1982) in 1982 for the treatment of a type II fracture. Anterior odontoid screw fixation is an osteosynthetic technique that provides immediate stability and exhibits a pressure effect on the fracture ends, which benefit fracture healing; the overall rate of fracture union has been reported to be 92.3% with fracture healing averaging 5.5 months (Etter et al. 1991). Fixation preserves rotatory function along the atlantoaxial joint and also avoids the dissection of the posterior neck muscles during the posterior approach; hence, it has now become the most widely used technique.

3.1 Indication

Indications for anterior odontoid screw fixation include type II fractures and especially Grauer subtype IIB, good fracture reduction, and alignment, as well as those who with IIA fracture are not resistant to external fixation.

3.2 Contraindication

Contraindications include type IIC fracture (anteroinferior to posterosuperior oblique fracture and comminuted fracture), severe osteoporosis, severe cervicothoracic kyphosis, short neck deformity, nonunions, nonreducible fractures, and ligament transverse rupture (Aebi et al. 1989; Agrillo et al. 2008; Henry et al. 1999).

3.3 Preoperative Preparation

Patients with odontoid fractures should take the standard trauma series consisting of high-quality anterior–posterior (AP), lateral, and open-mouth X-ray. Preoperative X-ray could provide information regarding the atlantoaxial relationship, atlantoaxial dislocation, atlantoaxial instability (interval between atlantoaxial more than 3-mm implies a ligament transverse rupture), and any deformity of the cervical spine. Thin-layer CT scan and 3D reconstruction provides the best resolution of the bony elements allowing for identification and characterization of an odontoid fracture. MRI should be obtained to assess injuries of the cervical cord and the transverse ligament. Three radiology examinations should provide detailed information regarding odontoid fracture and will help clinicians to choose the ideal treatment.

Concurrently, the general condition of the patient should be evaluated before operation, so as to eliminate any contraindications and ensure the safety of the surgical procedure. For cases with displaced fracture, preoperative traction should be given for reduction. A posterior approach for atlantoaxial fusion should be taken for unreducible fractures. During traction, bedside X-ray should be taken to evaluate the position of the fracture and to observe the general conditions of patients and timely detection the deterioration of nerve function.

Surgeons that plan to perform odontoid anterior screw fixation should master atlantoaxial anatomy and the cervical anterior approach and of posterior atlantoaxial fusion techniques. In patients who are unable to undergo the anterior approach, posterior fusion is a suitable alternative.

3.4 Procedures

Procedures of robot-assisted odontoid anterior screw fixation include:

1. Anesthesia. The operation is performed under intubation general anesthesia, with the patient's head fixed in a radiolucent Mayfield skull clamp. The patient is then transferred to the radiolucent Jackson table in the supine position.
2. Position. The Mayfield skull clamp is connected to Mayfield adapter on the table. Adjusting the Mayfield adapter, the Mayfield skull clamp is placed to reduce manipulation and to achieve reduction while keeping the head in traction and extension. Both upper limbs are tightly fixed on the both sides of the body. Patient positioning is critical to facilitate the trajectory of odontoid screw placement (Fig. 7.2).
3. The robot preparation. The patient is prepared and draped according to the routine sterile fashion. The patient tracker is settled on the Mayfield skull clamp to ensure the tracker is closed to operative regions (Fig. 7.3).

   Next, a 3D C-arm (Siemens Medical Solutions, Erlangen, Germany) is used to obtain AP and lateral plain radiographs to verify the relationship between the odontoid and axis basement, as well as the degree of extension (Figs. 7.4 and 7.5).

   Next, the robot is introduced, and the robotic arm is registered using special registration device (with the plate locator on it) (Fig. 7.6). The 3D C-arm is used to scan an operation region, and data is transferred to the robot system (Fig. 7.7).
4. Preoperative planning. Preoperative planning is carried out on the robot system, which includes the entry point, the trajectory of the screw, the length and the diameter of the screw, as well as the simulation of the screw positioning in the 3D image to further finely adjust the entry point and direction (Fig. 7.8). Next, the preoperative plan is sent to guide the robotic system.
5. The guide tube is connected. Based on the result of the robot system calculation, the

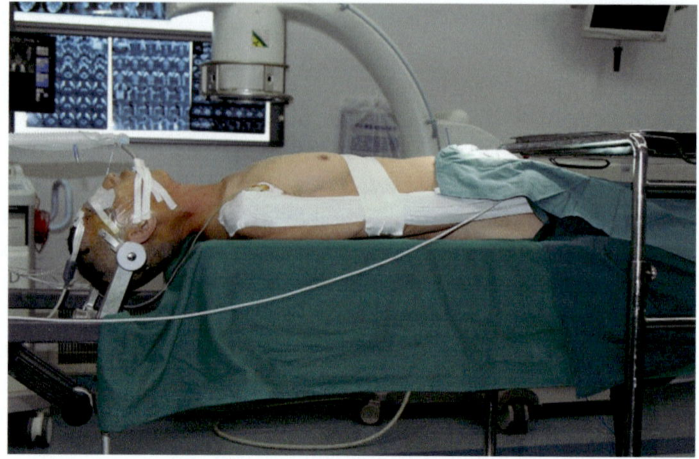

Fig. 7.2 Lateral view of patient position. The Mayfield skull clamp is used to position the neck in an extended position to facilitate the screw trajectory. While both upper limbs are slightly dragged and fixed on the both sides of body

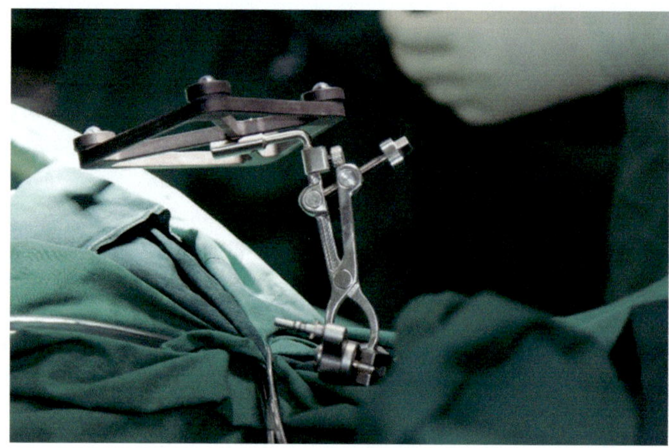

Fig. 7.3 The patient tracker is connected to the Mayfield skull clamp

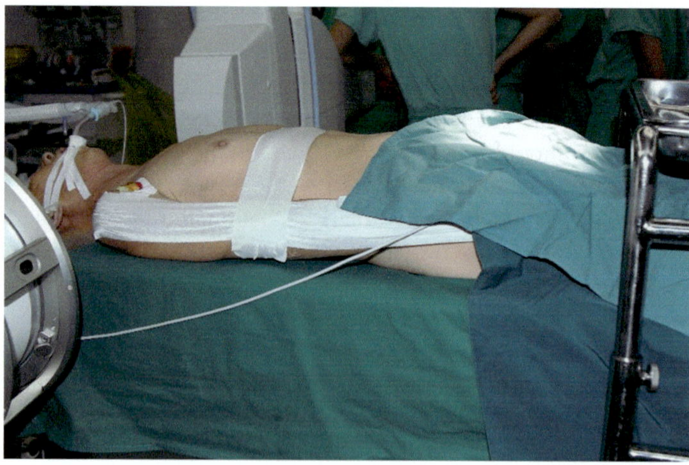

Fig. 7.4 Intraoperative fluoroscopy is used to confirm the position of the fractured fragments

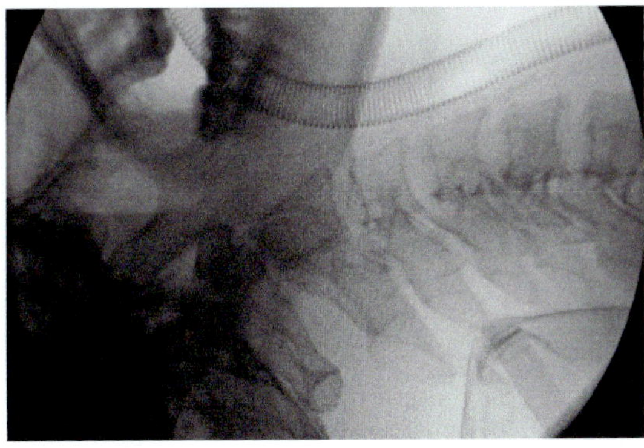

Fig. 7.5 Lateral view of cervical fluoroscopy after positioning

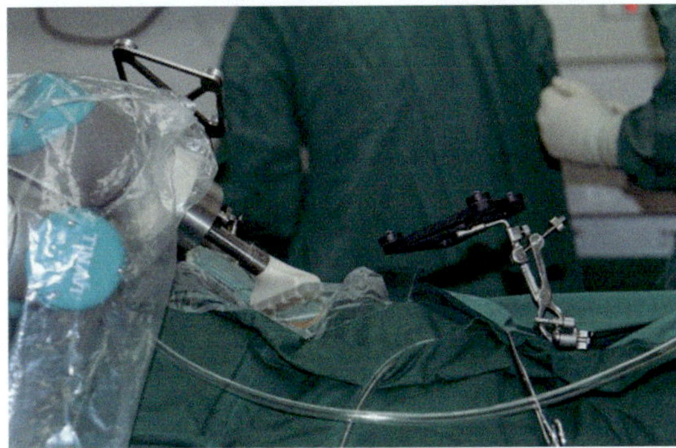

Fig. 7.6 The robotic arm is registered using the special registration device

ideal guide tube is chosen and installed in the robotic arm (Fig. 7.9).

6. Locate the skin incision. Next, the robotic arm spontaneously moves precisely to the required location based on the preoperative planning. The skin incision is located and marked on the skin (Fig. 7.10). Subsequently, the robotic arm is moved away.
7. Exposure. A 2–3 cm incision is made, and blunt dissection is carried out down to the center of the anterior inferior border of the C2 vertebra. Minimally invasive retractors or self-retaining retractors are used to retract the tissue and to expose the channel (Figs. 7.11 and 7.12).

   During the procedure, attention should be paid to the trachea, esophagus, blood vessels, and other important structures.
8. Enter point location. Once more, let the robotic arm spontaneously move to the required location and position the tip of the guide tube on the entry point on the anterior inferior edge of the C2 vertebra (Fig. 7.13). The robot system will calculate the value of error and ensure the value is within the range of allowable error (normally less than 0.5 mm). Next, the guide tube is mildly tapped to ensure close contact with the anterior and inferior border of the C2 vertebra (Fig. 7.14).

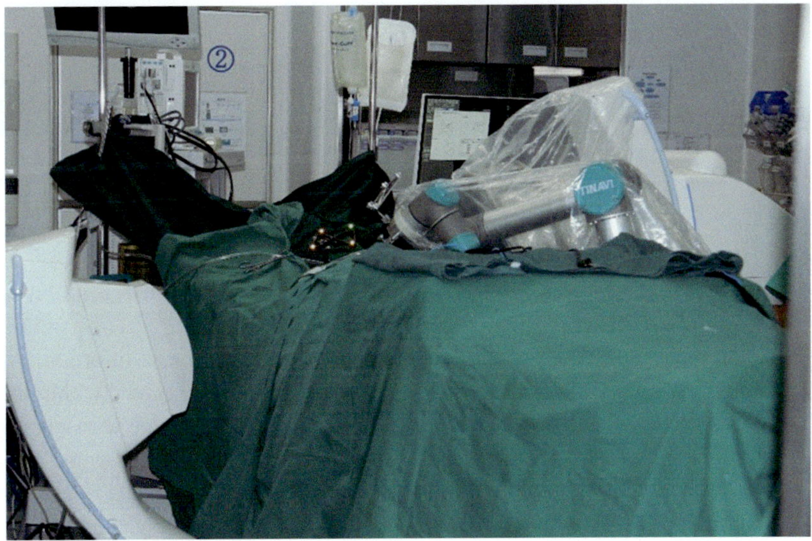

Fig. 7.7 The intraoperative 3D images are scanned using the 3D C-arm

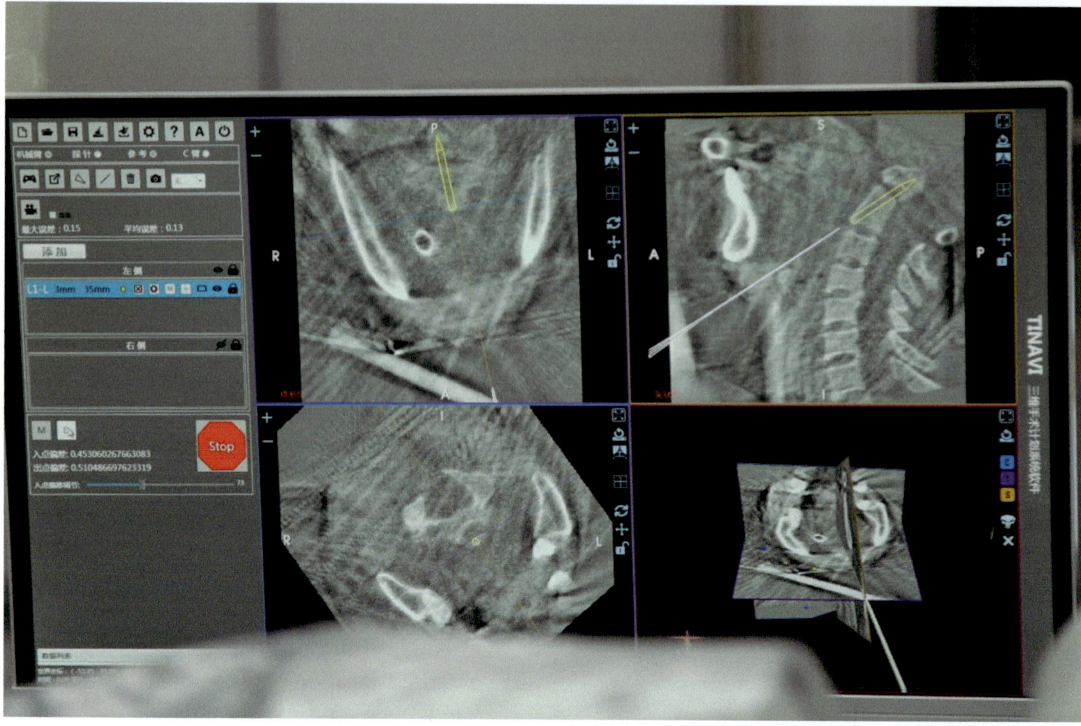

Fig. 7.8 Graphical user interface of the surgical plan in the TiRobot system. The surgeon can use intraoperative 3D images to determine the best screw trajectory

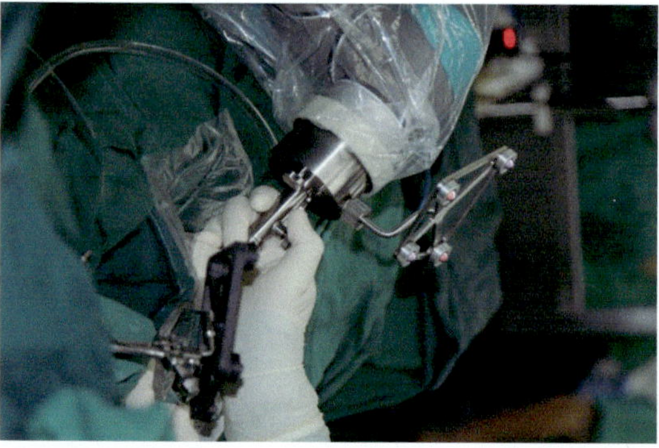

Fig. 7.9 The ideal guide tube is connected to the robotic arm

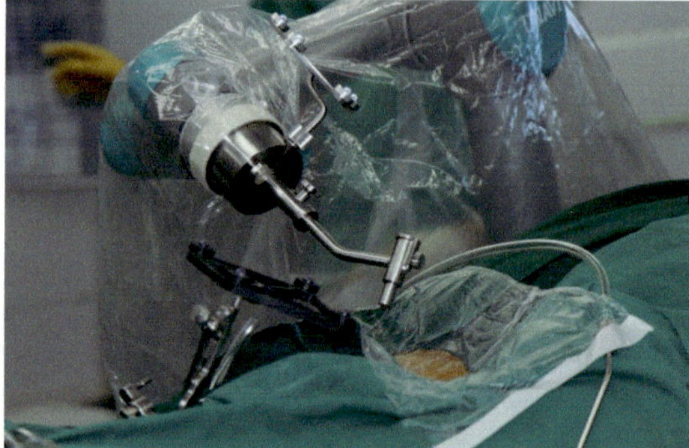

Fig. 7.10 The skin incision is located through the robotic arm spontaneously moving accurately to the required location based on preoperative planning

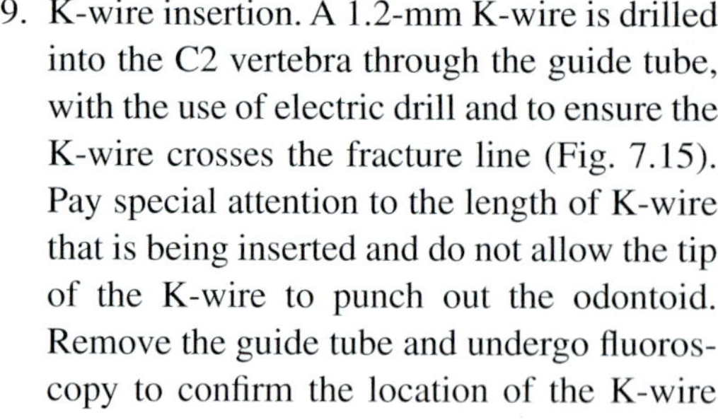

9. K-wire insertion. A 1.2-mm K-wire is drilled into the C2 vertebra through the guide tube, with the use of electric drill and to ensure the K-wire crosses the fracture line (Fig. 7.15). Pay special attention to the length of K-wire that is being inserted and do not allow the tip of the K-wire to punch out the odontoid. Remove the guide tube and undergo fluoroscopy to confirm the location of the K-wire and the relationship with the fracture line (Fig. 7.16).
10. Screw insertion. After confirming, the screw trajectory within the C2 vertebra and odontoid is made with a hollow drill, under the guidance of the K-wire. The cannulated screw, chosen according to preoperative planning, is inserted. Finally, the location of screw and fracture fragments are confirmed by fluoroscopy (Fig. 7.17).

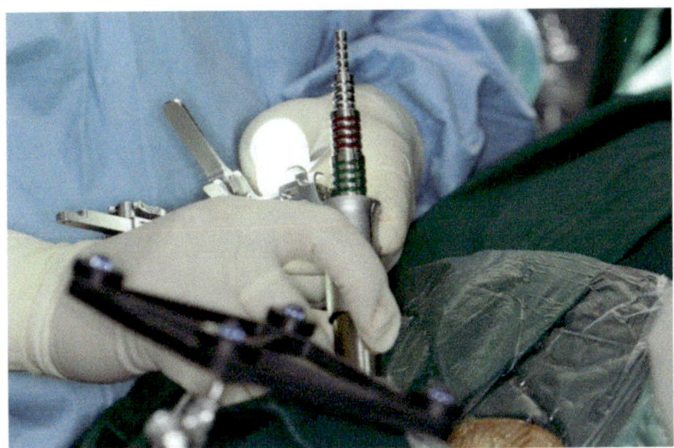

Fig. 7.11 The working channel is set up with the minimally invasive retractor

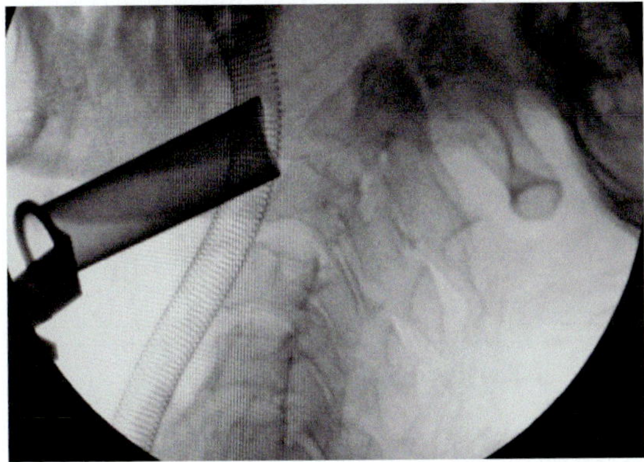

Fig. 7.12 Fluoroscopy is used to confirm the working channel

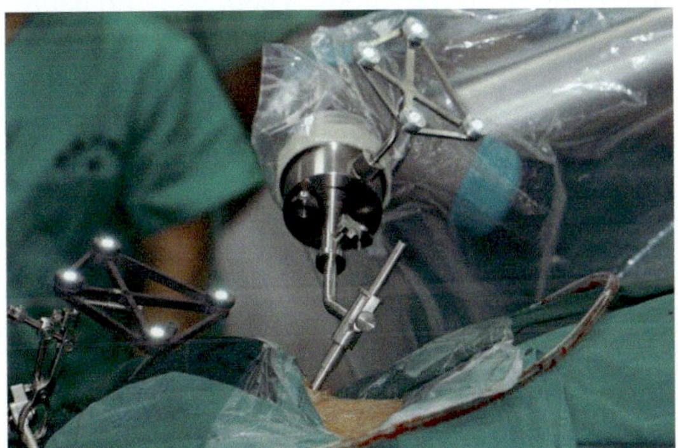

Fig. 7.13 A cannula is inserted through the robotic sleeve to reach the bone cortex, after which a K-wire is placed through the cannula (Citation with permission from Tian W, Wang H, Liu YJ. Robot-assisted Anterior Odontoid Screw Fixation: A Case Report. Orthopaedic Surgery 2016; 8(3): 400–4)

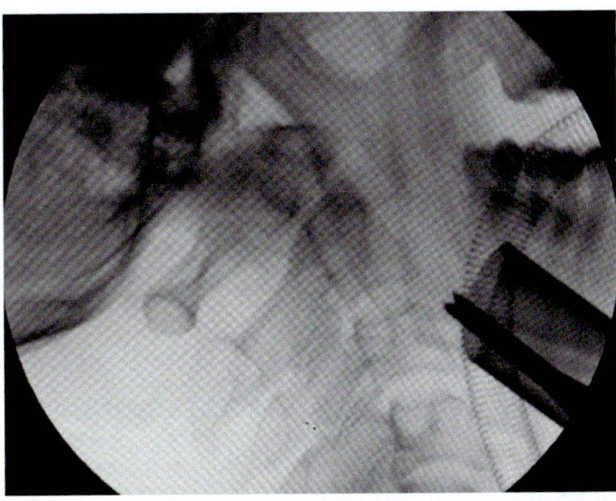

Fig. 7.14 Fluoroscopy is used to confirm the position of guide tube

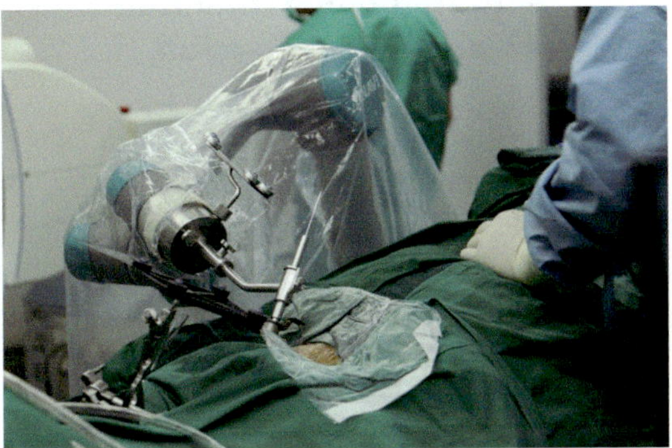

Fig. 7.15 A 1.2 mm K-wire is drilled into the C2 vertebra through the guidewire

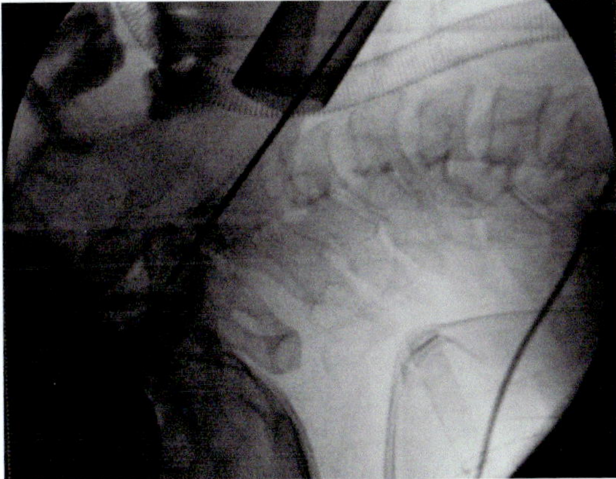

Fig. 7.16 The intraoperative fluoroscopy is used to confirm the location of K-wire and the relationship with fracture line

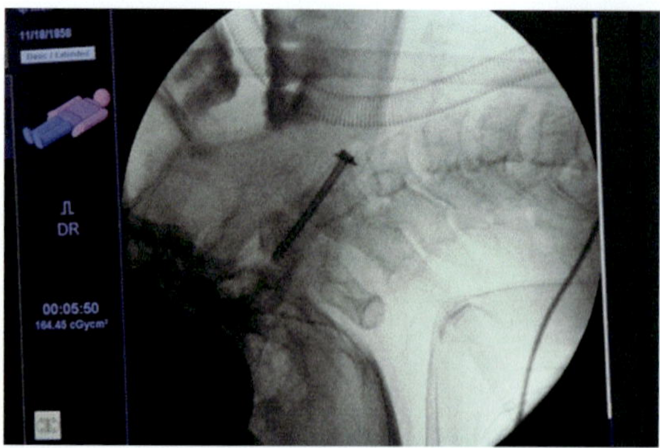

Fig. 7.17 Fluoroscopy is used to confirm the location of screw and fracture fragments

3.5 Advancement in Comparison with Traditional Odontoid Anterior Screw Fixation

During the traditional odontoid anterior screw fixation procedure, a G-arm or double C-arms are needed to provide an AP view and later view to confirm the position. The position of patient's head needs to be repeatedly adjusted in order to avoid interference from the teeth and the mandibular in fluoroscopic images, which may take a long time. In addition, there is no guide device for K-wire inserting; thus, operative time and X-ray expose time are prolonged to repeatedly check and confirm.

On the contrary, robot-assisted odontoid anterior screw fixation is a simple and accurate operation, less demanding of patient's position, and without the need for repeated fluoroscopy, and the K-wire could be accurately positioned at one attempt with the guidance of robot.

3.6 Tips

1. There are some pitfalls to be avoided in robot-assisted odontoid anterior screw fixation.
2. The K-wire might slip when it touches the hard cortex bone, which should be avoided during operation.
3. The guide tube should be maintained without any tension, because the large soft tissue tension will decrease the accuracy of the robot system.
4. The robotic arm should be within the surveillance scope of camera during the entire procedure of arm location, because shading will affect the accuracy of the operation.
5. Specialists should be present who are responsible for monitoring real-time error value calculated by robot system during K-wire placing. If the error value is more than 0.5 mm, the procedure should be paused to identify the reason and find a solution.
6. The operator should have the ability to find problem timely and sometimes use fluoroscopy to confirm the position in order to ensure the accuracy of the operation.

4 Typical Case[20]

A 61-year-old woman presented to the emergency department with upper neck pain after a fall. Physical examination showed tenderness in the upper cervical region and a decreased range of motion in all directions. There were no neurological deficits.

Cervical CT images showed a type IIB odontoid fracture, with 2-mm anterior displacement of the upper portion (Fig. 7.18).

Diagnosis: Odontoid Fracture (Type IIB).

TiRobot-assisted anterior odontoid screw fixation was performed (Figs. 7.19 and 7.20).

The patient was discharged on Day 5 with no operative complications. Postoperative CT scan showed the accuracy of the screw, with no perforation or loosening (Fig. 7.21). Two years after the surgery, the clinical follow-up showed that she had recovered full strength in her extremities.

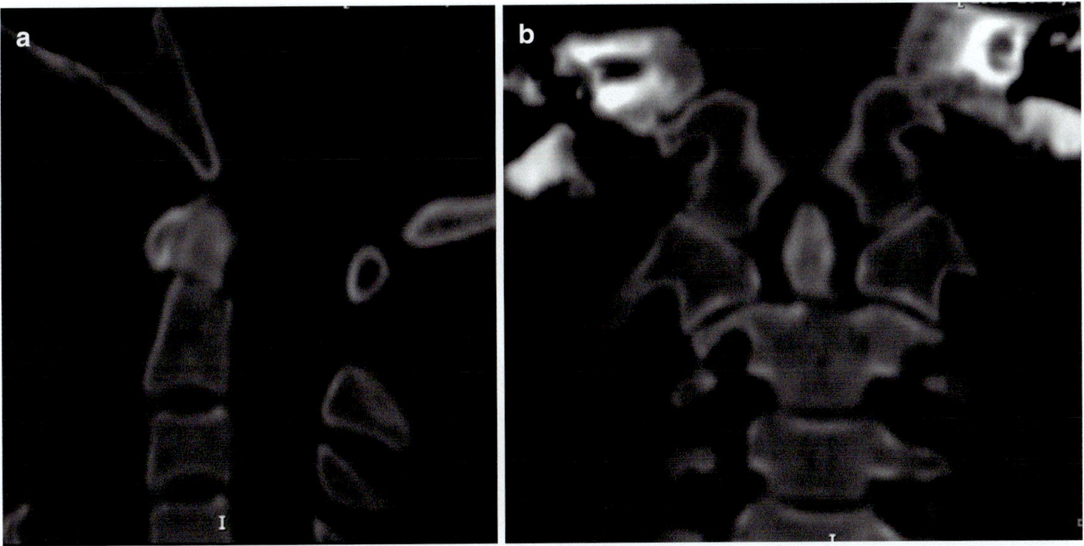

Fig. 7.18 Sagittal (**a**) and coronal (**b**) CT images showing a type IIB odontoid fracture

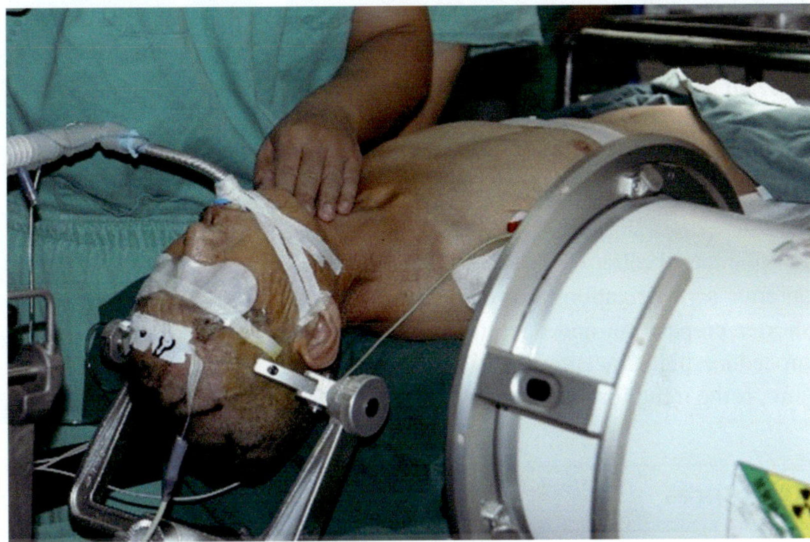

Fig. 7.19 The intraoperative position

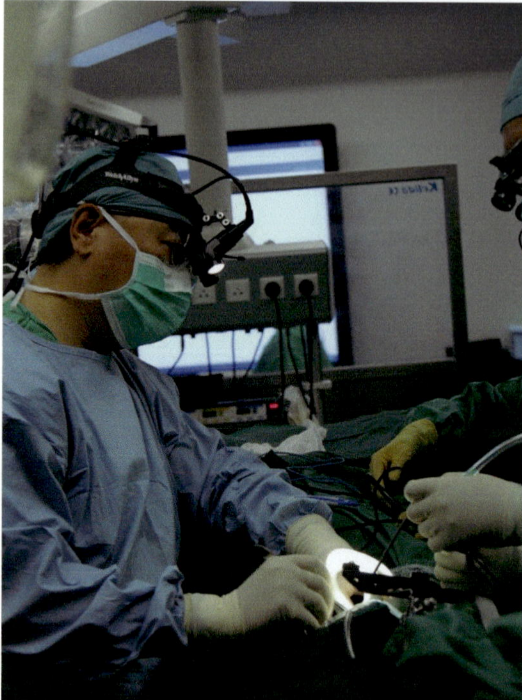

Fig. 7.20 Excision and soft tissue exposure

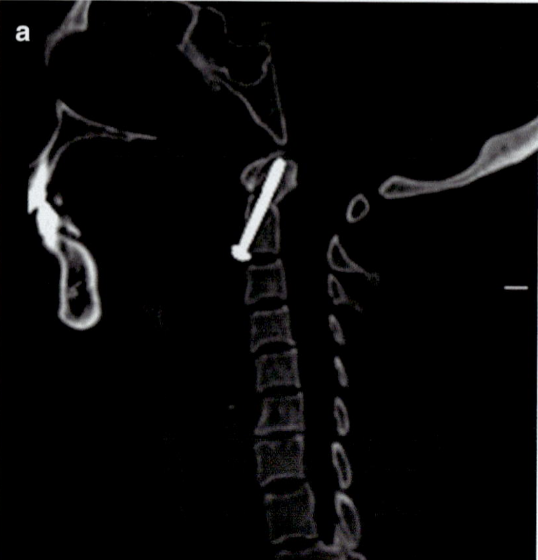

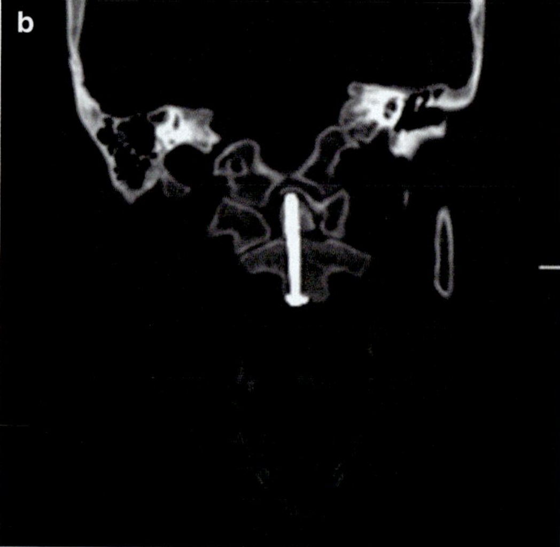

Fig. 7.21 Sagittal (**a**) and coronal (**b**) postoperative CT images showing the accurate position of the screw

5 Summary

In summary, robot-assisted odontoid fracture anterior screw fixation, with the advantages of shorter preparation and operation time, simpler procedure, higher accuracy, and low X-ray exposure, is the trend for the future.

References

Goldberg W, Mueller C, Panacek E, et al. Distribution and patterns of blunt traumatic cervical spine injury. Ann Emerg Med. 2001;38(1):17–21.

White AA 3rd. Clinical biomechanics of cervical spine implants. Spine (Phila Pa 1976). 1989; 14(10):1040–5.

Anderson LD, D'Alonzo RT. Fractures of the odontoid process of the axis. J Bone Joint Surg Am. 1974;56(8):1663–74.

Dumonski ML, Vaccaro AR. Treatment of odontoid fractures. Neurosurgery Quar. 2010;20(3):183–8.

Müller EJ, Schwinnen I, Fischer K, Wick M, Muhr G. Non-rigid immobilisation of odontoid fractures. Eur Spine J. 2003;12(5):522–5.

Osman A, Alageli NA, Short DJ, Masri WSE. Conservative management of odontoid peg fractures, long term follow up. J Clin Orthop Trauma. 2017;8(2):103–6.

Platzer P, Thalhammer G, Sarahrudi K, et al. Nonoperative management of odontoid fractures using a halothoracic vest. Neurosurgery. 2007;61(3):522–9. discussion 9-30

Govender S, Maharaj JF, Haffajee MR. Fractures of the odontoid process an angiographic and clinical study. J Bone Joint Surg British. 2000;82(8):1143.

Koivikko MP, Kiuru MJ, Koskinen SK, Myllynen P, Santavirta S, Kivisaari L. Factors associated with nonunion in conservatively-treated type-II fractures of the odontoid process. J Bone Joint Surge British. 2004;86(8):1146–51.

Grauer JN, Shafi B, Hilibrand AS, et al. Proposal of a modified, treatment-oriented classification of odontoid fractures. Spine J. 2005;5(2):123–9.

Hanigan WC, Powell FC, Elwood PW, Henderson JP. Odontoid fractures in elderly patients. J Neurosurg. 1993;78(1):32–5.

Lennarson PJ, Mostafavi H, Traynelis VC, Walters BC. Management of type II dens fractures: a case-control study. Spine (Phila Pa 1976). 2000;25(10):1234–7.

Joaquim AF, Patel A. Occipito cervical trauma: evaluation, classification and treatment. Contemp Spine Surg. 2010a;32:1–5.

Joaquim AF, Patel AA. C1 and C2 spine trauma: evaluation, classification, and treatment. Contemp Spine Surg. 2010b;11(3):1–7.

Bohler J. Anterior stabilization for acute fractures and non-unions of the dens. J Bone Joint Surg Am. 1982;64(1):18–27.

Etter C, Coscia M, Jaberg H, Aebi M. Direct anterior fixation of dens fractures with a cannulated screw system. Spine (Phila Pa 1976). 1991;16(3 Suppl): S25–32.

Aebi M, Etter C, Coscia M. Fractures of the odontoid process. Treatment with anterior screw fixation. Spine (Phila Pa 1976). 1989;14(10):1065–70.

Agrillo A, Russo N, Marotta N, Delfini R. Treatment of remote type ii axis fractures in the elderly: feasibility of anterior odontoid screw fixation. Neurosurgery. 2008;63(6):1145–50. discussion 50-1

Henry AD, Bohly J, Grosse A. Fixation of odontoid fractures by an anterior screw. J Bone Joint Surg Br. 1999;81(3):472–7.

Robot-Assisted C2 Pedicle Screw Placement for the Treatment of Hangman's Fracture

8

Bo Liu, Jingye Wu, Huadong Wang, and Wei Tian

Abstract

Hangman's fracture is the most frequent upper cervical fracture apart from odontoid fracture. The advantages of C2 instrumentation are early mobilization of the patient, preservation of rotational movement at C1–C2, and avoidance of prolonged traction or halo placement. However, the anatomy of the upper cervical spine is variable, and the presence of adjacent neurovascular structures makes pedicle screw fixations even more technically challenging. Robot-assisted C2 pedicle screw placement is indicated in Hangman's fracture, which permits safe and accurate instrumentations.

Keywords

Hangman's fracture · C2 pedicle screw · Robot · Traumatic spondylolisthesis of the axis · Screw fixation

1 Introduction

Hangman's fracture, also known as traumatic spondylolisthesis of the C2, is defined as a fracture involving the lamina, articular facets, pedicles, or pars interarticularis of the axis vertebra. Hangman's fracture was initially described by Schneider et al. in 1965 and is the most frequent upper cervical fracture apart from odontoid fracture.

Variable displacement of C2 on C3 is seen in these fractures. Hangman's fracture may result from a variety of mechanisms of injuries, including motor vehicle accidents and fall injuries. Classification of Hangman's fracture was proposed by Effendi et al. and modified by Levine and Edwards. According to the classification by Levine and Edwards, fractures with concomitant severe circumferential discoligamentous injuries (type II, type IIA, and type III) are thought to be unstable and require rigid immobilization. The advantages of C2 instrumentation are early mobilization of the patient, preservation of rotational movement at C1–C2, and avoidance of prolonged traction or halo placement.

Treatment goals in Hangman's fracture are to achieve anatomical reduction, maintain alignment, and maintain the patients' ability to live an active life without pain or disability. Several anterior approaches, such as the classical anterior cervical discectomy and fusion, and transoral or extraoral approach were applied with C2–C3 discectomy and segmental fixation with bony fusion. Anterior cervical discectomy and fusion addresses C2–C3 disk herniation and C2–C3 stabilization. Anterior approach, however, does not address the posterior fractured part of the C2. In addition, it may have the disadvantages of approach-related problems; the high anterior approach risks injury to vital

B. Liu · J. Wu · H. Wang · W. Tian (✉)
Department of Spine Surgery, Beijing Jishuitan Hospital, Fourth Clinical Hospital of Peking University, Beijing, China
e-mail: tianweijst@vip.163.com

W. Tian (ed.), *Navigation Assisted Robotics in Spine and Trauma Surgery*,
https://doi.org/10.1007/978-981-15-1846-1_8

structures, especially the facial and hypoglossal nerves, branches of the external carotid artery, contents of the carotid sheath, and the superior laryngeal nerve. The posterior approach, involving a simple exposure, can simultaneously fixate the posterior and anterior parts of the C2 vertebra. Among the different posterior approaches, several clinical studies report direct posterior fixation of the pedicles or pars fracture, with the advantage of motion preservation at C2–C3 joint. However, it is ineffective in patients with unstable fractures due to discoligamentous injury at C2–C3, as it fails to prevent loss of disc height, lordosis, and kyphosis. Treatment of Hangman's fracture after direct pars repair has been reported in various studies. In the biomechanical study by Duggal et al., posterior C2–C3 screw technique was more effective in the stabilization of Hangman's fracture than anterior cervical plating and C2 pars screw placement.

The anatomy of the upper cervical spine is variable, and the presence of adjacent neurovascular structures makes pedicle screw fixations even more technically challenging. Using biplanar fluoroscopy, misplacement of cervical pedicle screws is reported in up to 21.6% of such procedures. The advent of intraoperative three-dimensional (3D) navigation systems permits safe and accurate instrumentations of the cervical spine.

Pedicle screw placement is technically challenging because of the large individual variation in the pedicle dimensions and the course of the vertebral artery. The conventional techniques of screw placement described in the literature rely solely on the external anatomic landmarks to guide screw insertion. Yukawa et al. reported a grade 2 and grade 3 screw misplacement rate of 13.1% in 620 cervical pedicle screw fixations using a fluoroscopy-assisted technique, whereas the misplacement rate in C2 and C3 was even higher (21.6%). This high perforation rate may be partly attributable to the lack of landmarks and an accurate entrance to the cervical pedicles. With the use of continuous radioscopy with a two-dimensional (2D) view, potential complications for screw misplacement of C2 and C3 are still present even in the experienced hands. Real-time feedback of the proposed screw trajectory in the axial, sagittal, and coronal planes can be achieved by intraoperative 3D navigation. Richter et al. reported excellent results of cervical screw placement using computed tomography-based navigation in a cadaveric study (Tian et al. 2016). Tian et al. showed good accuracy with grade 2 misplacement of 7.84% and no grade 3 misplacement with intraoperative 3D fluoroscopy-based navigation; Ito et al. reported a misplacement rate of no more than 2 mm in 2.8% of 176 cervical pedicle screws using Iso-C 3D navigation Tian et al. (2012). Singh PK et al. reported that there was only one grade 2 misplacement (5%) of C2 pedicle screw in ten cases using O-arm-based navigation (Singh et al, 2014).

Robot-assisted C2 pedicle screw placement is indicated in Hangman's fracture. Patients with type I or type II fracture (Levine and Edwards) cannot tolerate prolonged external immobilization. Using percutaneous C2 pedicle screw placement can allow early mobilization of the neck and rehabilitation.

2 Surgical Procedure (C2/3 Fixation and Fusion or C2 Isthmic Screws Only)

2.1 Positioning the Patient

The patient was placed in prone position after induction of general anesthesia. Mayfield tongs were placed to manipulate to achieve reduction while keeping the head in traction and slight flexion (Fig. 8.1). Reduction of fracture can be confirmed by fluoroscopy.

2.2 Robot Registration and Intraoperative Planning

After prepping and draping, the sterilized patient tracker was then connected onto the Mayfield tongs. 3-D C-arm scanning is carried out and the images are transmitted into the TiRobot system. Using the robotic built-in software, surgeons can perform the trajectory planning on the screen monitor (Fig. 8.2a, b). Receiving the surgeons' instruction, the arm of the TiRobot then moved to the surgical field to guide the planned pins insertion (Fig. 8.3).

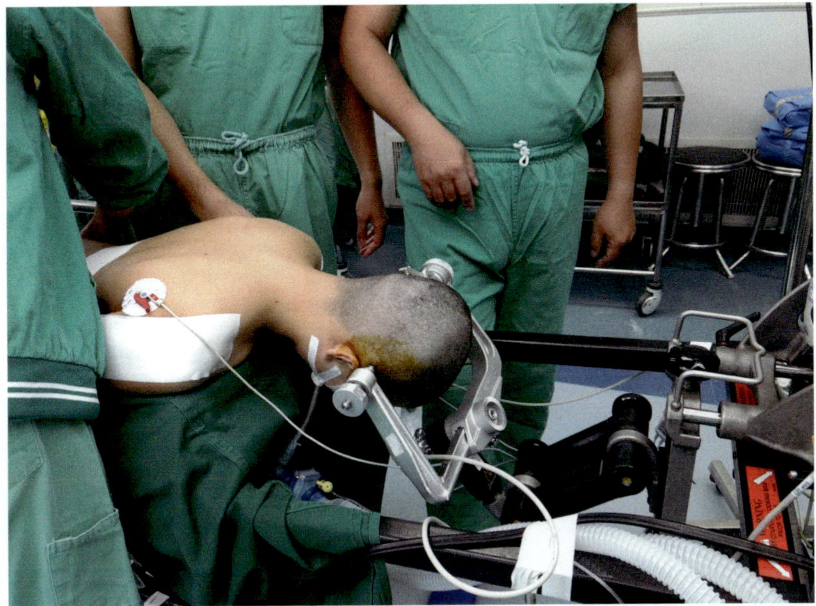

Fig. 8.1 Patient positioning

2.3 Exposure and Screw Insertion

A single midline incision to two-sided incision is acceptable during this procedure. Two-sided incision has the advantage of less soft tissue tension, permitting more lateral trajectory of pedicle screws of C2. Therefore, two-sided incisions are preferred in our center.

If only pedicle screw of C2 is planned, percutaneous techniques can be used. A left-sided and right-sided tiny skin incision was made under robotic guidance and exposure to the posterior-inferior border of the axis achieved. A cannula was inserted through the sleeve of the robotic arm, after which a Kirschner wire was drilled into the C2 pedicle. A 4-mm diameter cannulated screw was then inserted under K-wire guidance and the placement of the screw found to be satisfactory according to an intraoperative 3-D C-arm fluoroscopy scan (Figs. 8.4–8.9).

If C2/3 fixation and fusion are needed, Kirschner wire in C2 can be replaced by pedicle screws, and lateral mass screws were inserted in C3 and sometimes C4 with the guidance of robot, depending upon the severity of the discoligamentous injury, listhesis, and the need to correct the angulation. After screw placement, rods were inserted on both sides, and the screws were tightened. The facet joint of C2/3 is decancellated and cancellous bone graft is used to facilitate the fusion.

3 Conclusion

C2 pedicle screws can be put with precision under robot assistance, and intraoperative computed tomographic scan can confirm position of screws. Patients can be operated and mobilized early with negligible risk of screw misplacement, with preservation of motion at the C1–C2 joint.

4 Typical Case

A 13-year-old woman presented with neck pain for 9 days resulting from car accident. On physical examination, he had neck pain and limitation of motion of the neck, Hoffmann's sign (−), Romberg's sign (−), Tandem gait (−), Babinski's test (−), and sensation and muscle strength of limbs are normal.

Diagnosis: Hangman's fracture (Fig. 8.10a, b)

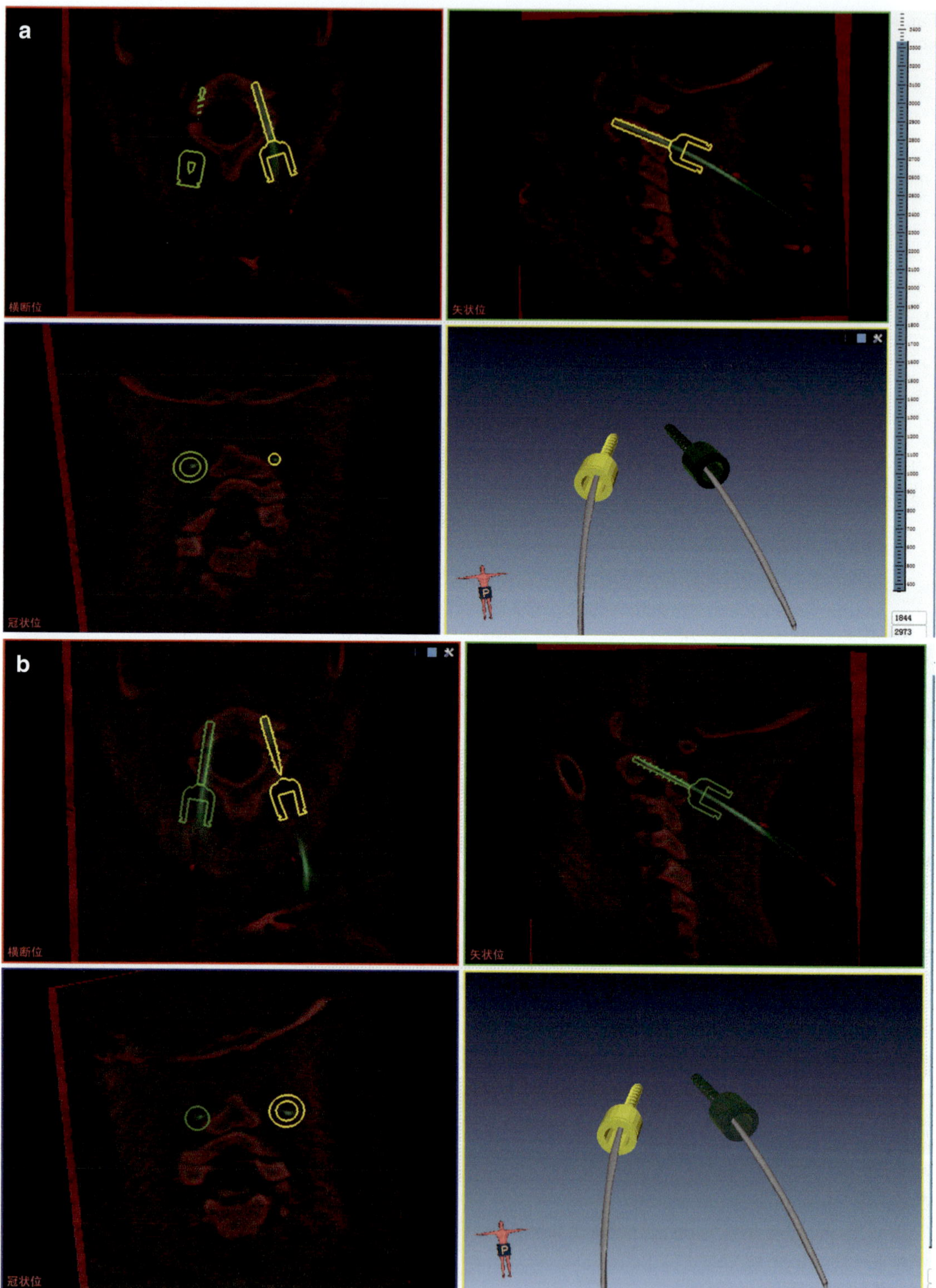

Fig. 8.2 (**a**, **b**) Trajectory planning of both sides of pedicle

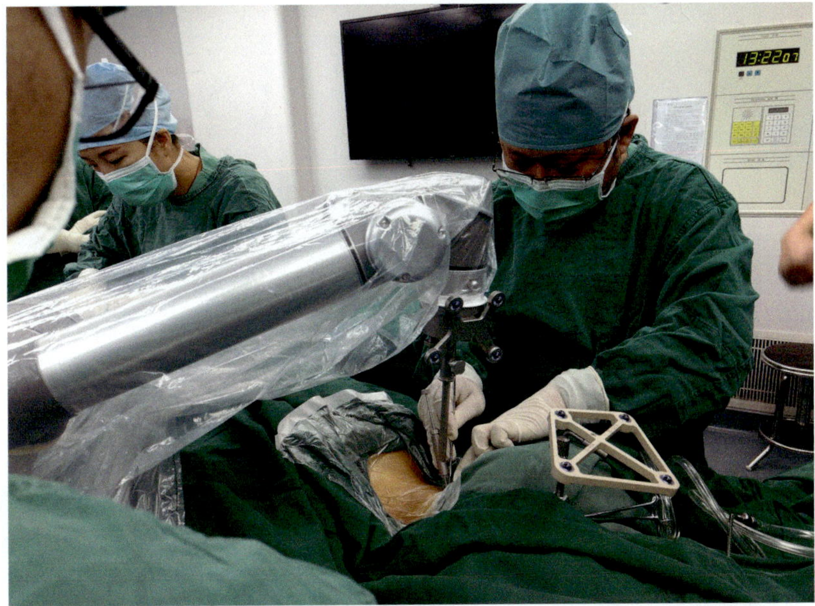

Fig. 8.3 K-wire insertion guided by robot arm

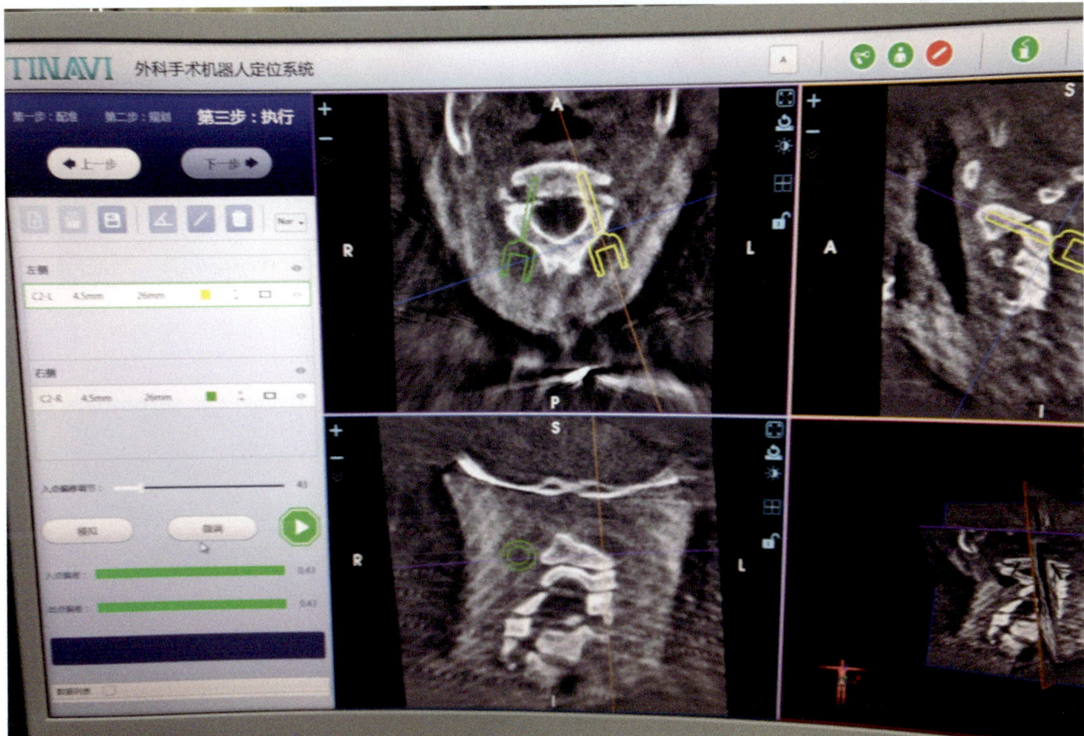

Fig. 8.4 Screw planning

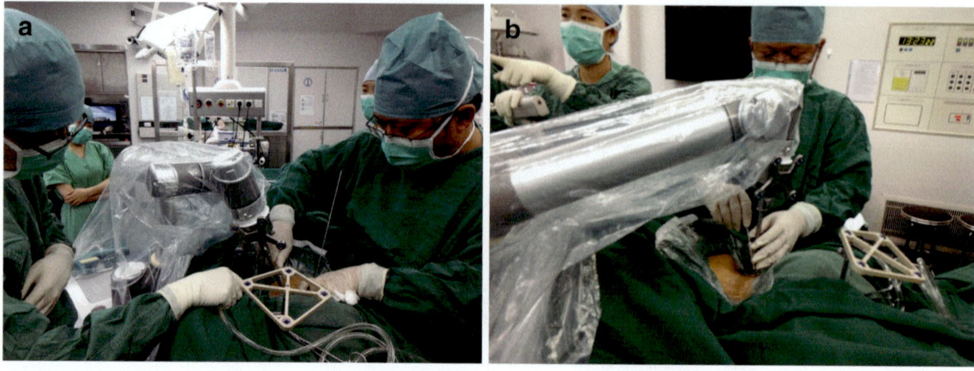

Fig. 8.5 (**a**, **b**) Insert the K-wires on both sides followed the pathways provided by the robot arm

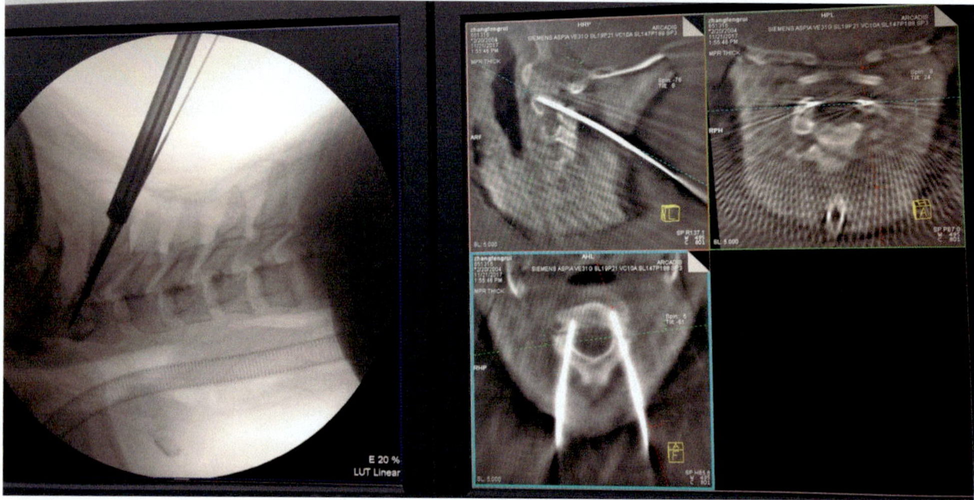

Fig. 8.6 Scan the positions of K-wires using intraoperative 3D C-arm

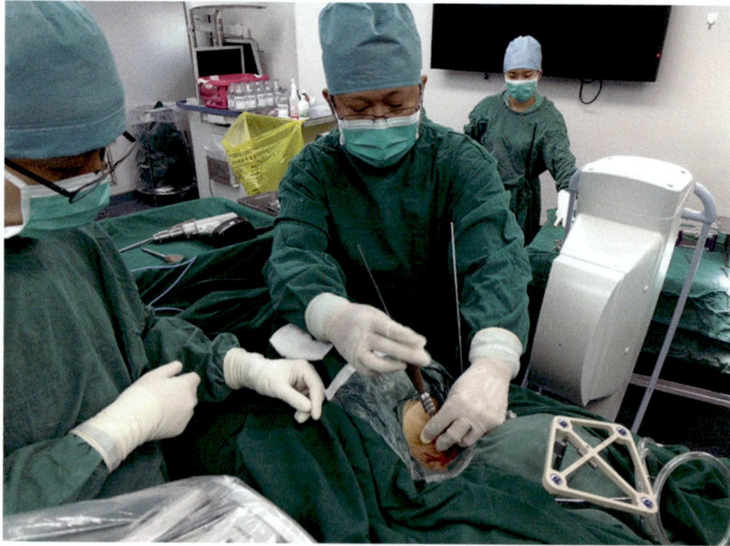

Fig. 8.7 Implant the cannulated screws under K-wire guidance

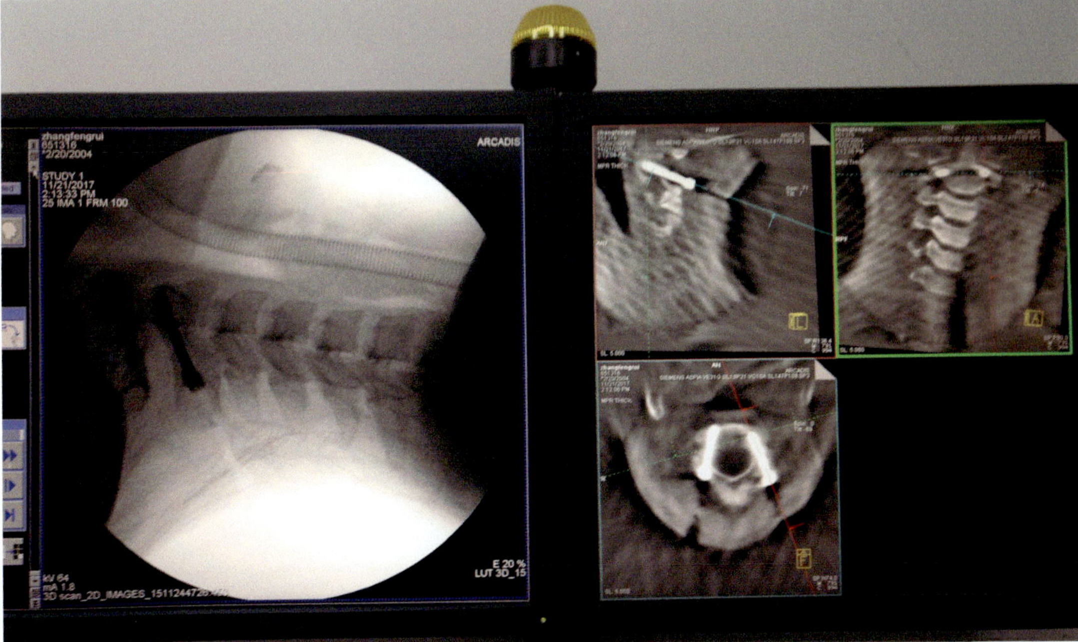

Fig. 8.8 The intraoperative 3D C-arm scanning of the screws

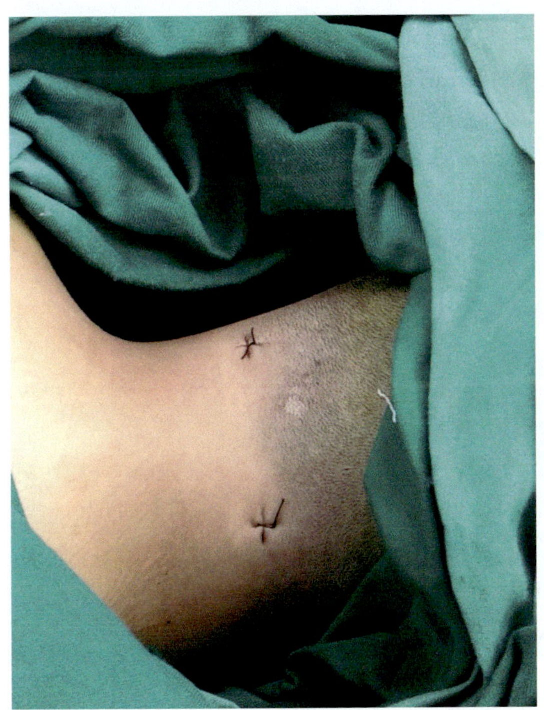

Fig. 8.9 The post-op minimal incisions

Robot-assisted C2 pedicle screw fixation was performed.

Postoperative CT scan showed the excellent position of C2 pedicle screws (Fig. 8.11a–c)

5 Tips

1. The patient tracker is connected to the Mayfield tong or the spinous process of the C2. For the accuracy requirements of the navigation system, the cervical spine should be rigid. However, the upper cervical spine is relatively mobile even though anchored with the Mayfield tong. Therefore, the manipulation force applied to the cervical spine should be minimal particularly during the initial phase of K-wire insertion; otherwise, the navigation system may be inaccurate.
2. At the initial phase of K-wire insertion guided by robotic system, the K-wire should be held still in a cannula with the same diameter of the K-wire; otherwise, it may slip at the bony sur-

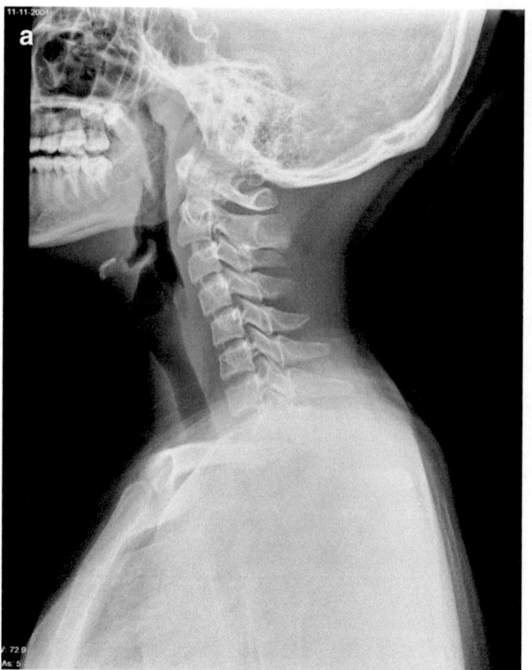

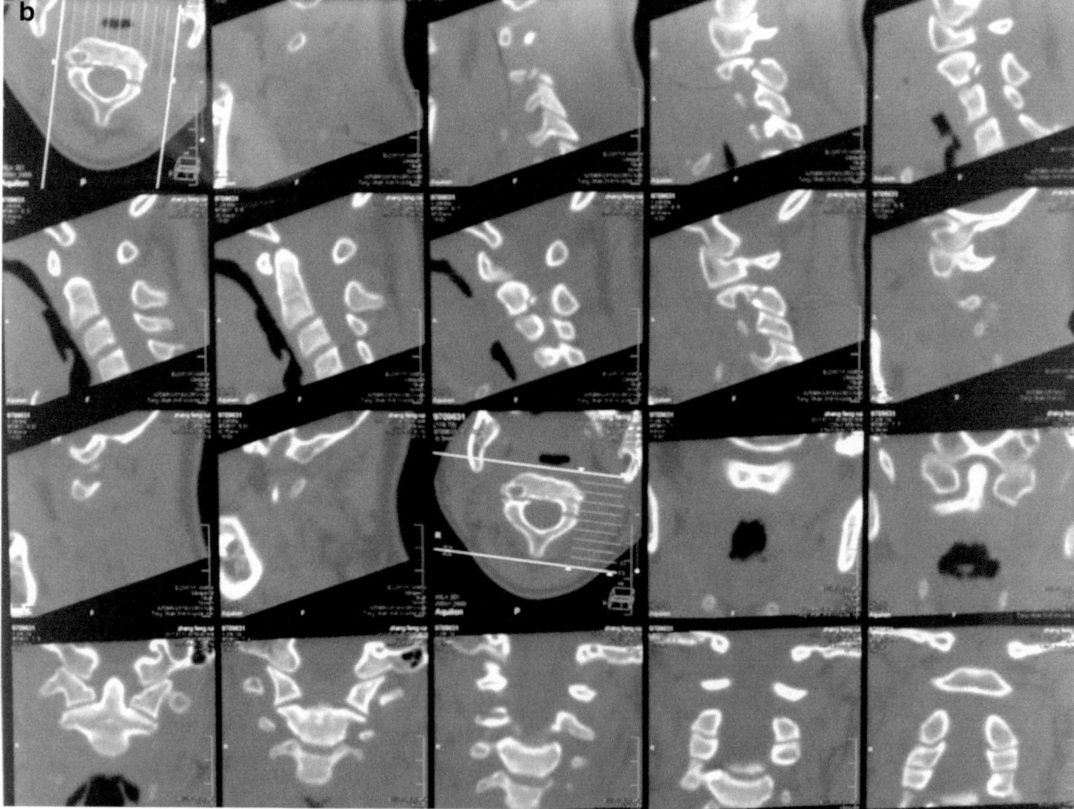

Fig. 8.10 (**a**) X-ray image of the patient; (**b**) CT images of the patient

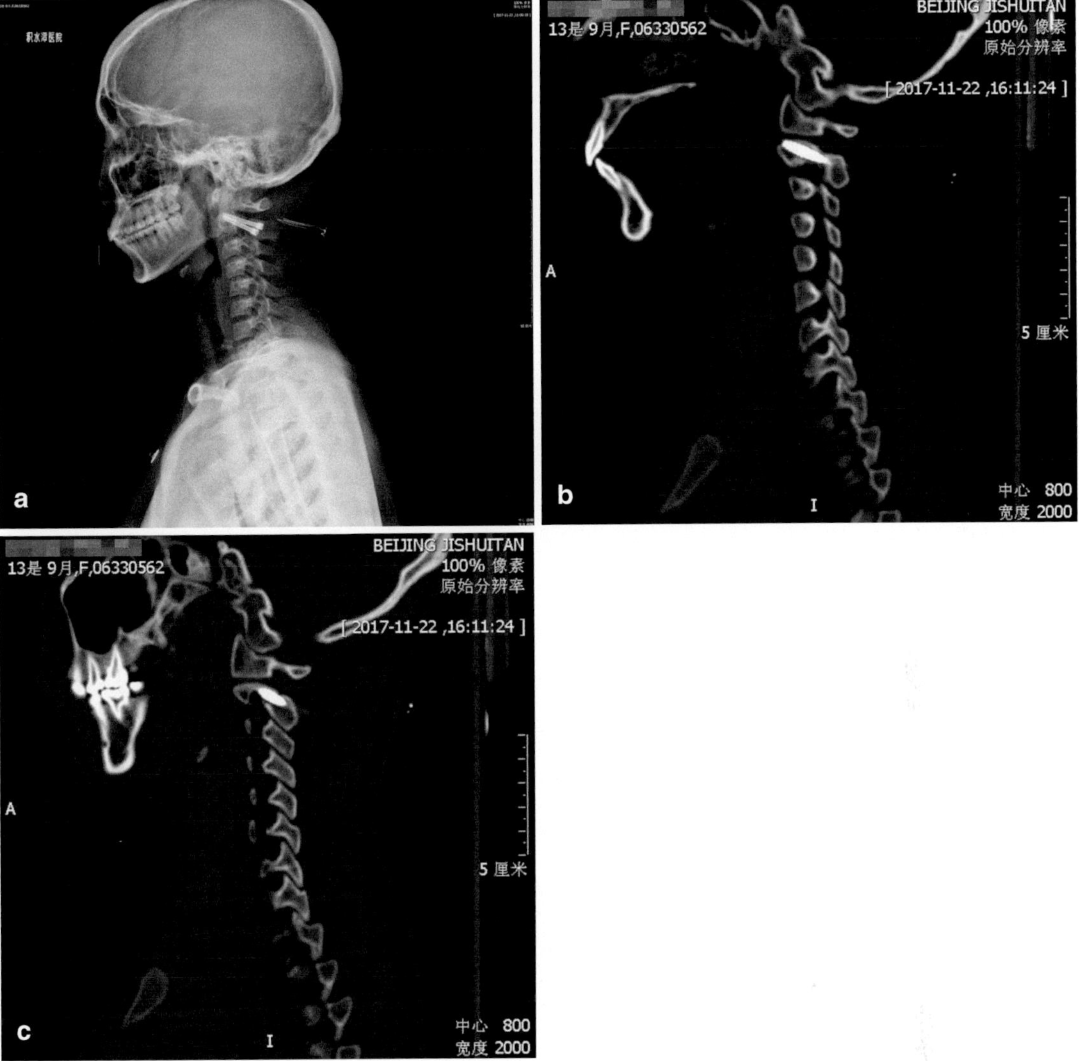

Fig. 8.11 (**a**) Postoperative X-ray image; (**b**, **c**) postoperative CT images

face especially at smooth or steep portion of the bone. Thus, the K-wire must be guided by the cannula or the sleeve of the robotic arm. During the trajectory planning, the surgeon can choose the trajectory able to avoid the steep portion of the bony surface. The larger the diameter of the K-wire, the more rigid it will be.

3. The trajectory of the pedicle screw at the C2 has more lateral angulation. During the insertion of the K-wire, the robotic arm bears a large amount of the soft tissue tension when using midline insertion. Thus, two-sided incisions are preferred, or two additional stab incisions are to be used for insertion of the pedicle screws.
4. The threaded portion of cannulate screws should sustain the opposite fragment. A compressive force can be generated as the mechanism of lag screws. The Herbert screw could be chosen as an alternative implant.

References

Singh PK, Gang K, Sawarkar D, et al. Computed tomography-guided C2 pedicle screw placement for treatment of unstable Hangman fractures. Spine. 2014;39(18):E1058–65.

Tian W, Weng C, Liu B, et al. Posterior fixation and fusion of unstable Hangman's fracture by using intraoperative three-dimensional fluoroscopy-based navigation. Eur Spine. 2012;21:863–71.

Tian W, Wang H, Liu YJ, et al. Robot-assisted anterior odontoid screw fixation: a case report. Orthop Surg. 2016;8(3):400–4.

9 Robot-Assisted Cervical Pedicle Screw Fixation

Da He, Xinfeng Wu, Shan Zheng, and Wei Tian

Abstract

The cervical pedicle screw fixation technique is a reliable technique for stabilization of the unstable cervical motion segments; at the same time, it is very risky. Even well-planned procedures may have severe complications because of the variation of anatomy. However, the CAMISS and robot-assisted cervical pedicle screw placement can achieve a higher precision in cervical pedicle fixation surgeries; meanwhile, complications are obviously reduced.

Keywords

Robot-assisted · Cervical spine · Pedicle screw fixation · Preoperative planning · 3D image · Precision · CAMISS

1 Introduction

Cervical pedicle screw fixation presents a superior stabilizing effect compared with other fixation procedures by biomechanical studies. Cervical pedicle screw fixation has been adopted into clinical use by the pioneers (Leconte 1964, Borne et al. 1984, Roy-Camille et al. 1989, Abumi et al. 1994, and Jeanneret et al. 1994). Abumi et al. expanded the indication of cervical screw fixation to nontraumatic lesions, reconstruction of the craniocervical junction, and correction of cervical kyphosis (Abumi and Kaneda 1997; Abumi et al. 1999a, b; Abumi 2015).

Cervical pedicle screw fixation is a reliable technique for stabilization of the unstable cervical motion segments and is especially beneficial to those patients who lack of posterior elements or who need to restore the physiological sagittal alignment of the cervical spine (Abumi et al. 2012). However, this technique has been considered too risky because of the limited space of the ideal trajectory between the spinal canal medially and the vertebral artery laterally. A little deviation may cause severe neurovascular complications including injury to the vertebral artery, nerve roots, and spinal cord.

Although complications associated with cervical pedicle screw fixation cannot be completely obviated, they can be minimized by a combination of sufficient preoperative imaging studies of the pedicles, thorough knowledge of the local anatomy, and meticulous surgical techniques of screw placement (Abumi et al. 2012). In recent years, increased use of computer-assisted image guidance and robot-assisted spinal surgery has improved precision for screw placement (Kostrzewski et al. 2012).

D. He · X. Wu · S. Zheng · W. Tian (✉)
Department of Spine Surgery, Beijing Jishuitan Hospital, Fourth Clinical Hospital of Peking University, Beijing, China
e-mail: tianweijst@vip.163.com

W. Tian (ed.), *Navigation Assisted Robotics in Spine and Trauma Surgery*,
https://doi.org/10.1007/978-981-15-1846-1_9

Professor Tian Wei proposed CAMISS and popularized robot-assisted spine surgery in China (Tian et al. 2011, 2017; Yuan et al. 2014; Lang et al. 2016; Tian 2016).

2 Preoperative Imaging and Planning

AP view, lateral view radiographs are needed, and computer tomography scan are especially important for surgical planning. All relevant preoperative imaging studies should be considered to design the appropriate trajectory and direction, as well as the length and diameter of pedicle screw.

3 Procedure

3.1 Positioning

The prone position is applied with flexed hips and knees on a Jackson table. The buttocks of the patient are fastened to the surgical table with a belt prevent slipping caudally (Fig. 9.1). The upper limb is fastened to the trunk for a good view of fluoroscopy during the operation. The head is immobilized with frame Mayfield or adhesive tape (Fig. 9.2).

3.2 Exposure

The best choice of surgical exposure is bilateral percutaneous incision, which can reduce the traction force of the muscle and improve the accuracy. Sometimes, midline incision is made for exposure of spinous process for putting on patient tracker (Fig. 9.3).

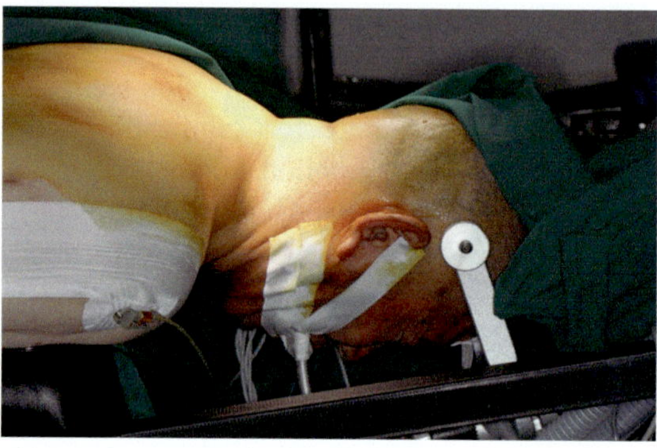

Fig. 9.2 Upper limb fasten to the trunk and head immobilized with frame Mayfield

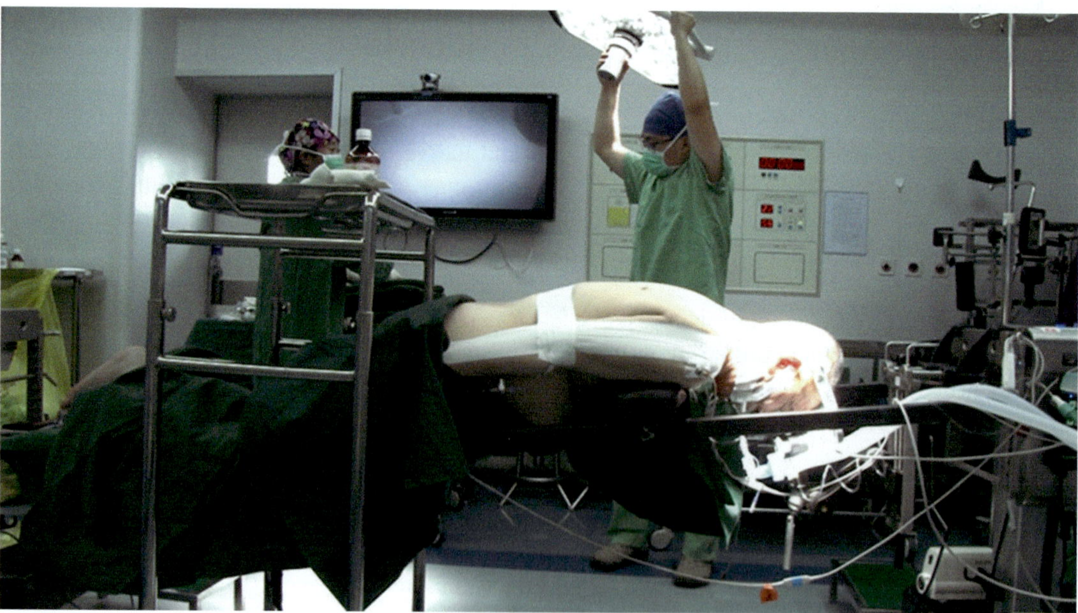

Fig. 9.1 Patient fastened in the prone position on a Jackson table

3.3 Surgical Procedure

3.3.1 Step 1

The patient tracker is fixed to the connecting link on Mayfield frame cranially or fixed to the spinous process inside the incision. A rigid fixation of patient tracker is a prerequisite for accuracy. Sheathe the robot arm by using the sterilization bag. Assemble the registration plate to the robot arm and move it to the appropriate position in the operative field (Fig. 9.4). Adjust the operation table and robot arm to ensure the registration plate can be seen on the AP view and lateral view of fluoroscopy. Then 3D images are harvested from motorized C arm.

3.3.2 Step 2

Transfer the images to the robot workstation from the C arm workstation. Specific software is used to design the entry point, orientation, and dimension of the screw (Fig. 9.5).

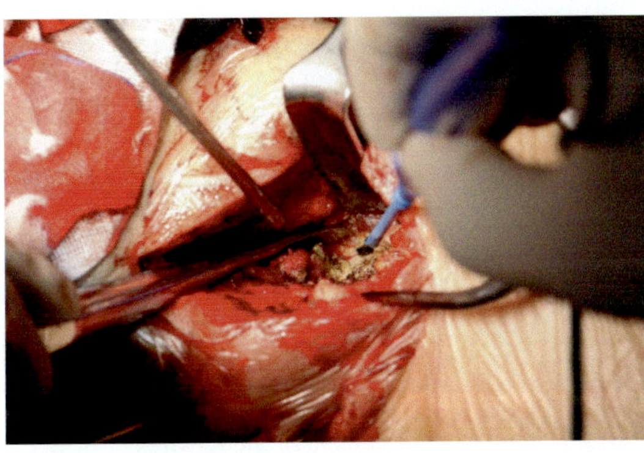

Fig. 9.3 Incision and exposure

3.3.3 Step 3

Remove the registration plate and assemble the guiding tube to the robot arm. Let the guiding tube slowly move to the target under the guidance of the robot. When the guiding tube is in place, along the axis of the pedicle, place the work tube into the guiding tube and ensure the tip of the work tube touches the bony element at the entry point of the pedicle. Finely adjust the robot arm to ensure the accuracy error below 0.5 mm. Next, place a K-wire along the guider into pedicle (Fig. 9.6). Repeat the procedure and finish the placement of the K-wires (Fig. 9.7). Confirm the position of the K-wire with fluoroscopy or 3D C arm scan (Fig. 9.8a, b).

3.3.4 Step 4

Tap the pedicle trajectory along the K-wires. Then, remove the tap and K-wire, screw in the pedicle screw, and confirm the position of the screws using fluoroscopy or the 3D C-arm scan (Fig. 9.9a, b).

4 Tips

1. Do not hesitate to readjust the patient tracker and reharvest the 3D image if there is any suspicion of displacement of the tracker.

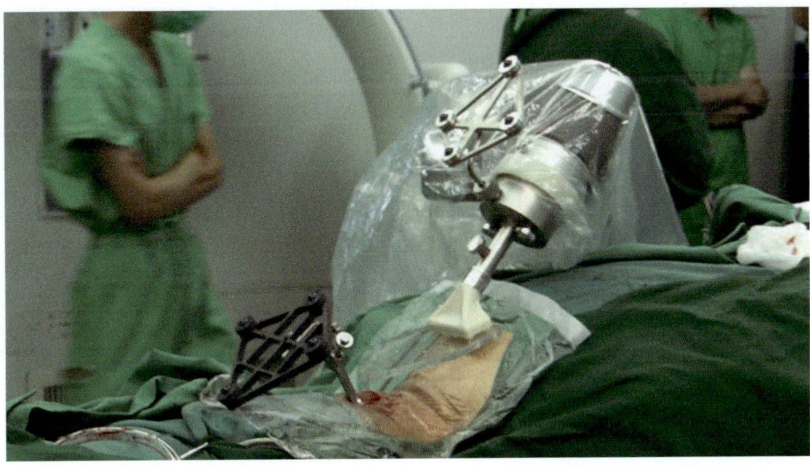

Fig. 9.4 The patient tracker is fixed to the spinous process inside the incision. The robot arm is sheathed with sterilization bag. The registration plate is assembled to the robot arm and moved to the appropriate position in the operative field

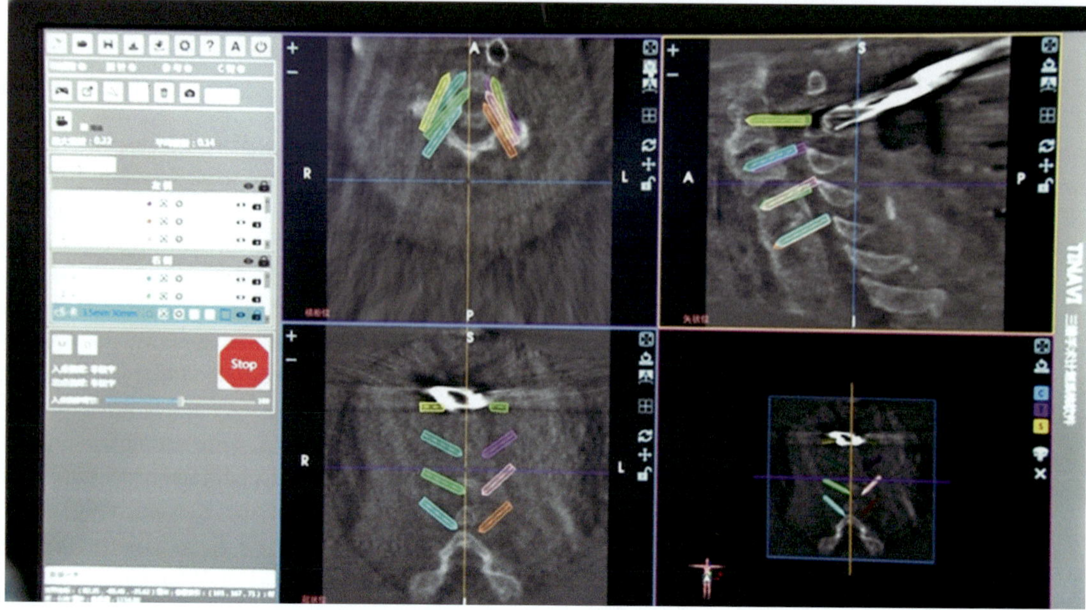

Fig. 9.5 Design the entry point, orientation, and dimension of the screws

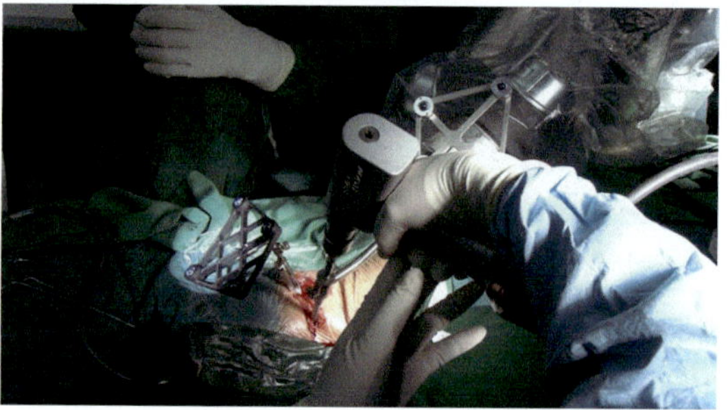

Fig. 9.6 With the guidance of the robot, drill a K-wire into pedicle

Fig. 9.7 Finish the placement of the K-wires

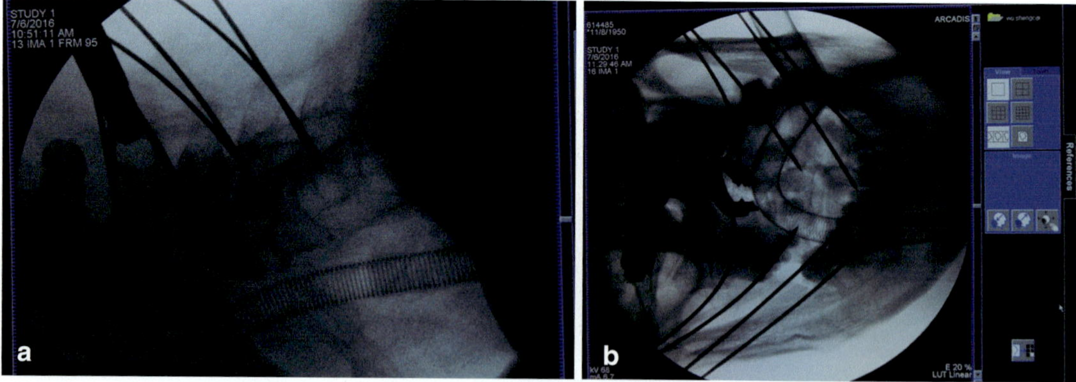

Fig. 9.8 (**a**) lateral view of cervical spine to confirm the position of the K-wire. (**b**) A-P view of cervical spine to confirm the position of the K-wire

2. Image shifting will emerge as a result of traction of the soft tissue, which will decrease accuracy.
3. When inserting the K-wire, decreasing the tide volume temporarily will improve accuracy.
4. Inserting the K-wire before decompression to avoid decreasing accuracy will result in relative displacement of bony structures.
5. Do not insert the K-wire too much to prevent injury of neurovascular structures and nearby organ. Specifically, do not let the K-wire go forward along the tap.
6. Grind the entry point of pedicle screw smoothly using the high-speed drill or ultrasonic osteotome to avoid sliding of the tip of K-wire.
7. The placement of pedicle screw will become easy if a relatively medial entry point and smaller convergence orientation are chosen in an open surgery.

5 Typical Case

Chief complaint: car accident with quadriplegia for 13 h.

Current history: 13 h prior, the patient was accidentally hit by a car. At that time, he felt neck pain and paralysis of legs and hands and could not stand or walk.

Physical examination: spine percussion pain(+), limited ROM, POM(+). Upper limb and Lower limb muscle strength Grade 0–2.

Imaging: X-ray, CT, and MRI: C2, C3 fracture.

Diagnosis: cervical fracture with spinal cord injury.

Operation: robot-assisted percutaneous minimally invasive cervical fracture reduction, pedicle screw internal fixation (Fig. 9.10).

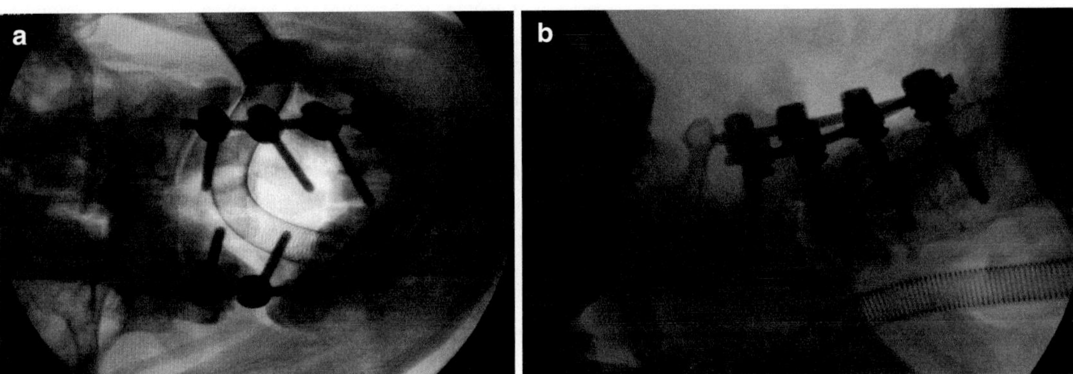

Fig. 9.9 (**a**) A-P of cervical spine to confirm the position of the pedicle screws. (**b**) lateral view of cervical spine to confirm the position of the pedicle screws

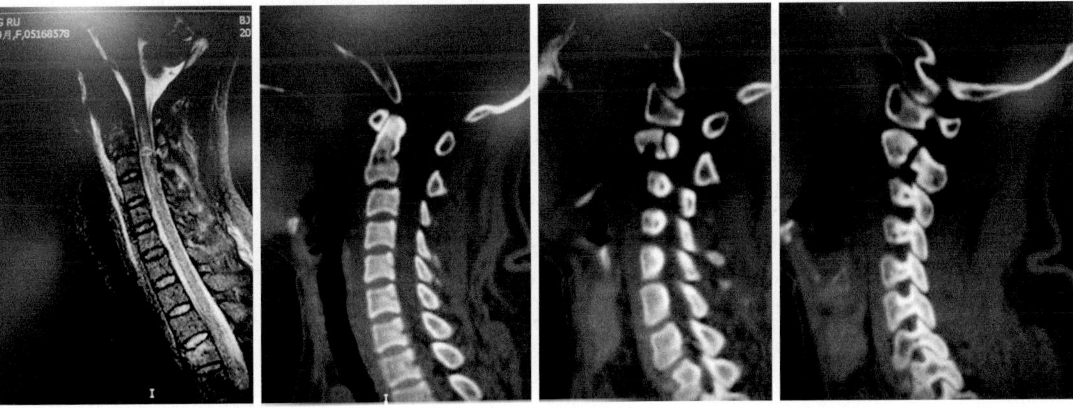

Fig. 9.10 A cases of robot-assisted percutaneous minimally invasive cervical fracture reduction and pedicle screw internal fixation. Preoperational CT and MRI as well as postoperational CT are illustrated

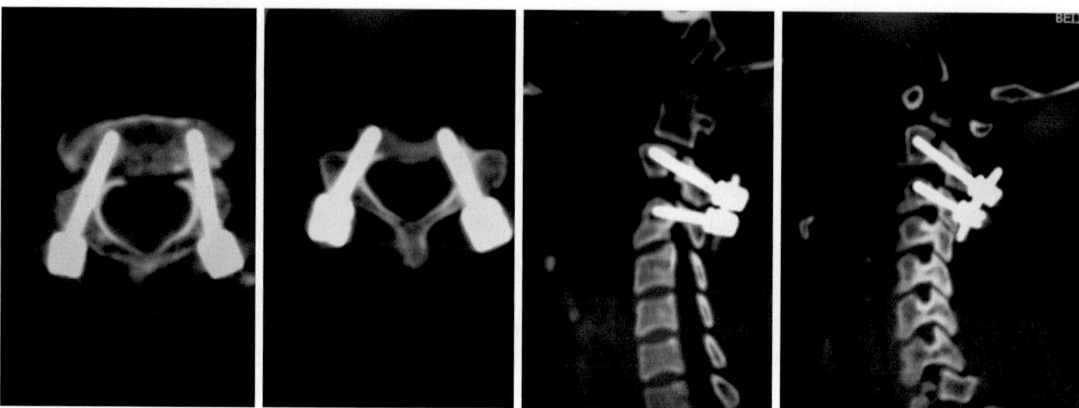

Fig. 9.10 (continued)

References

Abumi K. Cervical spondylotic myelopathy: posterior decompression and pedicle screw fixation. Eur Spine J. 2015;24(Suppl 2):S186–96.

Abumi K, Kaneda K. Pedicle screw fixation for nontraumatic lesions of the cervical spine. Spine (Phila Pa 1976). 1997;22(16):1853–63.

Abumi K, Ito H, Taneichi H, Kaneda K. Transpedicular screw fixation for traumatic lesions of the middle and lower cervical spine. Description of the techniques and preliminary report. J Spinal Disorder. 1994;7(1):19–28.

Abumi K, Shono Y, Taneichi T, Ito M, Kaneda K. Correction of cervical kyphosis using pedicle screw fixation systems. Spine (Phila Pa 1976). 1999a;24(22):2389–96.

Abumi K, Takada T, Shono Y, Kaneda K, Fujiya M. Posterior occipitocervical reconstruction using cervical pedicle screws and plate-rod systems. Spine (Phila Pa 1976). 1999b;24(14):1425–34.

Abumi K, Ito M, Sudo H. Reconstruction of the subaxial cervical spine. Using pedicle screw instrumentation. Spine. 2012;37(5):E349–56.

Borne GM, Bedou GL, Pinaudeau M. Treatment of pedicular fractures of the axis. A clinical study and screw fixation technique. J Neurosurg. 1984;60(1):88–93.

Jeanneret B, Gebhard JS, Magerl F. Transpedicular screw fixation of articular mass fracture-separation: results of an anatomical study and operative technique. J Spinal Disord. 1994;7(1):222–9.

Kostrzewski S, Duff JM, Baur C, Olszewski M. Robotic system for cervical spine surgery. Int J Med Robot. 2012;8:184–90.

Lang Z, Tian W, Liu Y, Liu B, Yuan Q, Sun Y. Minimally invasive pedicle screw fixation using intraoperative 3-dimensional fluoroscopy-based navigation (CAMISS technique) for Hangman fracture. Spine (Phila Pa 1976). 2016;41(1):39–45. https://doi.org/10.1097/BRS.0000000000001111.

Leconte P. Fracture et luxation des deux premieres vertebres cervicales. In: Judet R, editor. Luxation Congenitale de la Hanche. Fractures du Cou-de-pied Rachis cervical. Actualites de Chirurgie Orthopedique de l'Hospital Raymond-Poincare, vol. 3. Paris: Masson et Cie; 1964. p. 147–66.

Roy-Camille R, Salient G, Mazel C. Internal fixation of theunstable cervical spine by a posterior osteosynthesis with plates and screws. In: The Cervical Spine Research Society, editor. The cervical spine. 2nd ed. Philadelphia: B Lippincott; 1989. p. 390–403.

Tian W. Robot-assisted posterior C1-2 transarticular screw fixation for atlantoaxial instability: a case report. Spine (Phila Pa 1976). 2016;41(Suppl 19):B2–5.

Tian W, Han X, He D, Liu B, Li Q, Li ZY, Liu YJ, Li N. The comparison of computer assisted minimally invasive spine surgery and traditional open treatment for thoracolumbar fractures. Zhonghua Wai Ke Za Zhi. 2011;49(12):1061–6.

Tian W, Fan MX, Liu YJ. Robot-assisted percutaneous pedicle screw placement using three-dimensional fluoroscopy: a preliminary clinical study. Chin Med J. 2017;130(13):1617–8. https://doi.org/10.4103/0366-6999.208251.

Yuan Q, Zheng S, Tian W. Computer-assisted minimally invasive spine surgery for resection of ossification of the ligamentum flavum in the thoracic spine. Chin Med J. 2014;127(11):2043–7.

Robot-Assisted Thoracic Pedicle Screw Fixation Technique

10

Ning Yuan, Shuo Feng, and Wei Tian

Abstract

The incidence of thoracic disease is not prominent in the population compared with cervical and lumbar spine disease. However, because of its special anatomical structure and high surgical risk, the treatment of thoracic vertebra disease has become difficulty in the clinical work of spinal surgery. The robot-assisted thoracic pedicle screw fixation technique further improved the accuracy, stability, and repeatability of the screws. And almost all cases requiring the use of thoracic pedicle screws are applicable to robotics. Although there are still some problems such as complex facilities and high price, there remains a wide space for the technology of robot-assisted pedicle screw fixation.

Keywords

Orthopedic department · Spine · Surgical robot · Thoracic vertebra · Pedicle · Screw

The thoracic vertebra is a relatively stable part of the human body, with relatively little activity. The thoracic vertebra and the sternum and ribs form the thoracic cavity protect the heart and lungs, and the thoracic spine plays a protective role in the thoracic spinal cord. There are fewer possibilities of degenerative disease of the thoracic vertebrae due to its fewer activities. However, the incidence of thoracic deformities is high, and idiopathic scoliosis and congenital scoliosis are common in the thoracic spine. The incidence of thoracic trauma fractures is not low; hence, the incidence of thoracic surgery is not uncommon.

Thoracic surgery can be divided into the anterior and posterior approaches. Nowadays, spine surgeons are more likely to choose the posterior surgery. The posterior approach can be directly applied to the thoracic spine. This approach is suitable for interventions, such as vertebral disk decompression, internal fixation, and fusion. One of the important issues of posterior surgery is ensuring proper fixation. The emergence of thoracic pedicle screws has provided a good solution to this problem. Because of the high tensile strength of the cortical bone around the screw, reconstruction of the structure is better for correcting the deformity (Liljenqvist et al. 2002; Bess et al. 2007).

However, how to place the pedicle screw is a difficult technical issue. The lower thoracic vertebral pedicle has obvious anatomical markers as insertion points, and the vertebral pedicle is relatively thick; thus, it is relatively easy to use. However, the pedicle of the topper thoracic vertebras gradually thins, and the anatomical mark is no longer obvious. Although entering into the

N. Yuan · S. Feng · W. Tian (✉)
Department of Spine Surgery, Beijing Jishuitan Hospital, Fourth Clinical Hospital of Peking University, Beijing, China
e-mail: tianweijst@vip.163.com

W. Tian (ed.), *Navigation Assisted Robotics in Spine and Trauma Surgery*,
https://doi.org/10.1007/978-981-15-1846-1_10

spinal canal is rare, the occurrence of spinal cord injury can result in serious consequences. There is no fixed position on the outside. There is damage to the disk if the location is above the thoracic, and there is damage to the nerve roots if the location is under the thoracic and causes intercostal neuralgia (Kim et al. 2004). The FDA does not recommend T10 or more segments with pedicle screw fixation. Still some spine surgeons prefer pedicle screw fixation. In order to increase its safety, the C-arm is used to penetrate the screws. Although accuracy is improved, the radiation exposure of patients is increased. Moreover, it is difficult to see the upper thoracic vertebra clearly due to the occlusion by the scapula. In addition, the internal angle cannot be established, and it cannot avoid the deviation of the pedicle screw position, especially when the vertebral body is rotated. The so-called thoracic pedicle screws actually go from the outside through the thoracic and costal joint to the vertebral body, some of which are very difficult to be fixed on the outside. Can the thoracic vertebra be fixed with pedicle screws? The answer is yes. The robot can be used to assist the pedicle screw internal fixation technique (Tian et al. 2014).

1 Indications for Thoracic Robot-Assisted Surgery

Almost all of the thoracic abnormal bony structure or cases of thoracic pedicle screws can be used for robotics, but because of the limited equipment and expensive costs, indications are limited:

1. The thoracic vertebra has a serious lateral convex and rotating deformity, and the lateral angle of vertebral pedicle is difficult to grasp.
2. Due to the large tumor or hyperplasia of the joints, it is difficult to identify the bone structure.
3. Severe fracture, severe bone structure damage, increases the difficulty to grasp the entering position and the direction of screw.
4. Cases of osteoporosis, when hand feeling is weak.
5. Revision surgery or modification of pedicle screw path.
6. Preoperative CT shows that the pedicle is abnormal.

2 The Procedure of Robot-Assisted Thoracic Surgery

1. General anesthesia, prone position, place the patient on the four-point supported carbon operating table (Fig. 10.1), which is convenient for use in the 3D C-arm.
2. The thoracic posterior median incision is used to reveal the spinous process of the adjacent segment of the thoracic vertebra which needs to be fixed, and the tracer is installed on this spinous process, ensuring the tracer is installed firmly (Fig. 10.2).
3. The robot is placed to the side of the operating table, extending the robotic arm, installing the sterile sleeve, and the end of the robotic arm is close to the field (Fig. 10.3).
4. Enter the interface of robot-assisted surgery and adjust the direction of the infrared camera to the operation field.
5. The position of 3D C-arm and operating table is adjusted to ensure the surgical area is centered on the AP and lateral position of the fluoroscopy (Fig. 10.4). Rotate 190° for X-ray scanning.
6. After the fluoroscopy, the 3D data obtained is automatically transferred to the robot host. After the procedure, the local fault images and the 3D images can be displayed on the screen.
7. In the 3D image, pedicle screw insertion point should be planned, and the orientation of the screw and the appropriate screw length is selected (Fig. 10.5).
8. The installation guide sleeve (Fig. 10.6) is placed at the end of the robot arm manipulator in accordance with the planning of pedicle screw position and is automatically run to a fixed position, in accordance with the operation; choose the midline incision or minimally invasive incision in the robot

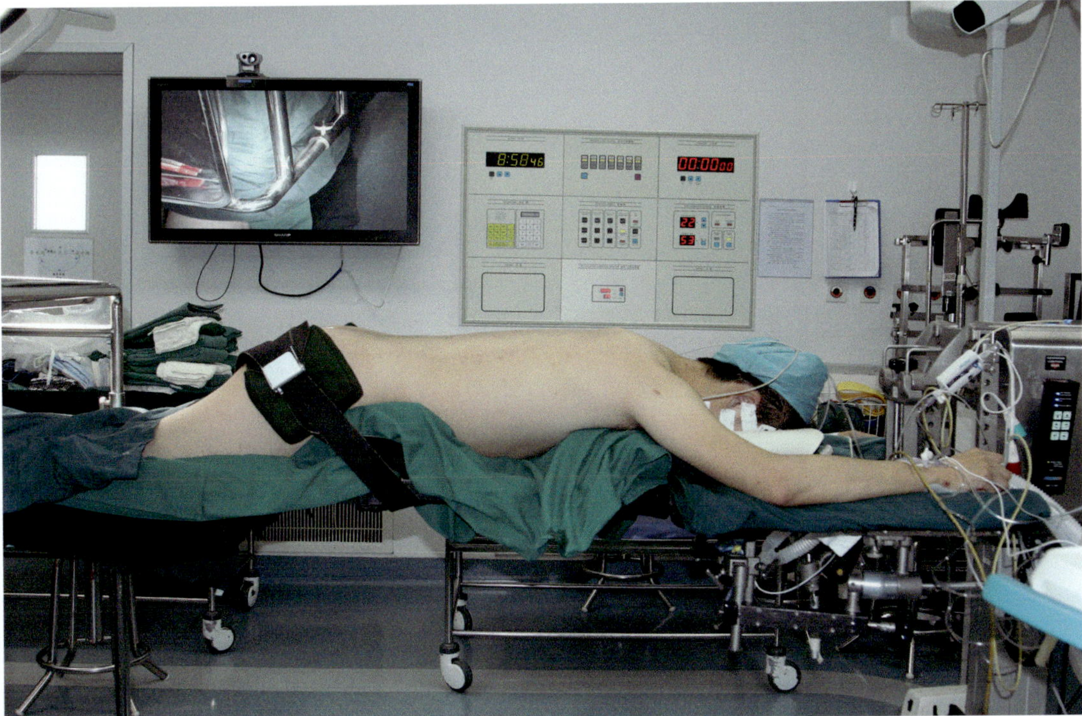

Fig. 10.1 Carbon operating table

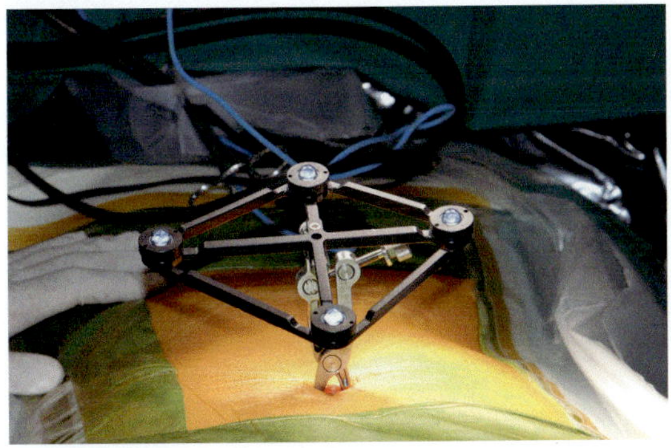

Fig. 10.2 The tracer is installed on this spinous process

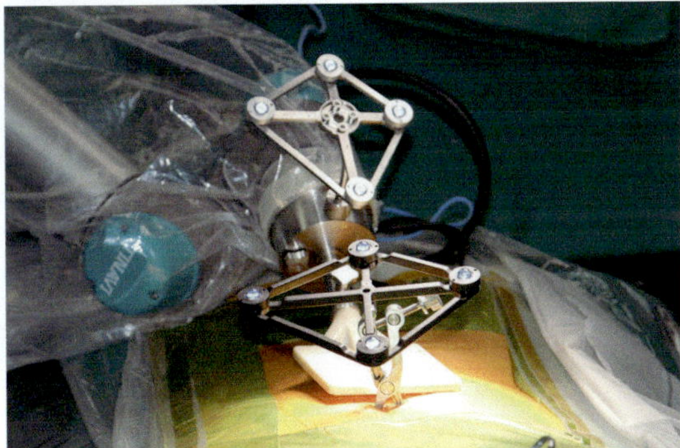

Fig. 10.3 The end of the robotic arm is close to the field

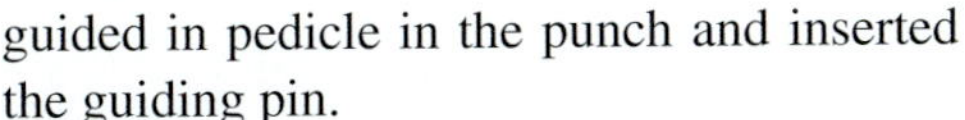

guided in pedicle in the punch and inserted the guiding pin.

9. After all the guiding pins are positioned (Fig. 10.7), remove the mechanical arm and insert the pedicle screw into the guide pin (Fig. 10.8).
10. It is possible to identify the position of decompression, vertebral osteotomy, tumors, or ossification excision under the guidance of the robot.

3 Techniques and Experience with Robot-Assisted Thoracic Pedicle Screw Placement

The fixation of upper thoracic pedicle or other complex deformities is best supported by robots. The lower thoracic vertebra can be inserted by hand. Plan well before surgery. The position of robot and camera is expected to avoid signal

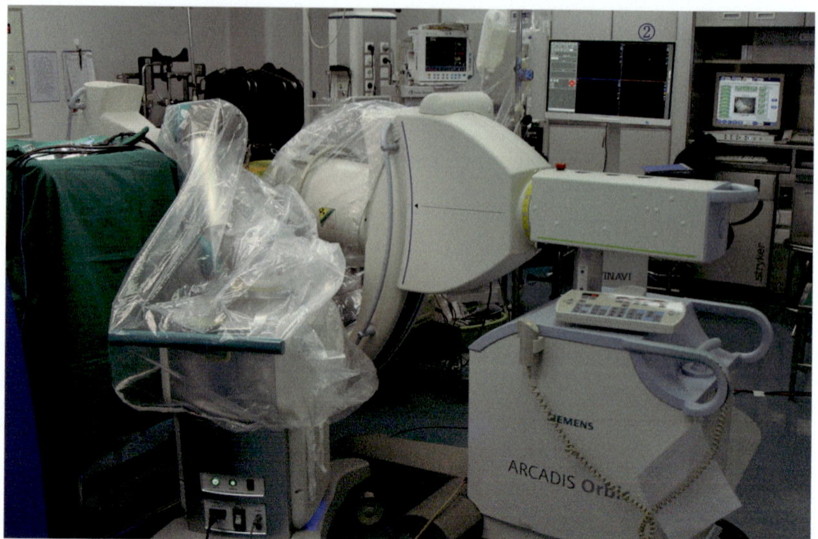

Fig. 10.4 3D C-arm and operating table

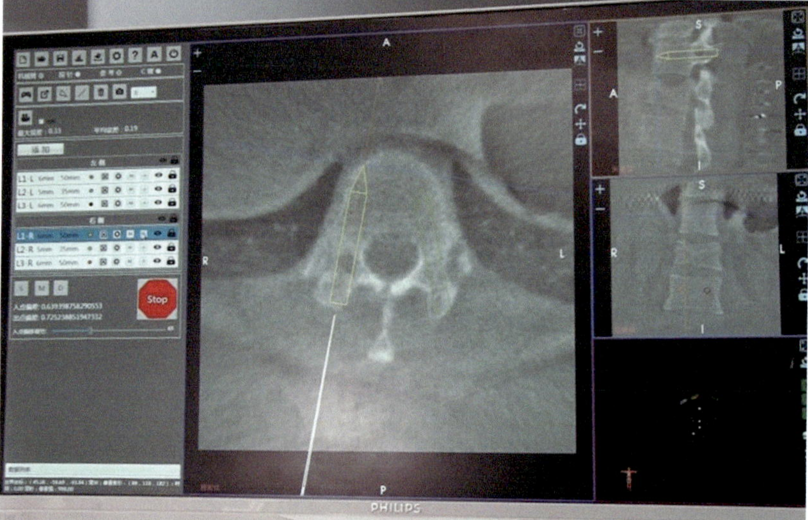

Fig. 10.5 Plan of the pedicle screw insertion point and orientation in the 3D image

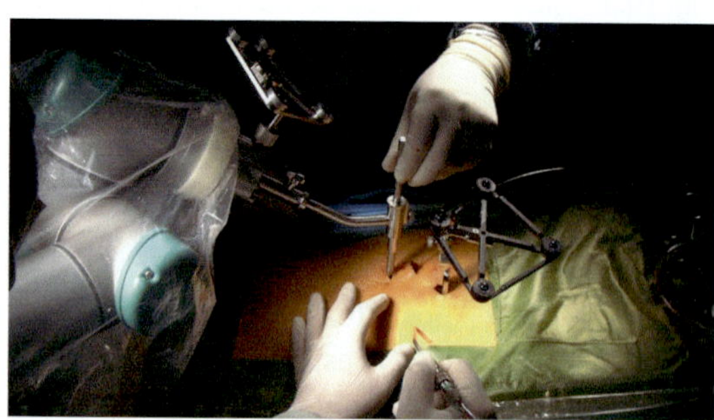

Fig. 10.6 Installation of the guide sleeve

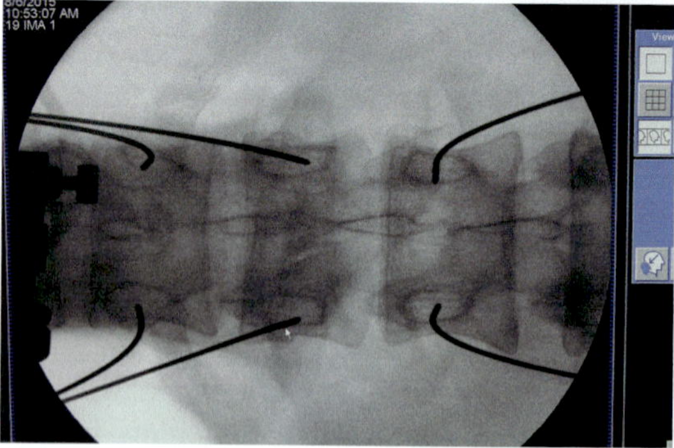

Fig. 10.7 All the guiding pins are put in

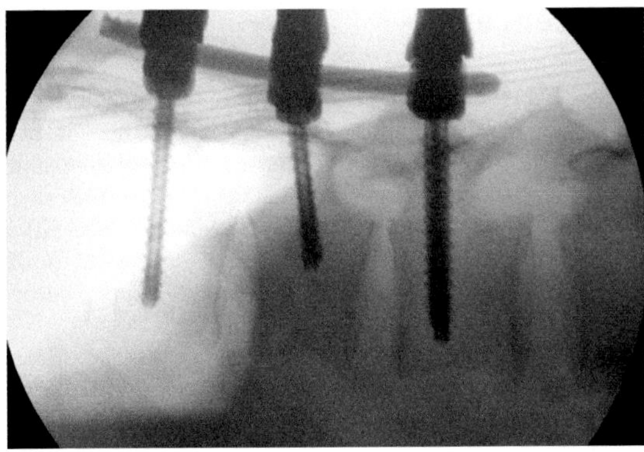

Fig. 10.8 Insertion of the pedicle screw

occlusion and other interference. The patient's tracer is firmly fixed, and the patient's tracer is prevented from colliding with the C-arm scan. The robot system needs to be calibrated. The operation needs to be as earnest and gentle as possible. In the early stage when doctors are not skilled, after the screws are completed, the 3D scan can be used for reconfirm.

In addition, the image collection is not more than five vertebral bodies at one time, and it may be necessary to collect images several times when applying multiple segments. At the same time, the image quality needs to be improved, but it is enough to meet the needs of pedicle screws. The application of robotic assistance in tiny pedicle can greatly help the surgeon to determine the specific conditions of pedicle. If we can pedicle screw fixation, it avoids the error of placing the pedicle screw into a vertebral body that cannot be fixed using a pedicle screw. The operation time will be reduced, and the risk of spinal cord nerve injury will be lowered.

The first operation of the spinal surgery application robot-assisted pedicle screw at the Beijing Jishuitan hospital was a minimally invasive internal fixation operation for thoracic vertebral fracture. At present, due to the application of a digital operating room and the gradual improvement of supporting facilities, image acquisition and transmission time are reduced. More and more applications have made the use of technology more skillful; the time difference between the screw and the X-ray is very similar, but the accuracy is greatly increased (Tian et al. 2017).

Although the pedicle screw technique has been widely used, because of the specificity of the anatomy of the thoracic vertebra, the incidental incidence of pedicle screw placement is higher. Compared with previous surgical methods (including navigation), robotic-assisted surgery further improved the accuracy, stability, and repeatability of the screws. The error caused by manual operation is almost avoided, and the accident rate is significantly reduced. A disadvantage is that the surgical method increases the cost and requires certain professional equipment: including orthopedic robot, 3D C-arm machine, carbon scanning bed, among others. It should be noted that orthopedic robot technology itself also requires a specific learning curve, and there may be some issues such as registration deviation during the operation. Therefore, it is necessary to master the technique of hand-to-hand pinning and carefully and repeatedly compare it in the operation to ensure the safety of the operation.

Typical Case.

28-year-old male patient.

Chief complaint: falling down lead to back pain and limited activity for 1 day.

Current history: the patient accidentally fell from a height of 4 m 1 day ago. At that time, he felt pain in his back and could not stand or walk.

Physical examination: spine percussion pain (+), limited range of motion (ROM), POM (+). Lower limb muscle strength was normal, euesthesia.

Imaging examination:

X-ray: The T11 vertebral body becomes wedge-shaped change.

CT and MRI: T11 vertebral compression fracture.

Diagnosis: thoracic vertebra compression fracture (T11).

Operation: robot-assisted percutaneous minimally invasive thoracic vertebra fracture reduction, pedicle screw internal fixation.

The operation was smooth, and there was less blood loss during the operation (Fig. 10.9). The patient walked with the brace on the first postoperative day, and the waist and back pain were relieved. CT examination showed that the thoracic

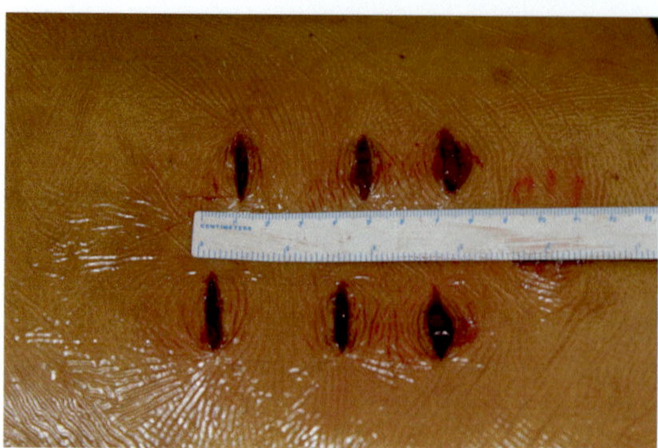

Fig. 10.9 Surgical incisions were very small. There was less blood loss

fracture was well restored and the position of the pedicle screw was good. Three months after the operation, the fracture healed.

References

Liljenqvist U, Lepsien U, Hackenberg L, Niemeyer T, Halm H. Comparative analysis of pedicle screw and hook instrumentation in posterior correction and fusion of idiopathic thoracic scoliosis. Eur Spine J. 2002;11(4):336–43.

Bess R, Lenke LK, Cheh G, Mandel S, Sides B. Comparison of thoracic pedicle screw to hook instrumentation for the treatment of adult spinal deformity. Spine. 2007;32(5):555–61.

Kim YJ, Lenke LG, Bridwell KH, Cho YS, Riew KD. Free hand pedicle screw placement in the thoracic spine: is it safe? Spine. 2004;29(3):333–42. discussion 342

Tian W, Han X, Liu B, Liu Y, Hu Y. A robot-assisted surgical system using a force-image control method for pedicle screw insertion. PLoS One. 2014;9(1):e86346.

Tian W, Fan MX, Liu YJ. Robot-assisted percutaneous pedicle screw placement using three-dimensional fluoroscopy: a preliminary clinical study. Chin Med J. 2017;130(13):1617–8.

11 Robot-Assisted Spine Surgery in Spinal Deformities

Bin Xiao, Kai Yan, and Wei Tian

Abstract

The advancements of spine deformity correction in this century include 3D understanding and evolution of surgical instruments and implants. The most advanced technique recently is robot-assisted orthopedics technique, which can accurately locate and control the direction of the insertion of screws in real time during the operation so as to reduce deviations caused by the surgeon's hand, especially in cases of severe deformity. Related surgical strategy and technical tips are described in this chapter.

Keywords

Spinal deformities · Robot-assisted orthopedics technique · Accurate insertion of screws · Real time · Reduced deviations · Surgical strategy

1 Introduction

The advancement of spine deformity correction technique in the twenty-first century is distinguished by the following two aspects:

1. The continued deeper understanding of deformity, from coronal to sagittal, from 2D to 3D, from the local to the whole, and from bony structure to soft tissue balance (Ilharreborde 2018).
2. The development of surgical instruments and implants, from Harrington to Luque, from the C–D segmental hook–rod system to the pedicle screw, which appeared at the end of the last century (Tambe et al. 2018).

Common spine deformities include adolescent idiopathic scoliosis, congenital scoliosis, lumbar spondylolytic spondylolisthesis, adult degenerative scoliosis, and sagittal imbalance.

The advantage of robot-assisted orthopedics technique is that it can accurately locate and control the direction of the insertion of screws in real time during the operation, so as to reduce deviations caused by the surgeon's hand. The technique can help surgeons to insert pedicle screws accurately in cases of severe deformity and even percutaneously. The principles and methods of robot-assisted orthopedics have been described in the previous chapters. In this section, an adolescent idiopathic scoliosis case is used to introduce the application of robot-assisted orthopedics technique in spine deformity correction.

2 Case Presentation

A 12-year-old girl presented asymmetry in the back for about 1 year. The deformity progressed recently. The girl has not reached

B. Xiao · K. Yan · W. Tian (✉)
Department of Spine Surgery, Beijing Jishuitan Hospital, Fourth Clinical Hospital of Peking University, Beijing, China
e-mail: tianweijst@vip.163.com

W. Tian (ed.), *Navigation Assisted Robotics in Spine and Trauma Surgery*,
https://doi.org/10.1007/978-981-15-1846-1_11

menarche yet. Her height is 148 cm, and body weight is 38 kg.

Clinical images of the patient are shown in Fig. 11.1 (posterior aspect), Fig. 11.2 (lateral aspect), and Fig. 11.3 Adam's forward bending test. The preoperative plain radiographs are shown in Fig. 11.4 (lateral bending view on the left side), Fig. 11.5 (PA view), Fig. 11.6 (lateral bending view on the right side), and Fig. 11.7 (lateral view).

Coronal parameters were as follows:

PT: T2–T4 35°(16°).

MT: T5–T11 78°(38°).

TL/L: T11–L4 71°(27°).

C7PL-CSVL: −14 mm, RSH: −5 mm, TTS:7 mm, T-AVT: 40 mm, L-AVT: 44 mm.

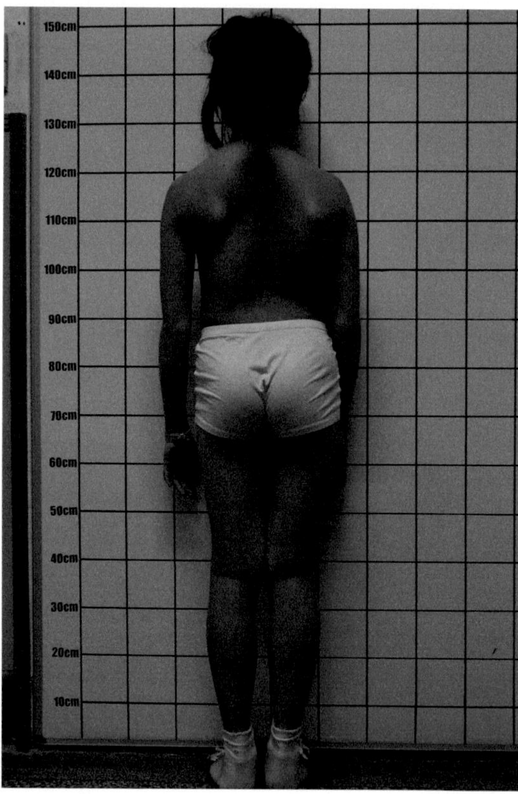

Fig. 11.1 Back view of the patient

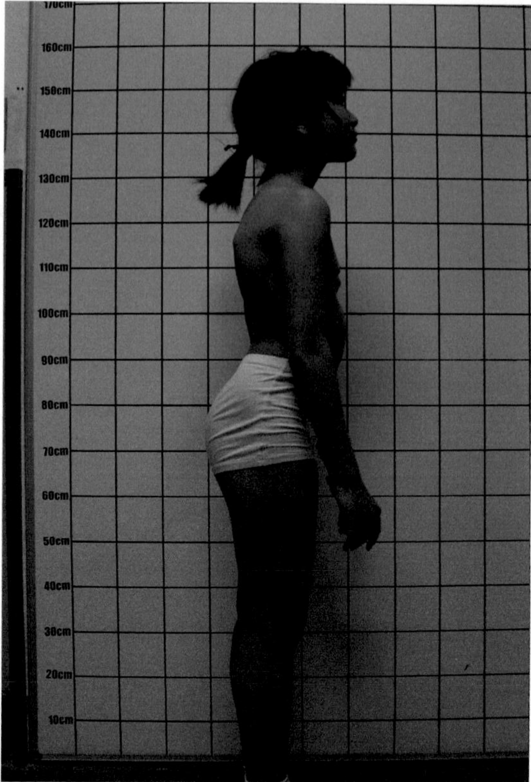

Fig. 11.2 Lateral view of the patient

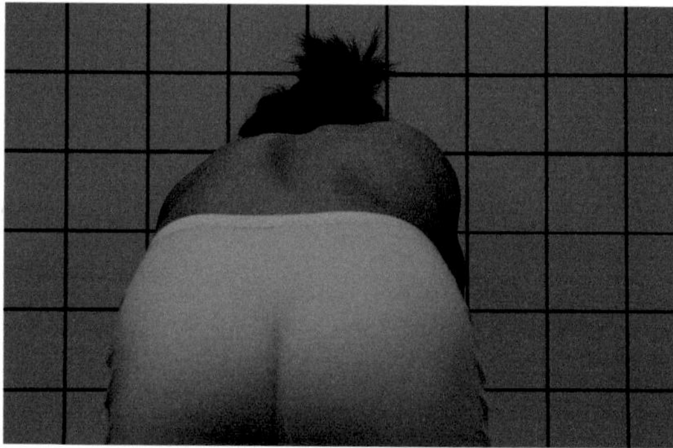

Fig. 11.3 Adam's forward bending test

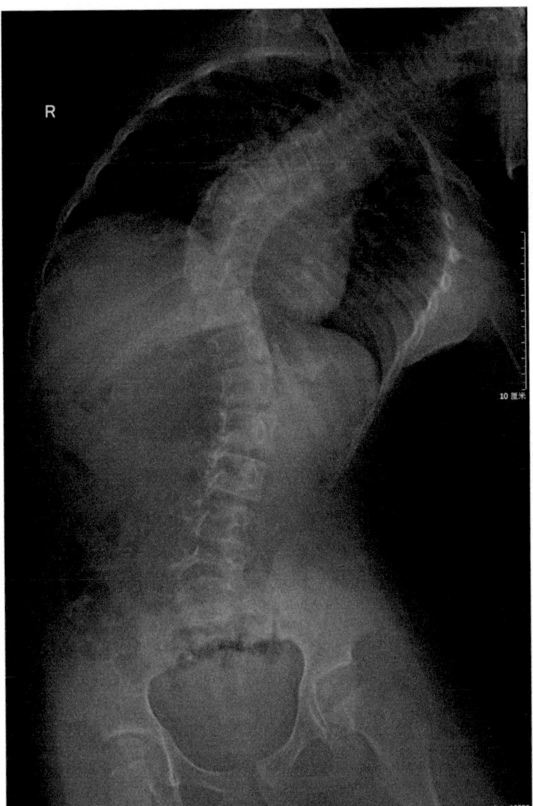

Fig. 11.4 Left side bending

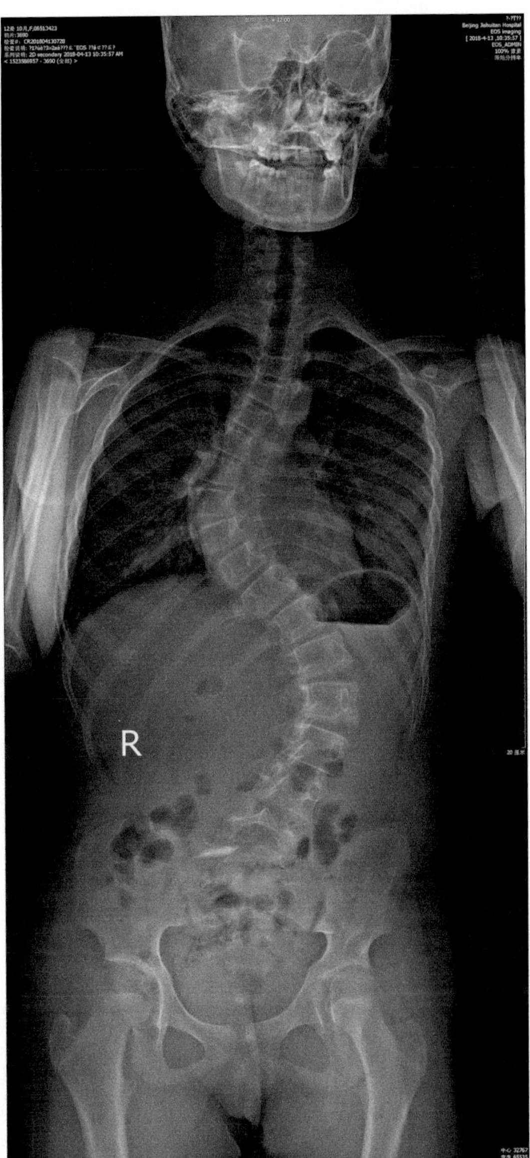

Fig. 11.5 PA view of X-ray

Sagittal parameters were as follows:

TK: 21°, LL: −55°, TLK: −3°.

T/L AVR: 12°/9° (scoliometer).

Risser Grade 2.

The distal radius and ulna classification (DRU) (Luk et al. 2014; Cheung and Luk 2017): R8U5.

MRI(−).

Diagnosis: AIS Lenke 3CN.

3 Surgical Strategy

The surgical strategy for posterior spinal fusion from T5 to L3 with multiple Schwab Grade 1 osteotomies (Schwab et al. 2015) used was the following:

Step 1: Skin incision, dissection of subcutaneous tissue, and paravertebral muscles were performed to expose the posterior surface of the vertebrae.

Step 2: All the pedicle screws were inserted as planned from the upper to the lowest instrumented vertebra using the robot.

Step 2.1: The robotic patient tracker frame was placed on the spinal process, the intraoperative 3D images were obtained using Siemens ISO-C Arcadis, and then were transferred to the robotic system (Fig. 11.8).

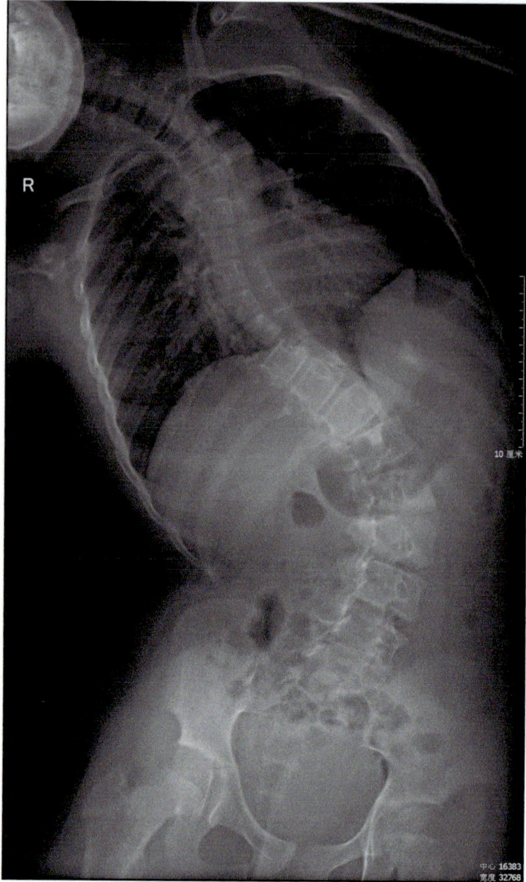

Fig. 11.6 Left side bending

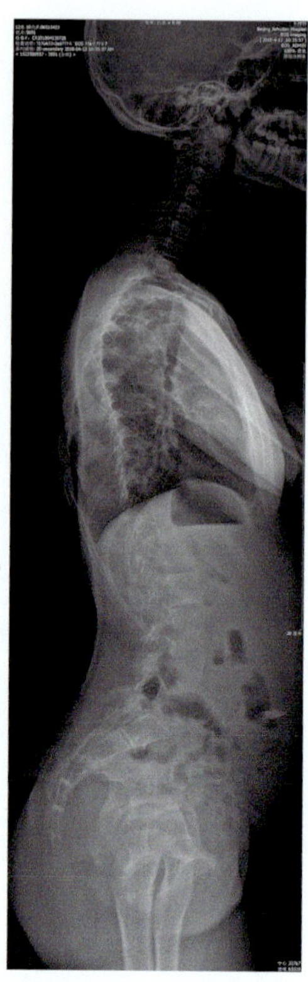

Fig. 11.7 Lateral view of the X-ray

Fig. 11.8 TiNAVI robot (left) and Siemens ISO-C Arcadis (right)

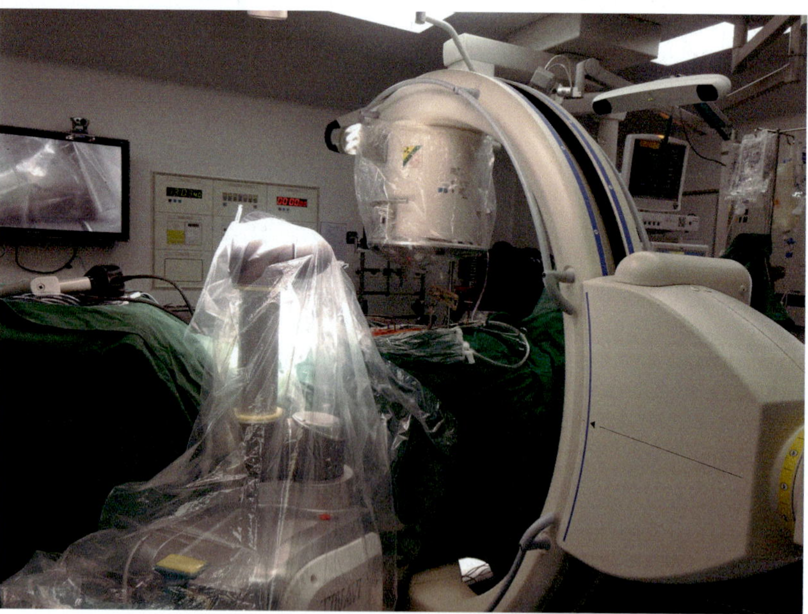

Step 2.2: The pedicle screws' path was planned in the robotic system (Fig. 11.9).

Step 2.3: The accuracy of the robot was checked and adjusted, and the K-wire was inserted in the pedicle through the mechanical arm using the drill. For one scan, an 8–10 K-wire insertion was performed (Fig. 11.10).

Step 2.4: The walls of the path were tapped and checked using the feeler.

Step 2.5: The pedicle screws were inserted and conformed to the position.

Step 3: Facetectomies were released (Schwab Grade 1 or 2 osteotomies) (Schwab et al. 2015).

Step 4: The contour rods were corrected following the insertion of the first rod, translation, en bloc derotation, and in situ. Next, the second rod was inserted, and the cantilever maneuver was used. Compression and distraction were performed, followed by segmental derotation (Fig. 11.11).

Step 5: Corticotomies of the posterior vertebral laminae and transverse processes and morselized laying of local bone grafts were achieved.

Step 6: Closure was performed following drainage close the fascia, subcutaneous tissue, and skin.

Figures 11.12 and 11.13 show the postoperative images

	Pre-OP	Post-OP	Correction
PT: T2–T4	35°	26°	25%
MT: T5–T11	78°	27°	65%
TL/L: T11–L4	71°	17°	76%
C7PL-CSVL	−14 mm	4 mm	

Tips

1. All the methods for correction should follow the routine rules.
2. Surgeons can use the robotic system in the apical area and freehand method in other area. Robot and navigation could reduce pedicle perforation rates (Chan and Kwan 2017; Tian et al. 2017; Macke et al. 2016).

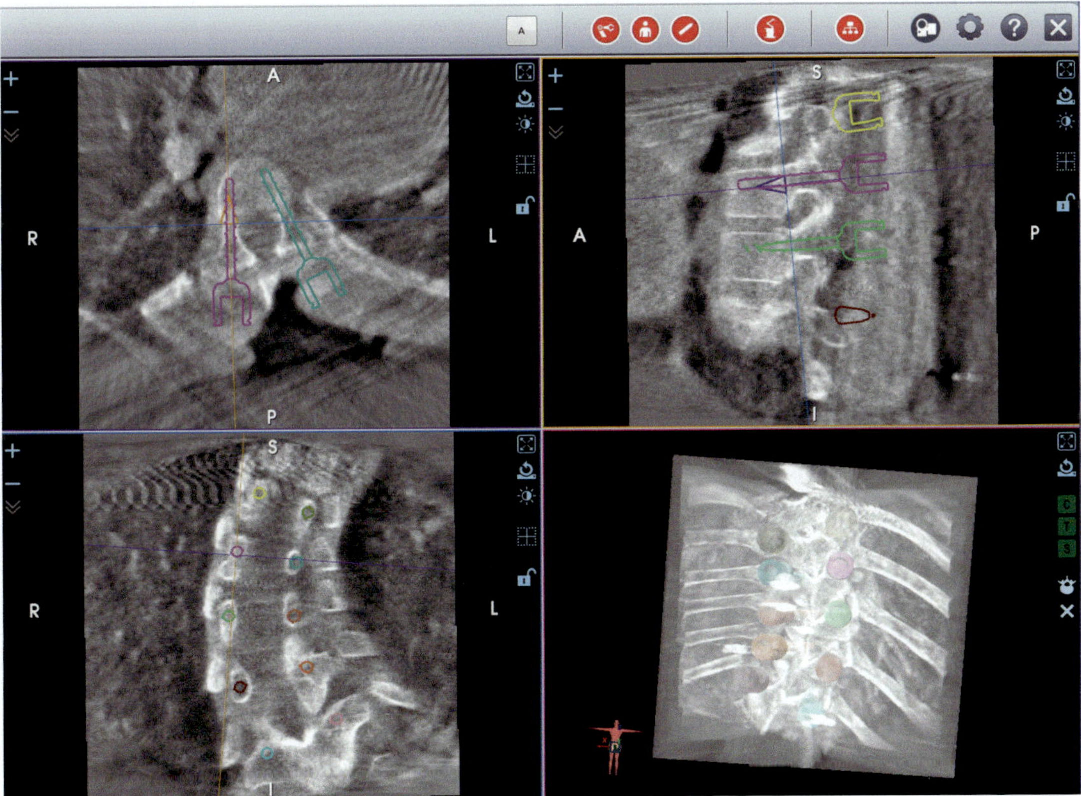

Fig. 11.9 Pedicle screws planning

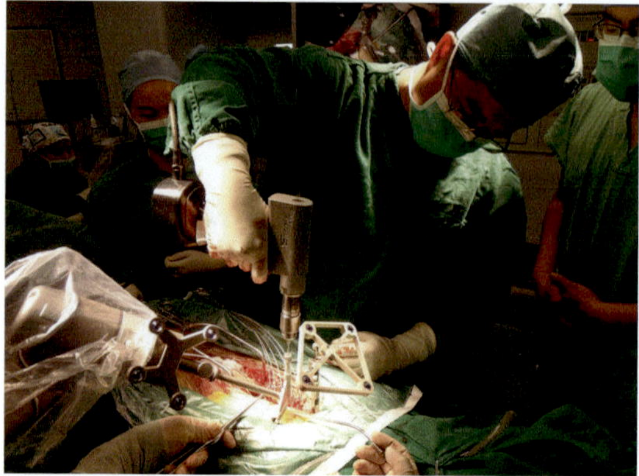

Fig. 11.10 Insertion of the K-wire using the robot

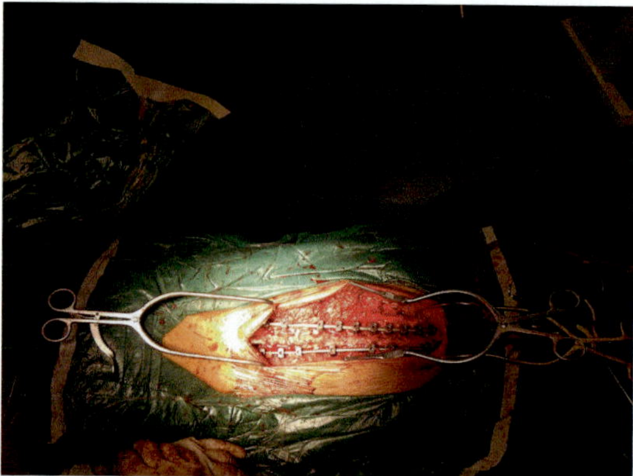

Fig. 11.11 Intraoperative picture after the correction

3. A cannulated tap and pedicle feeler should be used before screw insertions.
4. If the pedicle is too narrow to insert the screw, hook, sublaminar wire/tape, or in–out–in screw insertion is an alternative method for anchoring.
5. To date, the robot may help surgeons insert screws accurately in the malformed spine. Other applications are being studied.
6. Some surgeons use low-dose CT scan with robot-assisted spinal surgery, which could reduce the radiation exposure of the patients (Sensakovic et al. 2017).

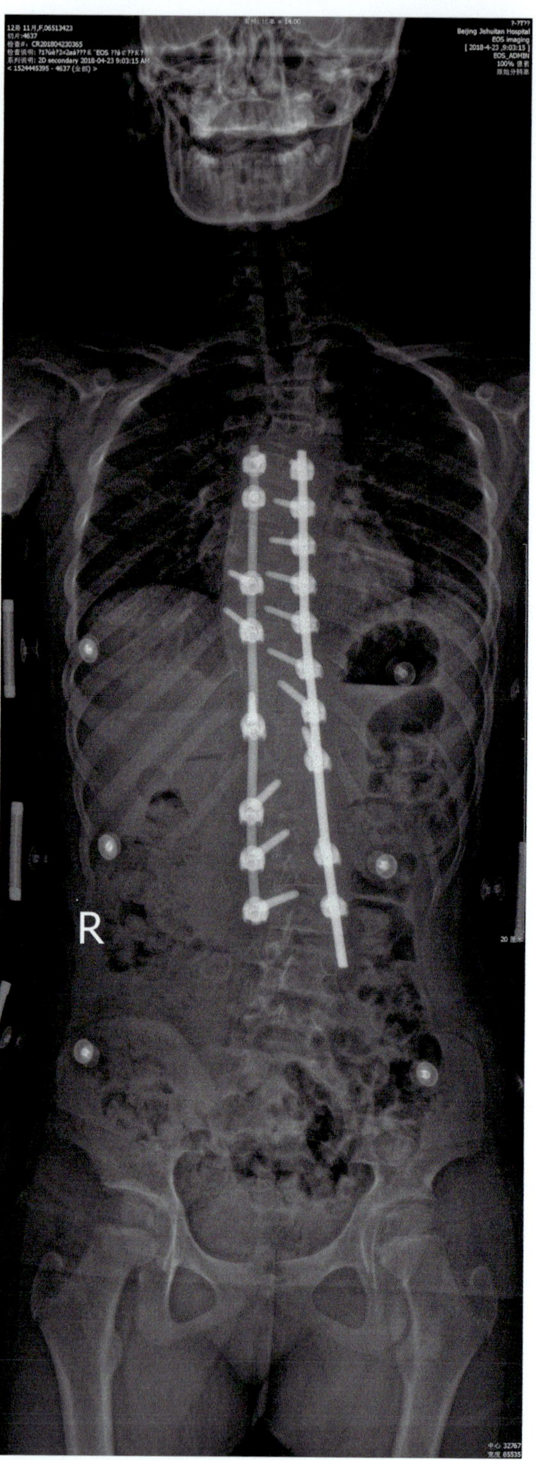

Fig. 11.12 Postoperative PA view

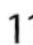

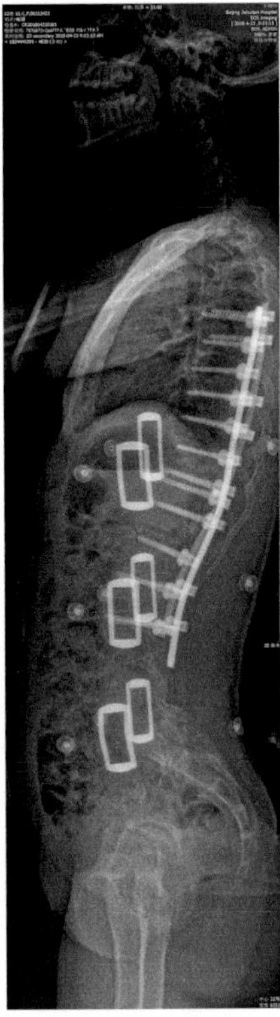

Fig. 11.13 Postop lateral view

7. The rate of successfully placed pedicle screws improves with increasing experience. The frequency of screw malposition was reported to be similar over the learning curve (Hu and Lieberman 2014).

References

Ilharreborde B. Sagittal balance and idiopathic scoliosis: does final sagittal alignment influence outcomes, degeneration rate or failure rate? Eur Spine J. 2018;S1:48–58.

Tambe AD, Panikkar SJ, Millner PA, et al. Current concepts in the surgical management of adolescent idiopathic scoliosis. Bone Joint J. 2018;100-B(4):415–24.

Luk KD, Saw LB, Grozman S, et al. Assessment of skeletal maturity in scoliosis patients to determine clinical management: a new classification scheme using distal radius and ulna radiographs. Spine J. 2014;14(2):315–25.

Cheung JPY, Luk KD. Managing the pediatric spine: growth assessment. Asian Spine J. 2017;11(5):804–16.

Schwab F, Blondel B, Chay E, et al. The comprehensive anatomical spinal osteotomy classification. Neurosurgery. 2015;76(Suppl 1):S33–41.

Chan CYW, Kwan MK. Safety of pedicle screws in adolescent idiopathic scoliosis surgery. Asian Spine J. 2017;11(6):998–1007.

Tian W, Zeng C, An Y, et al. Accuracy and postoperative assessment of pedicle screw placement during scoliosis surgery with computer-assisted navigation: a meta-analysis. Int J Med Robot. 2017;13(1) https://doi.org/10.1002/rcs.1732.

Macke JJ, Woo R, Varich L. Accuracy of robot-assisted pedicle screw placement for adolescent idiopathic scoliosis in the pediatric population. J Robot Surg. 2016;10(2):145–50.

Sensakovic WF, O'Dell MC, Agha A, et al. CT radiation dose reduction in robot-assisted pediatric spinal surgery. Spine (Phila Pa 1976). 2017;42(7):E417–24.

Hu X, Lieberman IH. What is the learning curve for robotic-assisted pedicle screw placement in spine surgery? Clin Orthop Relat Res. 2014;472(6):1839–44.

12 Robot-Assisted Lumbar Pedicle Screw Fixation

Zhiyu Li, Zhao Lang, and Wei Tian

Abstract

The pedicle screw fixation technique is challenging. However, with the help of the robot, the lumbar pedicle screw placement can achieve a higher accuracy both in open and percutaneous surgeries compared with freehand fluoroscopy-guided technique. To ensure the safety of screw placement, a thorough understanding of the pertinent spinal anatomy, detailed preoperative planning, and gentle and appropriate manipulation intraoperatively should be highly considered.

Keywords

Robot-assisted · Lumbar spine · Pedicle screw fixation · Preoperative planning · 3D image · Accuracy · Percutaneous technique

1 Introduction

In 1970, Roy-Camille promoted the use of the pedicle as a point of fixation for thoracolumbar segmental instrumentation (Roy-Camille et al. 1970). Since then, pedicle screw fixation has been demonstrated to be biomechanically superior to hook and sublaminar wire constructs (Abumi et al. 1989), providing opportunities for the use of shorter constructs and for earlier post-operative recovery.

1.1 Indications

In the following situations, the robot-assisted technique is believed to be much more helpful:

1. Severe deformity with obvious vertebral rotation.
2. Severe degeneration or spondylolisthesis making identification of the entry point difficult.
3. Cement augmentation in osteoporosis.
4. Minimally invasive surgery.

1.2 Contraindication

Almost all patients who need posterior lumbar spine fixation could be candidates of robot-assisted lumbar pedicle screw placement after excluding the anatomical variation, which will hinder the availability of appropriate trajectory.

Z. Li · Z. Lang · W. Tian (✉)
Department of Spine Surgery, Beijing Jishuitan Hospital, Fourth Clinical Hospital of Peking University, Beijing, China
e-mail: tianweijst@vip.163.com

W. Tian (ed.), *Navigation Assisted Robotics in Spine and Trauma Surgery*,
https://doi.org/10.1007/978-981-15-1846-1_12

2 Difficulties of Traditional Methods and the Advantages of Robotic Surgery

The pedicle screw fixation technique is challenging with regard to accurate placement of the screws through a narrow invisible trajectory into the vertebral body, especially when percutaneous techniques with limited exposure of the spinal anatomy are applied (Nevzati et al. 2014). The concern about the neurovascular damage due to misplacement of pedicle screws promoted the application of navigation and robotics to enhance the accuracy of screw placement. Recent studies showed that robot-assisted technique can achieve a higher accuracy of screw placement both in open and percutaneous surgeries compared with freehand fluoroscopy-guided technique (Keric et al. 2017; Kim et al. 2017).

3 Preoperative Imaging and Planning

Posteroanterior, lateral standing radiographs, and computer tomography scan are necessary imaging modalities preoperatively. The surgeon should have a thorough understanding of the pertinent spinal anatomy and carefully and accurately interpret all relevant preoperative imaging studies. Appropriate trajectory and the dimension of pedicle screw should be determined. If there is no appropriate trajectory, other methods of screw insertion should be considered. For aged patients, bone mineral density must be evaluated, so as to determine the necessity of cement augmentation.

4 Surgical Technique

1. Positioning. The patient is prone on the Jackson table with the abdomen free of any compression to reduce venous congestion. The thigh is neutral or slightly extended.
2. Exposure. For open surgery, the standard midline incision with subperiosteal exposure of the pertinent posterior osseous elements may be performed. Alternatively, the surgical exposure may be achieved by the Wiltse paraspinal approach to reduce the traction force of the muscle. For percutaneous surgery, minimally invasive approaches using a muscle-splitting technique could be applied (Fig. 12.1).
3. The patient tracker is placed to the spinous process of one to two vertebrae cranial to the operative segments to avoid interfering with the manipulation. Ensure the rigid fixation of patient tracker, so as to not lose the accuracy.
4. Sheathe the robot arm by using the sterilization bag. Assemble the registration plate to the robot arm and place it to the appropriate position in the operative field (Fig. 12.2).

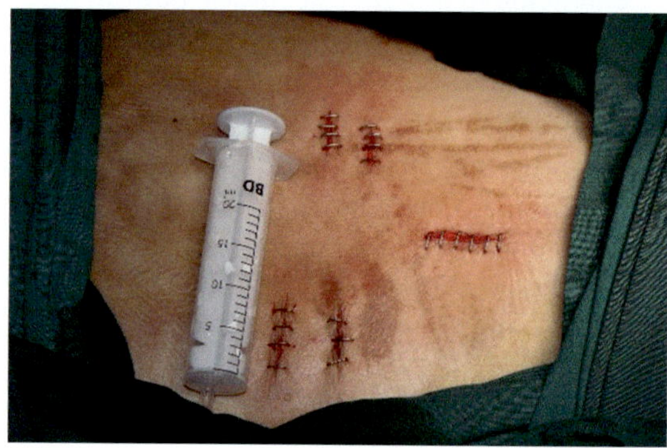

Fig. 12.1 Minimally invasive approach for lumbar pedicle screw fixation is applied in percutaneous surgery

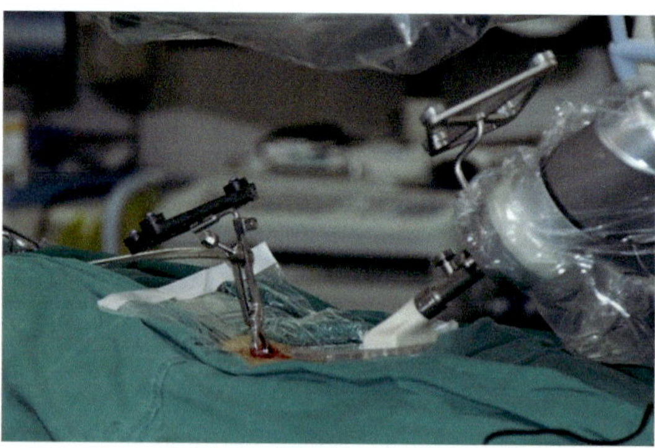

Fig. 12.2 Place the registration plate to the appropriate position in the operative field

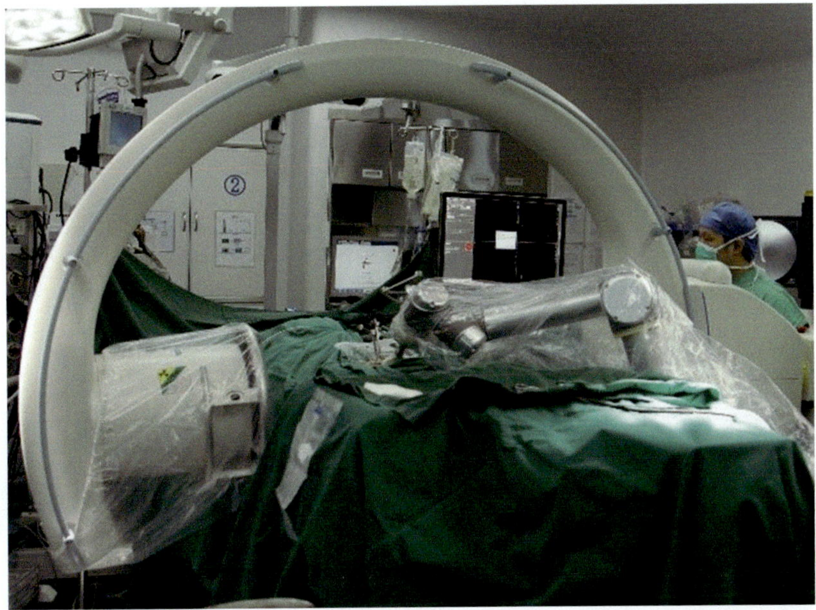

Fig. 12.3 Three dimension image is harvested using motorized C arm

Adjust the operation table and robot arm to ensure the registration plate can be seen on the biplanar view of fluoroscopy.

5. The 3D image is harvested using motorized C-arm (Fig. 12.3). Do not hesitate to refix the patient tracker and re-obtain the 3D image if there is any suspicion of displacement of the tracker.
6. Transfer the images from the C-arm workstation to the robot workstation. Accomplish the screw placement planning using the specific software (Fig. 12.4). When choosing the entry point and convergence orientation of the screw, the exposure approach should be taken into account. The placement of pedicle screw will become difficult if a relatively lateral entry point and larger convergence orientation are chosen in an open surgery.
7. Assemble the guiding tube to the robot arm after disassembling the registration plate. Then under the guidance of navigation, the guiding tube is slowly moved to the target place (Fig. 12.5).
8. When the guiding tube is correctly positioned along the axis of the pedicle, place the guider into the guiding tube and ensure the tip of the guider touches the bony element at the entry point of the pedicle (Fig. 12.6).
9. Finely adjust the robot arm to decrease the accuracy error below 0.5 mm. Next, place a K-wire along the guider into the vertebra (Fig. 12.7). Do not insert too much K-wire to avoid any damage of internal organs. In order to avoid the sliding of the tip of K-wire, the surgeon could prepare the entry point of pedicle screw using a high-speed drill or an ultrasonic osteotome.
10. Repeat the procedure and finish placement the K-wire. Confirm the position of the K-wire under fluoroscopy or using the motorized C-arm scanning (Fig. 12.8a, b).
11. Place pedicle screws along the K-wires, taking care not to let the K-wire advance with the screw (Fig. 12.9). Then, remove the K-wire and confirm the position of the screws using the C-arm (Fig. 12.10a, b).

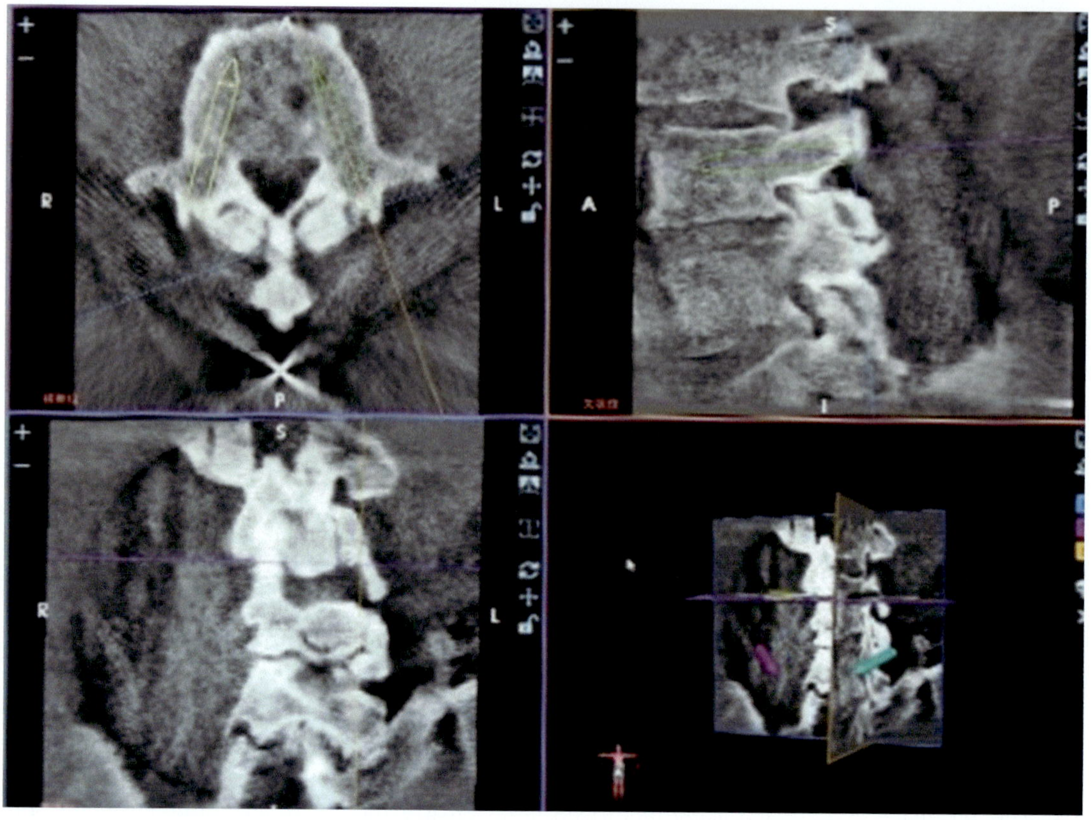

Fig. 12.4 Carry out screw placement planning in the work station

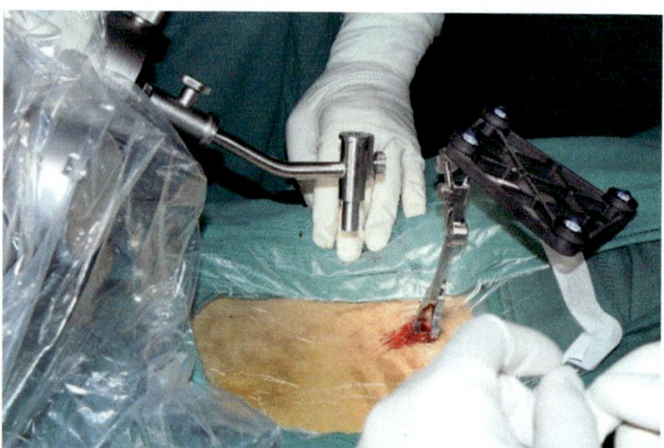

Fig. 12.5 Under the guidance of navigation, the guiding tube slowly moves to the target place

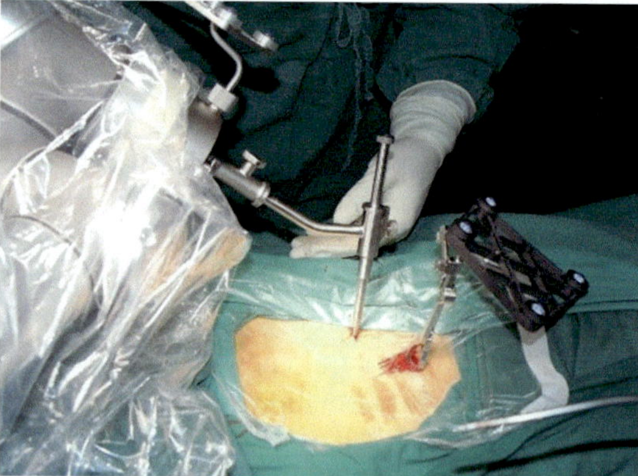

Fig. 12.6 Place the guider into the guiding tube along the axis of the pedicle when the guiding tube is at the right place

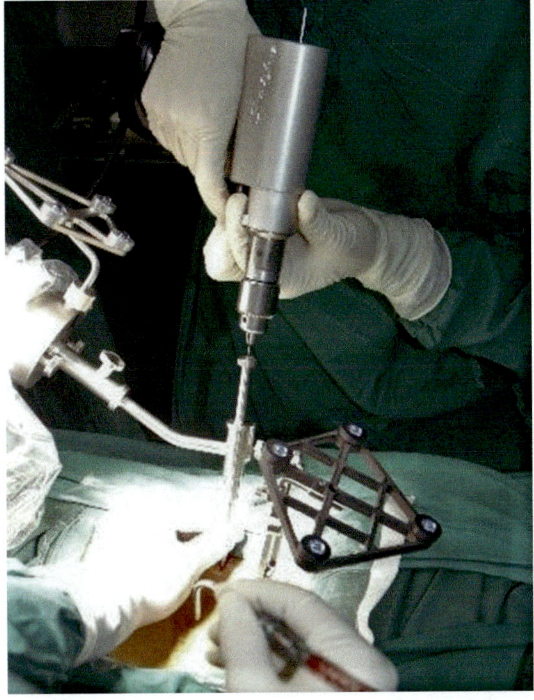

Fig. 12.7 Place a K wire along the guider into the vertebra

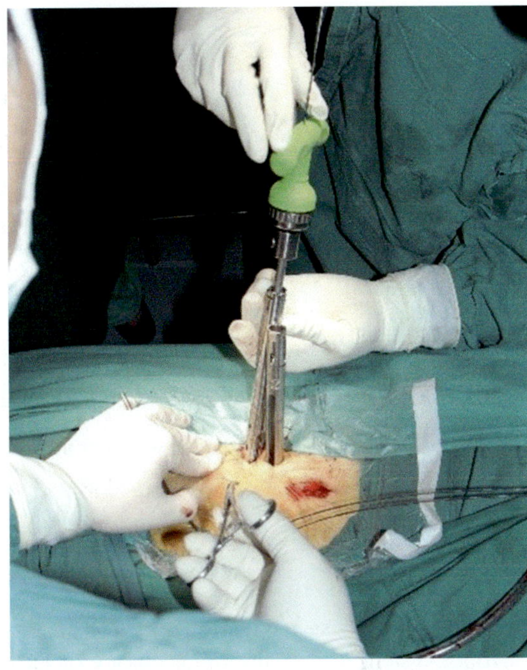

Fig. 12.9 Place lumbar pedicle screws along the K wires

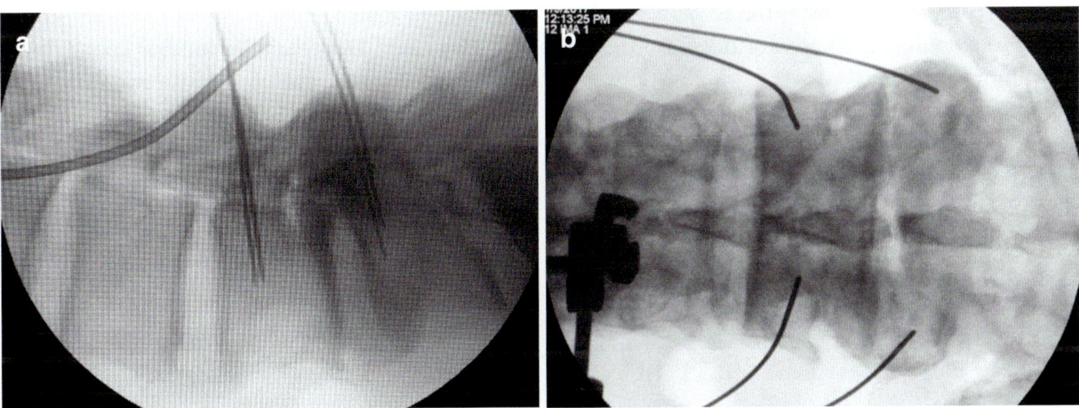

Fig. 12.8 Confirm position of the K wire under fluoroscopy. (**a**) lateral view. (**b**) anteroposterior view

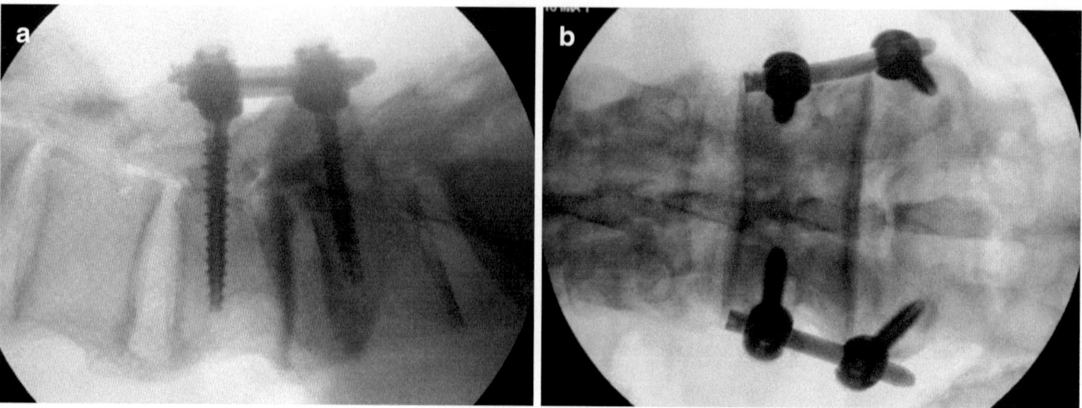

Fig. 12.10 Confirm position of the screws under fluoroscopy. (**a**) lateral view. (**b**) anteroposterior view

5 Tips

1. Surgeons can use navigation function in the robot system to reassure the accuracy of harvested images.
2. Do not tract the soft tissue too hard, which will result in image shifting. When using the drill to insert the K-wire, fully release the traction of soft tissue.
3. When preparing to insert the K-wire, it is better to stop the ventilation or decrease the tide volume temporarily.
4. To avoid sliding, drill but do not advance the K-wire on the surface of the bone at first and slowly insert the K-wire then.
5. Insert the K-wire before decompression is performed, so as to avoid decreasing the accuracy resulting from relative displacement of bony structures.

6 Typical Case

A 61-year-old female presented with low back pain and left low limb numbness for 5 years and progressive claudication for 6 months. Physical examination: MMT – left ankle plantar flexion 4/5. Sensation: lateral side hypoesthesia of left foot. Bilateral knee tendon reflex and ankle tendon reflex (+). Babinski's test (−). Left straight leg raise (+), 40°.

Diagnosis: Degenerative lumbar spondylolisthesis (L5/S1, Meyerding classification Grade 2) (Figs. 12.11a, b and 12.12a, b).

Robot-assisted lumbar pedicle screw fixation was performed with laminectomy and transforaminal lumbar interbody fusion (Fig. 12.13a–d).

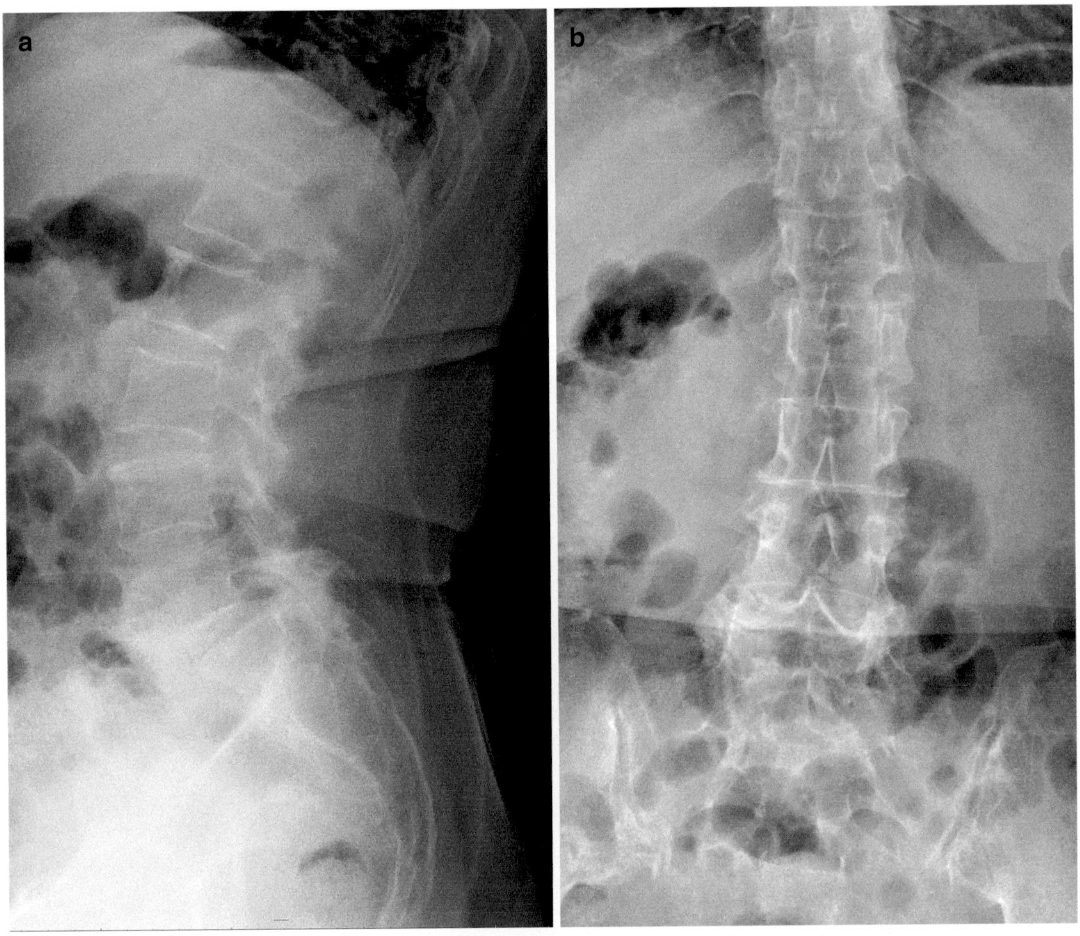

Fig. 12.11 An old lady presenting low back pain and left low limb numbness has degenerative lumbar spondylolisthesis (L5/S1). (**a**) lateral view. (**b**) anteroposterior view

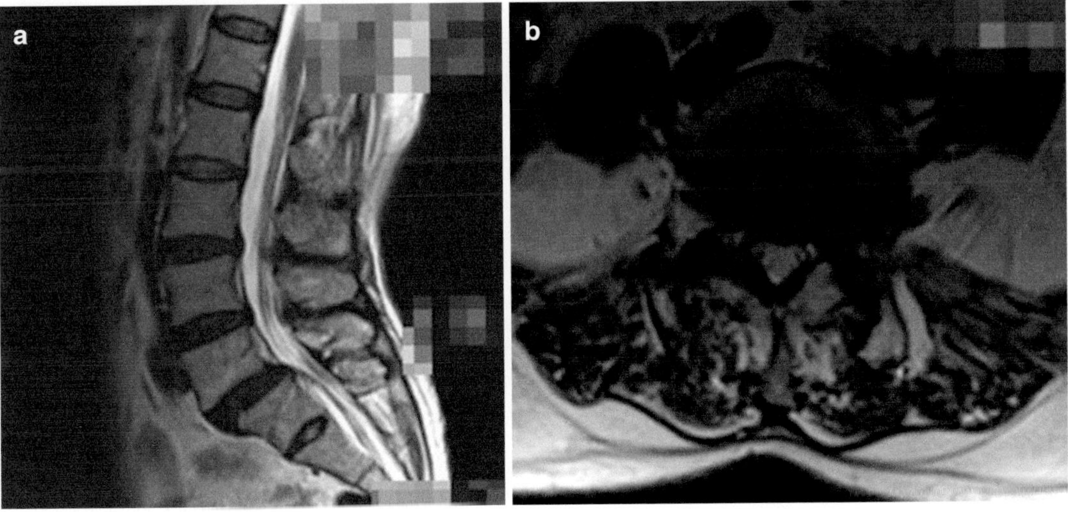

Fig. 12.12 Preoperative MRI scanning. (**a**) lumbar spondylolisthesis in L5/S1 in sagittal view. (**b**) lumbar stenosis in axial view

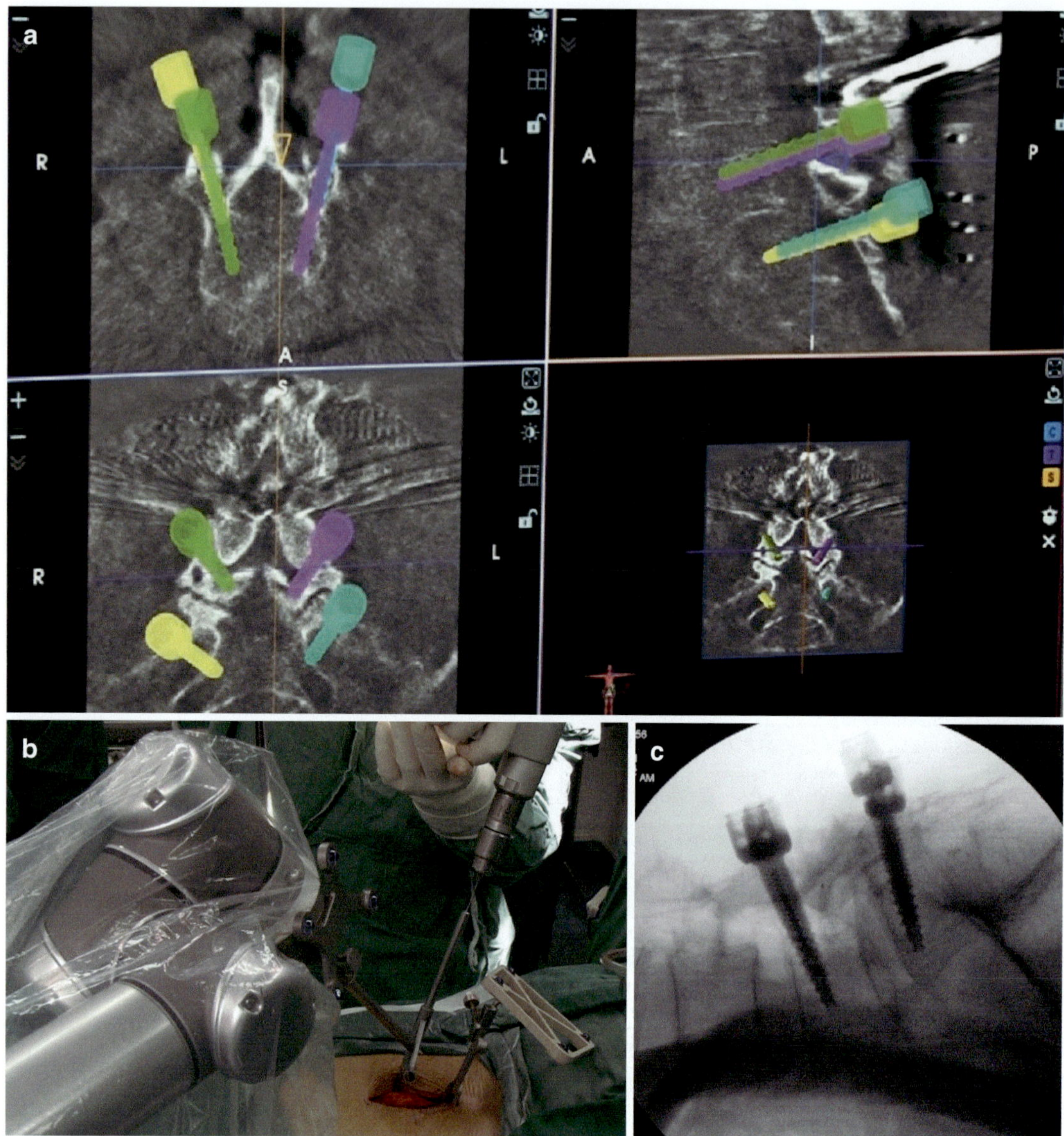

Fig. 12.13 Lumbar pedicle screw fixation using an open approach. (**a**) preoperative screw placement planning. (**b**) a muscle-splitting technique is used after making an incision in the fascia. (**c**) lateral view of the screws. (**d**) anteroposterior view of the screws

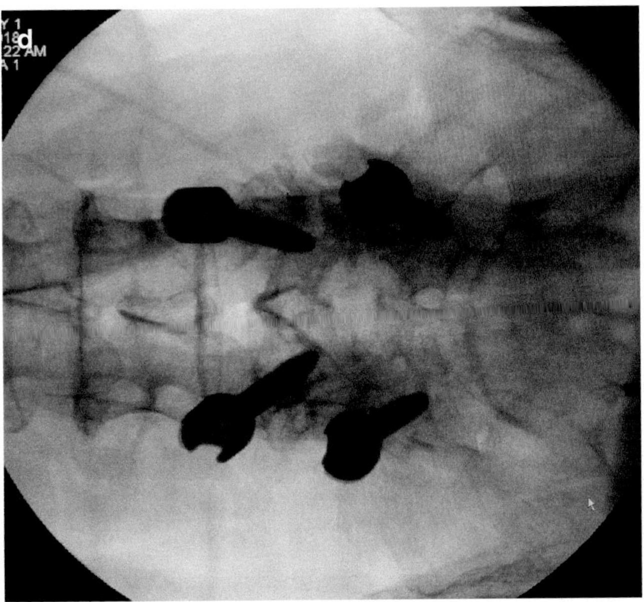

Fig. 12.13 (continued)

References

Roy-Camille R, Roy-Camille M, Demeulenaere C. Osteosynthesis of dorsal, lumbar, and lumbosacral spine with metallic plates screwed into vertebral pedicles and articular apophyses. La Presse Medicale. 1970;78:1447–8.

Abumi K, Panjabi MM, Duranceau J. Biomechanical evaluation of spinal fixation devices. Part III. Stability provided by six spinal fixation devices and interbody bone graft. Spine (Phila Pa 1976). 1989;14:1249–55.

Nevzati E, Marbacher S, Soleman J, Perrig WN, Diepers M, Khamis A, Fandino J. Accuracy of pedicle screw placement in the thoracic and lumbosacral spine using a conventional intraoperative fluoroscopy-guided technique: a national neurosurgical education and training center analysis of 1236 consecutive screws. World Neurosurg. 2014;82(5):866–71.

Keric N, Eum DJ, Afghanyar F, Rachwal-Czyzewicz I, Renovanz M, Conrad J, Wesp DM, Kantelhardt SR, Giese A. Evaluation of surgical strategy of conventional vs. percutaneous robot-assisted spinal trans-pedicular instrumentation in spondylodiscitis. J Robot Surg. 2017;11(1):17–25.

Kim HJ, Jung WI, Chang BS, Lee CK, Kang KT, Yeom JS. A prospective, randomized, controlled trial of robot-assisted vs freehand pedicle screw fixation in spine surgery. Int J Med Robot. 2017;13(3) https://doi.org/10.1002/rcs.1779.

13 Vertebroplasty in Osteoporotic Spine

Xiao Han, Yan An, and Wei Tian

Abstract

The navigation-assisted robots for PKP can significantly improve the accuracy and safety of surgery, simplify the surgical procedure, and reduce the radiation hazards and surgical complications with a positive effect. When PKP is used to treat osteoporotic vertebral compression fractures with multiple fractures (≥3 vertebrae), fractures in the upper-middle thoracic spine, severe fracture compression, or severe osteoporosis, the use of robot navigation aids should be considered.

Keywords

Surgical operations · Robot-assisted surgery · Spinal fractures · Kyphosis · Osteoporosis

1 Indications for Surgery

The incidence of osteoporosis in elderly women aged 60–69 years in China is as high as 50–70% and that of older men is 30% (Guixing 2005). Xu Ling reported that the prevalence of vertebral fractures in women over 50 years of age in Beijing, China, was 15% (Ling et al. 1995) and increased to 36.6% in women over 80 years of age. In fractures associated with osteoporosis, vertebral fractures should be given special attention, not only because of its high incidence but also because of kyphosis, pain, and loss of labor. With conservative treatments (bed rest and medication), vertebral fractures can lead to weeks of dysfunctional pain. This pain can result in loss of labor and exercise capacity. Nearly 40% of patients continue to see no improvement and may suffer from pulmonary atelectasis, pneumonia, deep vein thrombosis, pulmonary embolism, bedsores, and urinary infections. Kado et al. (1999) reported that the mortality rate of women over 65 years of age with osteoporotic vertebral compression fractures was 23% higher than that of the control group.

Percutaneous vertebroplasty (PVP) can fix the fractured vertebral and relieve pain. The mechanical environment of the kyphosis caused by fractures can easily cause new fractures (Harry et al. 2006). In order to correct kyphosis, it is often necessary to reset the fractured vertebral body. Percutaneous kyphoplasty (PKP) addresses these problems, so that PVP can restore normal physiological curves of the spine and arrest pain. Nevertheless, nerve damage or nerve burn may also be caused by the leakage of bone cement caused by operative technique

X. Han · Y. An · W. Tian (✉)
Department of Spine Surgery, Beijing Jishuitan Hospital, Fourth Clinical Hospital of Peking University, Beijing, China
e-mail: hanxiaomd@vip.163.com; tianweijst@vip.163.com

W. Tian (ed.), *Navigation Assisted Robotics in Spine and Trauma Surgery*,
https://doi.org/10.1007/978-981-15-1846-1_13

errors (Nussbaum et al. 2004). Because interventional operations lack anatomical landmarks, sometimes the most ideal entry point cannot be found with fluoroscopic guidance or by palpation alone. Thus, in the relatively thin upper thoracic pedicle, when severe fracture compression is associated with unclear images caused by osteoporosis, puncture failure is more likely to occur.

Indications of robot-assisted surgery with navigation in vertebroplasty or kyphoplasty include the following:

1. Multiple fractures (≥3 vertebrae). Only one 3D scan is needed to acquire the data of four adjacent vertebral bodies; hence, the effect of reducing radiation dose is more pronounced in multi-segment patients. Moreover, a single-sided approach surgery with navigation assistance can be safely performed on the multi-segment patient, which can simplify surgical procedures.
2. The upper thoracic spine. Because the pedicle of the upper thoracic spine is relatively thin and the lateral fluoroscopic view is often unclear, traditional fluoroscopic methods make it difficult to determine the point of entry and direction. Although some researchers have solved this problem by changing the needle path from the costovertebral joints to the vertebral body, the risk of leakage and injury has also increased significantly (Bronek et al. 2005).
3. In severe compression fractures cases, due to excessive loss of vertebral height, procedures relying on fluoroscopic guidance alone cannot ensure the safety space of the puncture needle into the vertebral body (Hyeun et al. 2007). In particular, in cases with over 50% compression of the upper thoracic spine, and over 75% compression of the lumbar spine, traditional fluoroscopic surgery may not be safe (Barr et al. 2000).
4. Patients with severe osteoporosis have unclear images under fluoroscopy with poor anatomical landmarks. It is also an indication for robot-assisted surgery with navigation.

2 Operation Difficulties and Advantages of Robot-Assisted Surgery with Navigation (Including Related Anatomy)

Once an error has occurred during the PVP or PKP procedure, it may cause nerve damage or the puncture of the pedicle with cement leakage that may lead to nerve compression or nerve burn (Nussbaum et al. 2004). Because interventional operations lack anatomical landmarks, sometimes the most ideal entry point cannot be found under fluoroscopic guidance or by palpation alone. Specifically in the relatively thin upper thoracic pedicle, combined with severe fracture compression or unclear images caused by osteoporosis, a puncture failure is more likely to occur. Therefore, many methods have been attempted to improve the accuracy of PKP surgery.

Many authors take preoperative computed tomography (CT) measurements to locate the best entry point and puncture point (Shi-jun and Li-ming 2009; Wang et al. 2008). However, based on our experience, preoperative CT measurements are not very reliable for spinal surgery operations, and there are significant differences in accuracy compared with that of the navigation method (Ya-jun and Wei 2005).

Many authors have also suggested the use of CT-guided puncture methods (Jun et al. 2003; Zhong-liang et al. 2002). The accuracy of this method is better than that of fluoroscopy, but since it is not a real-time image, it cannot guarantee the success of puncture, nor can it monitor the situation of bone cement injection in real time, and thus it cannot detect and prevent its leakage (Zhong-liang et al. 2002). In addition, compared with the traditional fluoroscopic method, in the CT-guided method, patients receive more radiation, and the operation takes longer.

The 2D navigation (En-zhi et al. 2009; Li-ming et al. 2006; Han et al. 2012) can provide real-time images and reduce the radiation dose, which has obvious advantages compared with traditional fluoroscopic methods, but it still has inadequate accuracy (Ya-jun and Wei 2005).

Although its 3D image is not clearer than the CT image, the intraoperative 3D image navigation can meet the need for accurate positioning of the bony structure as the 3D tomographic image is not significantly different from the CT image as guidance for operation. According to the SFDA registration data, the accuracy of Stryker's computer-assisted navigation system, where active optical tracking based on infrared light is 0.3 mm, is sufficient for kyphoplasty. There have also been reports describing the accuracy of vertebroplasty using other navigation devices with a precision level of 2.5 ± 1.5 mm (van de Kraats et al. 2006), which is suitable for kyphoplasty (Xiao et al. 2010). The use of intraoperative 3D scanning can significantly reduce the chance of needle adjustment for intraoperative puncture (Sembrano et al. 2015).

Steinmann et al. (2005) biomechanically assessed in vitro changes in strength, stiffness, and height of fractured vertebral body by unilateral balloon kyphoplasty and bilateral balloon kyphoplasty. The two approaches found no significant differences in the results, providing a theoretical basis for unilateral balloon kyphoplasty. Studies (Papadopoulos et al. 2008; Stephen et al. 2003) have also reported that unilateral puncture could achieve good results. Although the entry point and direction of the single-sided approach demand better precision than the traditional two-sided approach, a single-sided approach can be used in all procedures thanks to the accurate location provided by navigation. Thus, surgical operation steps, surgical injury, and operation time can be reduced.

Synowitz et al. (2006) studied X-ray doses received by left and right hands of PVP surgeons, with the left hand wearing protective gloves. The average X-ray exposure was (0.49 ± 0.4) mSv for the left hand and (1.81 ± 1. 31) mSv for the right hand, suggesting that wearing protective gloves during surgery could reduce the radiation dose by 75%. It also indicated that the X-ray dose received by PVP operators and patients was large. Since navigation-guided punctures and procedures for insertion into the channel do not require fluoroscopic assistance, robot-assisted surgery with navigation can reduce the operators' exposure to radiation by half compared with that of conventional surgery. The radiation dose for a single lumbar spine 3D scan of the Siemens Arcadis Orbic 3D C-arm is only 1.82 times that of a single chest radiograph and only 16.1% of that of the 64-row CT scan of the lumbar spine. Therefore, it does not increase the patient's radiation dose. Intraoperative real-time navigation helped both doctors and patients reduce radiation dose (zadpanah et al. 2009).

In conclusion, the advantages of robot-assisted PVP or PKP with navigation are as follows. The universal registration tool for puncture needles and sockets makes operations safer with a higher level of precision. Thanks to the precise location provided by navigation assistance, the unilateral pedicle approach can be applied to simplify the surgical operation procedures, reduce surgical injury, and shorten the operation time. The intraoperative real-time navigational helps both doctors and patients reduce exposure to radiation. However, a disadvantage of robot-assisted surgery with navigation is the additional a 1-cm incision required to place the tracer. The registration and 3D data collection require an additional 5–7 min, which lengthens the operation time for patients of single-segment surgery.

3 Preoperative Imaging Assessment and Surgical Planning

In general, fractures can be diagnosed by radiography, and fracture time and progression can be evaluated by comparing imaging results taken in different periods.

When it is impossible to perform magnetic resonance imaging (MRI) for various reasons, bone scan can be used as a suitable alternative examination to detect bone metabolic activity, which is extremely helpful in determining the fracture time. The presence of bone metabolic activity often suggests fresh fractures and/or nonunion fractures.

MRI can indicate the presence of fresh fractures and provide evidence of spinal edema and serious alterations. The T2 fat-suppression sequence can make the results more pronounced. An MRI scan of the upper and lower vertebrae of the intended surgical segment also helps to determine whether multiple simultaneous fractures exist.

The CT scan and reconstruction of the fracture can determine the degree of involvement of the posterior bone block on the spinal canal. Patients with posteriorly displaced fractures exhibiting over 30% central stenosis of the spinal canal are generally not eligible for PVP or PKP surgery. Sagittal reconstruction CT is better able to determine the degree of compression of different parts of the vertebral body. The position of the vertebral fracture line, which is also the location where the bone cement may leak during surgery, can be observed by axial and sagittal CT reconstruction. Doctors should avoid this position when planning the surgical needle entry point and channel path.

Bone mineral density testing can provide supportive evidence for an osteoporosis diagnosis, but it cannot directly determine whether a patient with fractures is eligible for vertebroplasty.

4 Traditional Surgical Procedures

PVP or PKP surgery is a minimally invasive surgery. The surgical intervention for L1 vertebral fracture with puncture from the right side is considered as an example below.

The patient is placed in a prone position, and the operating bed is adjusted so that the L1 vertebrae are perpendicular to the ground. Before the procedure, the position of the bilateral pedicles of L1 is confirmed under G-arm fluoroscopy and marked on the skin with a marker pen.

1. Routinely sterilize the drape. After the local anesthesia, cut a small incision at the previously marked entry point under the guidance of fluoroscopy. Use a puncture needle to be inserted at 2 o'clock over the projection of the right L1 pedicle. Select the direction of the needle guided by the lateral fluoroscopy, so that the puncture needle tip reaches about 1 cm beyond the posterior edge of the vertebral body. Then remove the needle core and insert the guide pin. The puncture needle is pulled out once fluoroscopy confirms that the direction of the guide pin is satisfactory. Insert the socket with the help of the guide pin, confirm the direction of the socket in fluoroscopy, and ensure the edge of the socket has reached approximately 1 cm beyond the posterior edge of the vertebral body. Remove the guide pin, use a special hand drill to open a path in the vertebral body, and ensure, with the help of the fluoroscopy, that the hand drill does not break through the anterior cortex of the vertebral body.
2. Extract the contrast agent Omnipaque using an appropriate syringe and vent the air, connect the airbag and pressure gauge, insert the socket, confirm the position of the airbag under fluoroscopy, and then slowly apply a pressure of 50 psi to the needle. Remove the guidewire. Continue to apply pressure to the needle plug until the balloon is inflated to 5 mL. During the entire process, ensure that the pressure does not exceed 300 psi. Observe the position and shape of the balloon after inflation and ensure that the shape of the vertebral body is satisfactory after expansion. Ask the patient whether he is experiencing low back pain and verify the activity of the lower limbs. If the patient can tolerate the pain and the activity of both lower limbs is good, keep the airbag inflated for about 5 min. Then withdraw the contrast agent and remove the balloon.
3. Stir the bone cement. After the bone cement is solidified to moderate viscous state, use a specific bone cement-filling needle to collect the bone cement. Next, fill the vertebral body cavity with the corresponding amount of bone cement. Confirm the shape of bone cement filling and the satisfaction of the vertebral body formation under fluoroscopy. Ask the patient whether he is experiencing any low back pain and verify the patient's lower limb activity. Once the cement is solidified, remove the socket and close the incision with a skin tape.

5 Procedure of Robot-Assisted Surgery with Navigation

Taking the Tianji Surgical Robot as an example, the following is a brief description of surgical procedure with the help of the navigation robot. To perform the operation safely, the Tianji Surgical Robot has a complete set of operational procedures. The process can be roughly divided into five parts, including robot settings, 3D image acquisition and automatic registration, path planning, robot-assisted needle insertion, and image verification. Before surgery, the Tianji robot system must be covered with aseptic plastic covers and placed along the side of the operating table to ensure that the robot arm can completely cover the entire surgical area.

1. Anesthesia: General anesthesia with endotracheal intubation is recommended, while patients with high pain tolerance can also be treated with lidocaine.
2. Position: The patient lies on the OSI carbon surgery bed. Confirm the location of fracture guided by fluoroscopy and routinely disinfect the drape.
3. Equipment setting and registration. The computer navigation infrared receiver arm is placed over the patient's head. A patient tracer with a reference frame is attached to the skin surface of the patient with a protective film (Fig. 13.1). Use ARcADISOrbic 3D scanning system to obtain 3D image data of the patient. Complete the automatic registration of the 3D images and the workspace of robotic arm system.
4. Registration. Set the PKP needle entry path and simulate robotic arm operation. After confirmation, start the robot system. The robotic arm system autonomously runs according to the planned path with fine-tuning (Fig. 13.2).
5. Robot-assisted surgery. Surgical operation is performed under the guidance of robot, and a single-sided approach is selected to inject the needle from the lateral heavier compression side. The specific procedure is the same as that of conventional PKP operation. Confirm the penetration point and direction of the puncture needle as well as the position and depth of the working channel with the help of robot guide socket (Fig. 13.3).

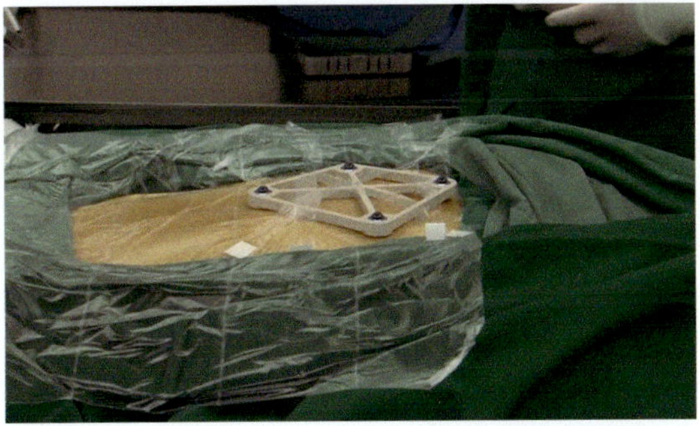

Fig. 13.1 A patient tracer with a reference frame is attached to the skin surface of the patient

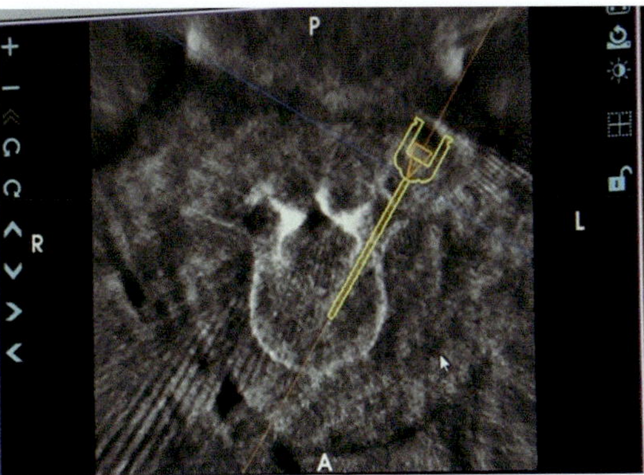

Fig. 13.2 Set the PKP needle entry path in the robot system

None of the above steps rely on fluoroscopy. Since the position of the vertebral body will change due to the balloon distraction process, a socket should be first placed on each vertebral body during the multi-segmental surgery, and then the balloon may be expanded (Fig. 13.4). When expanding the balloon and injecting bone cement, confirm the condition by G arm fluoroscopy. About 3–6 mL of bone cement is injected into each vertebral body (Fig. 13.5).

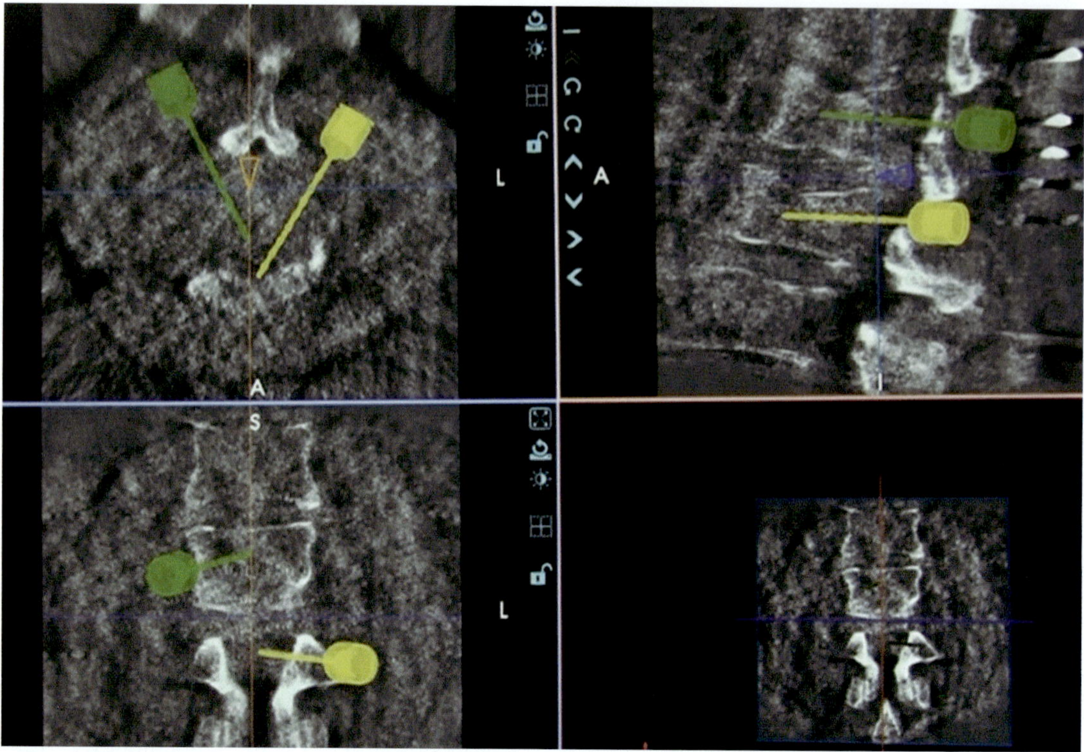

Fig. 13.3 Confirm the penetration point and direction of the puncture needle as well as the position and depth of the working channel with the help of robot guide socket

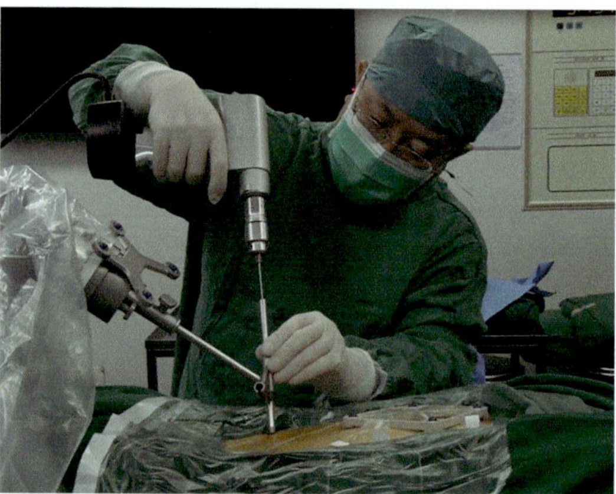

Fig. 13.4 Placing the socket

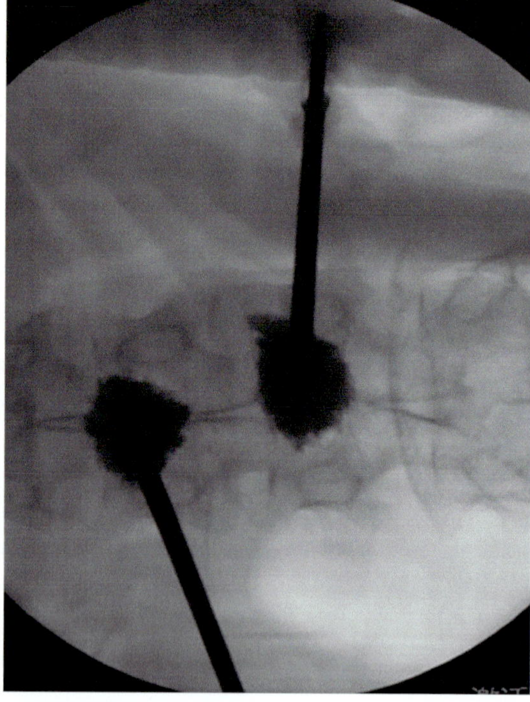

Fig. 13.5 During balloon expanding and bone cement injecting, confirm the condition by G-arm fluoroscopy

6 Key Points and Techniques of Robot-Assisted Surgery

When using robots with navigation assistance, the following points should seriously be considered:

1. The position of the navigator is very important (Wei 2004).
2. The patient's tracer should be firmly fixed. Once the navigator is activated during surgery, the patient tracer must not move.
3. Intraoperative operations should conform to traditional experience. If all operations are correct, confidence should be placed on the guidance by the robot.

7 Typical Case

Female patient, 63 years old, an outpatient suffering from low back pain for about 3 months, later admitted as an inpatient.

The patient complained of low back pain with no obvious injury 3 months prior, and there was no link between the pain and weather changes. The pain aggravated after exertion and improved slightly after resting. The patient received no special treatment. Prior to admittance to the hospital, the patient felt that the symptoms of low back pain were worsening and affected her quality of life. MRI at the local hospital indicated vertebral fractures at T9, T11, and L1. The patient was admitted into our hospital for further treatment.

The patient had a healthy medical record previously with no past experience with illness. She was a nonsmoker with no remarkable drinking habits. Menstruation first occurred at age 15 and menopause occurred at age 45.

Physical examination: The patient stepped into ward with normal gait. There was thoracolumbar kyphosis. Pain emerged when knocking thoracic and lumbar parts and on waist movements and with limited activity. Muscle strength was normal in both lower limbs. Deep and superficial reflexes could be stimulated normally in both lower limbs.

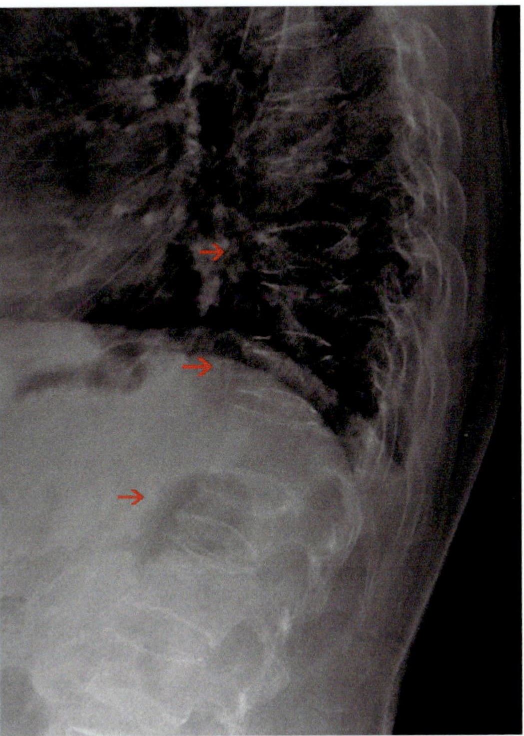

Fig. 13.6 Preoperative lateral X-ray

Preoperative lateral radiographs showed vertebral compression fractures at T9, T11, and L1 (Fig. 13.6).

Preoperative T1 MRI imaging showed low signals in the vertebral body of T9, T11, and L1 (Fig. 13.7).

Preoperative fat suppression MRI imaging showed high signals in the vertebral body of T9, T11, and L1 (Fig. 13.8).

The patient underwent robot-assisted kyphoplasty under general anesthesia. After the operation, the lower back pain was completely relieved. Lateral radiographs showed that the bone cement was placed in good position, and the thoracolumbar kyphosis was restored (Fig. 13.9). Postoperative CT indicated that the cement was evenly distributed within the fractured vertebra (Fig. 13.10). The patient was discharged 4 days later.

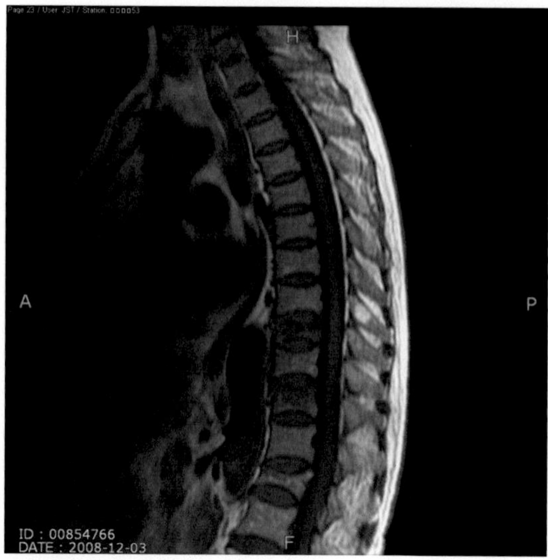

Fig. 13.7 Preoperative T1 MRI image

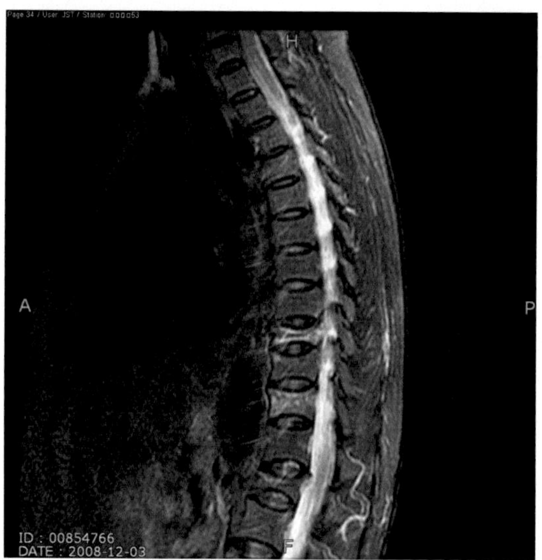

Fig. 13.8 Preoperative fat suppression T2 MRI image

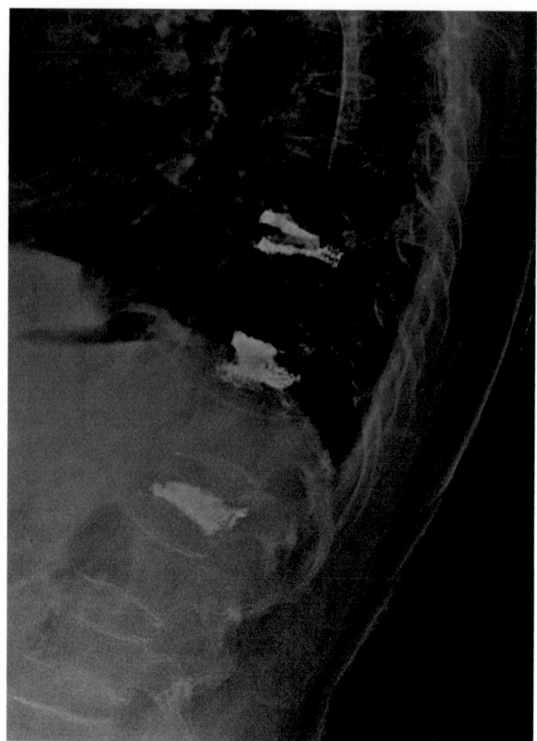

Fig. 13.9 Postoperative lateral X-ray

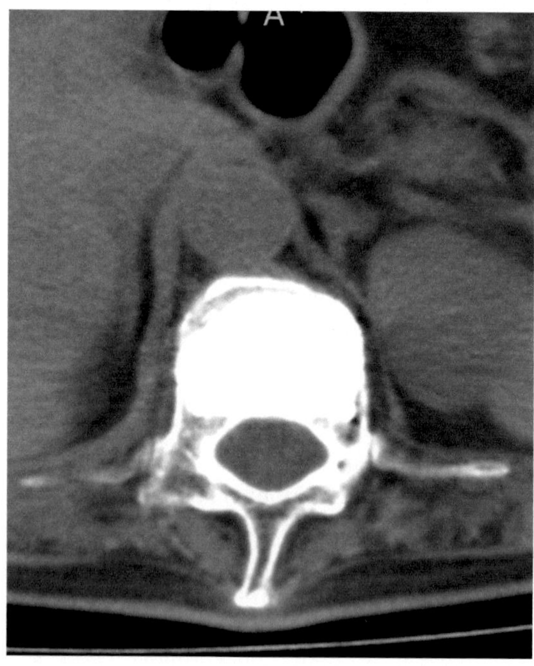

Fig. 13.10 Postoperative CT image

References

Gui-xing Q. Osteoporotic fracture–the neglected health killer. Natl Med J China. 2005;85(11):730.

Ling XU, Cummings SR, Ming-wei Q, et al. Vertebral osteoporosis of women in Beijing, China. Chin J Osteoporosis. 1995;1(1):81–4.

Kado DM, Browner WS, Palermo L, et al. Vertebral fractures and mortality in older women: a prospective study. Arch Intern Med. 1999;159(11):1215–20.

Harry N, Steven R, Frank J, et al. Rothman-simeone the spine. 5th ed. USA: Elsevier; 2006. p. 1341–2.

Nussbaum DA, Gailloud P, Murphy K. A review of complications associated with vertebroplasty and kyphoplasty as reported to the Food and Drug Administration medical device related web site. J Vasc Interv Radiol. 2004;15(11):1185–92.

Bronek MB, Michael B, Stefan H, et al. Transcostovertebral kyphoplasty of the mid and high thoracic spine. Eur Spine. 2005;14(6):992–9.

Hyeun SK, Chang IJ, Seok WK, et al. Balloon kyphoplasty in severe osteoporotic compression fracture: is it a contraindication? Neurosurgery. 2007;60(5):1–6.

Barr JD, Barr MS, Lemley TJ, et al. Percutaneous vertebroplasty for pain relief and spinal stabilization. Spine. 2000;25(8):923–8.

Shi-jun MI, Li-ming WU. Imaging measurement-based unilateral puncture entry point and path for vertebroplasty. J Clin Rehabil Tiss Eng Res. 2009;13(17):3237–40.

Wang Y, Xiao-dong G, Zhi-feng W, et al. Application of eFilm workstation in the preoperative plan, intraoperative and postoperative evaluation of PVP and PKP. Chin J Spine Spinal Cord. 2008;18(6):425–8.

Ya-jun L, Wei T. Pedicle screw fixation of cervical spine assisted by CT-based navigation system. Chin J Orthop Trauma. 2005;7(7):630–3.

Jun L, Hai-tao Z, Gui-xiang Z. Percutaneous vertebroplasty guided by CT. Chin J Med Imag Technol. 2003;19(8):1052–4.

Zhong-liang D, Wei-bo X, Guang-jun R. CT-guided percutaneous vertebroplasty. Chongqing Med. 2002;31(12):1159–60.

En-zhi L, Dong-ming G, Wei-shan C. Improved computer-assisted fluoroscopic navigation to guide percutaneous kyphoplasty to treat multiple osteoporotic spinal compression fractures. Clin Med China. 2009;25(7):762–4.

Li-ming W, Zhong Y, Jian-chao G. Percutaneous vertebroplasty assisted by infrared fluoroscopic navigation for 28 cases of vertebral osteoporotic compression fractures. Chin J Minim Invas Surg. 2006;6(7):490–3.

Han Y, En-zhi L, Dong-ming G, et al. Percutaneous kyphoplasty guided by modified imaging-assisted navigation for the treatment of multiple osteoporotic spinal compression fraction. Acad J Guangzhou Med College. 2012;40(6):29–1.

van de Kraats EB, van Walsum T, Verlaan JJ, et al. Three-dimensional rotational X-ray navigation for needle guidance in percutaneous vertebroplasty: an accuracy study. Spine. 2006;31(12):1359–64.

Xiao H, Wei T, Bo L, et al. Percutaneous kyphoplasty assisted by intraoperative three-dimensional navigation system. Chin J Orthop Trauma. 2010;12(2):109–12.

Sembrano JN, Yson SC, Polly DW Jr, et al. Comparison of nonnavigated and 3-dimensional image-based computer navigated balloon kyphoplasty. Orthopedics. 2015;38(1):17–23.

Steinmann J, Tingey CT, Cruz G, et al. Biomechanical comparison of unipedicular versus bipedicular kyphoplasty. Spine. 2005;30(2):201–5.

Papadopoulos EC, Edobor-Osula F, Gardner MJ, et al. Unipedicular balloon kyphoplasty for the treatment of osteoporotic vertebral compression fractures. J Spinal Disord Tech. 2008;21(8):589–96.

Stephen T, Michael G, Richard H, et al. Unilateral pedicular kyphoplasty for treatment of vertebral compression fractures. Spine. 2003;3(5):67–171.

Synowitz M, Kiwit J. Surgeon's radiation exposure during percutaneous vertebroplasty. J Neurosurg Spine. 2006;4:106.

zadpanah K, Konrad G, Südkamp NP, et al. Computer navigation in balloon kyphoplasty reduces the intraoperative radiation exposure. Spine. 2009;34(12):1325–9.

Wei T. Fixation assisted by computer navigation for spinal fracture and instability. Chin J Orthop Trauma. 2004;6(11):1218–9.

14 Robot-Assisted Translaminar Lag Screw Fixation of Spondylolysis

Guanyu Cui, Han Wang, and Wei Tian

Abstract

Translaminar lag screw fixation of spondylolysis is an effective but problematic surgery without image guidance. The application of robot can make directly fixing the thin pars interarticularis a procedure of high safety and practicability. Without wide dissection of soft tissue and damage to the blood supply in a minimally invasive robot-guided surgery, the union of spondylolysis and a good long-term result will be more convincing.

Keywords

Robot · Spondylolysis · Pars interarticularis · Isthmus · Lag screw

1 Introduction

The purpose of translaminar lag screw fixation is to both maintain physiologic motion and limit excessive motion of the lumbar spine. Thus, it can alleviate radicular pain by indirectly decompressing the intervertebral foramen. Concurrently, it can prevent the development of spondylolisthesis. Compared with traditional procedures, translaminar lag screw fixation can restore anatomic structure without any fusion (Johnson and Thompson 1992).

There are problems with this procedure (Dai et al. 2001; Buck 1970). Pars interarticularis is a thin structure, even in healthy individuals. With a possible underdevelopment in spondylolysis, surgeons will face difficulties in determining the entry point, direction, and length of screws. A wide dissection is made in an open procedure for detecting landmarks for entry point and bone graft region, causing a compromised blood supply to the isthmus and possible nonunion. Inaccurate insertion of screws may cause repetitive pinning and decreased pullout strength, predisposing screw loosening. Excessive screw length and perforation may result in nerve root irritation (Trout et al. 2015; Szypryt et al. 1989).

Robot-assisted translaminar lag screw fixation can achieve a better result. A minimally invasive procedure with accurate screw pinning will make the surgery easier and more effective.

2 Indications

1. Severe low back pain with or without radiculopathy; pain is not relieved after conservative treatment for more than 6 months.
2. No segmental disk herniation or obvious degeneration (disk height more than 2/3 that of normal).

G. Cui · H. Wang · W. Tian (✉)
Department of Spine Surgery, Beijing Jishuitan Hospital, Fourth Clinical Hospital of Peking University, Beijing, China
e-mail: tianweijst@vip.163.com

W. Tian (ed.), *Navigation Assisted Robotics in Spine and Trauma Surgery*,
https://doi.org/10.1007/978-981-15-1846-1_14

3. Translation of adjacent vertebral bodies less than 3 mm.
4. Pain alleviation is achieved after isthmus block preoperatively.

3 Surgical Planning

3.1 Radiological Investigations

X-ray, computed tomography (CT) scan, magnetic resonance imaging (MRI), and SPECT are all investigations used to confirm the diagnosis. CT scan can demonstrate the exact position and direction of the spondylolysis, but it can also indicate hyperplasia of fibrocartilage tissue on pars interarticularis. MRI can reveal the degree of intervertebral disc degeneration and the degree of intervertebral foramina stenosis.

3.2 Robot

The TianJi Robot was designed for orthopedic surgeries. Components of the robot include a main engine, a robotic arm, surgical planning and control software, an optical tracing system, a main console, and a navigation toolkit.

TianJi Robot receives intraoperative 3D images using a C-arm. After transmission and automatic registration, surgeons can design the trajectory of screws on the user interface. The robotic arm, driven by the software and the tracing system, will then move independently to the exact position of lag screw insertion.

4 Open Procedure

The surgical procedure involved is detailed below:

1. GA, prone positioning of patient, spinous process localization, disinfection, and draping are performed. A posterior midline incision is made at the level of the spondylolysis, and the spinous process, lamina, and superior facet joint of the affected vertebra are exposed (attention should be paid not to damage the posterior structure and the facet capsule) (Figs. 14.1 and 14.2).
2. The spondylolysis fracture line is verified (approximately 3.0 mm distal to the inferior facet of the proximal adjacent vertebra). Flexion position by lumbar bridge is used, and the spinous process is lifted to obtain a better view. An obvious fracture line is usually

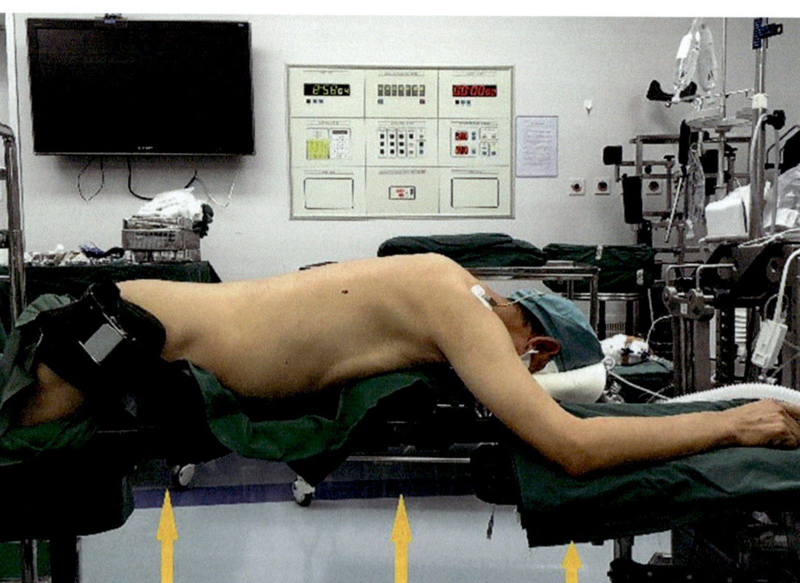

Fig. 14.1 Patient fastened in the prone position

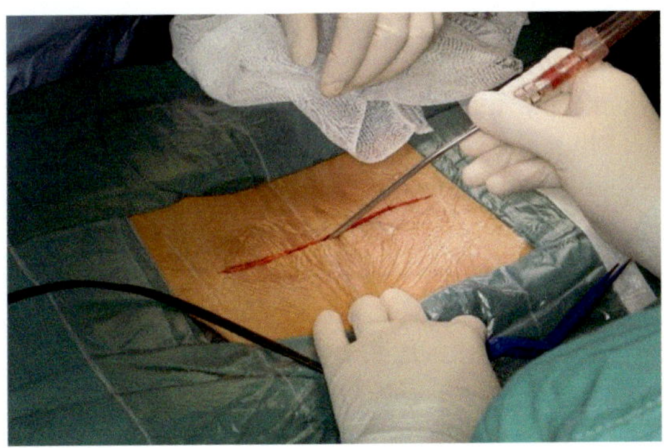

Fig. 14.2 Longitudinal incision

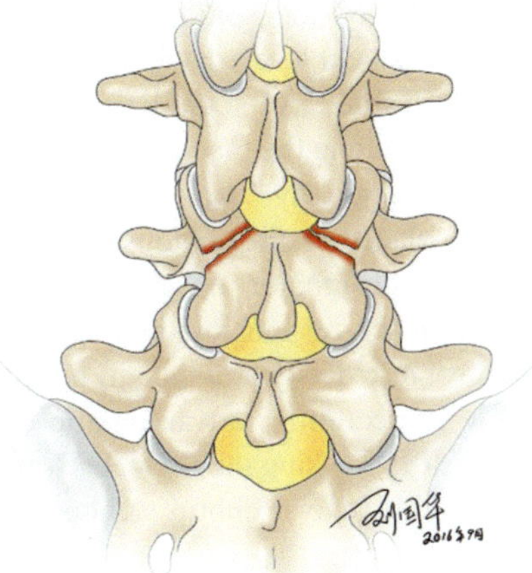

Fig. 14.3 Approach. (From W Tian, YJ Liu, D He, et al.: Operative techniques of navigation assisted spine surgery [M], 2017)

visible in fresh spondylolysis. However, most gaps of spondylolysis are filled with fibrocartilage tissue. The gaps are cleaned with a curette or burr in the direction ventrally and caudally until fresh trabeculae is exposed. Determine whether the ligamentum flavum and lateral side of facet capsule should be cleaned to decompress the nerve root as determined by symptoms of nerve root agitation and MRI results (Fig. 14.3).

3. Cancellous bone graft is acquired and cut into chips to insert into the gaps. The gaps will clamp the graft tightly by relieving the flexion position of lumbar bridge (Fig. 14.4).
4. Cut a little cortical bone with rongeur on the distal margin of lamina, about 0.8–1.0 cm away from the spinous process. The trajectories should be 30° laterally, forward, and superiorly according to the laminar position. A small skin incision is then cut in this trajectory. Drill a 2.5-mm hole through the guide. Under direct vision, the drill should pass through distal isthmus, bone graft, proximal isthmus, up to the cortex at pedicle–superior facet junction in the end (Fig. 14.5).

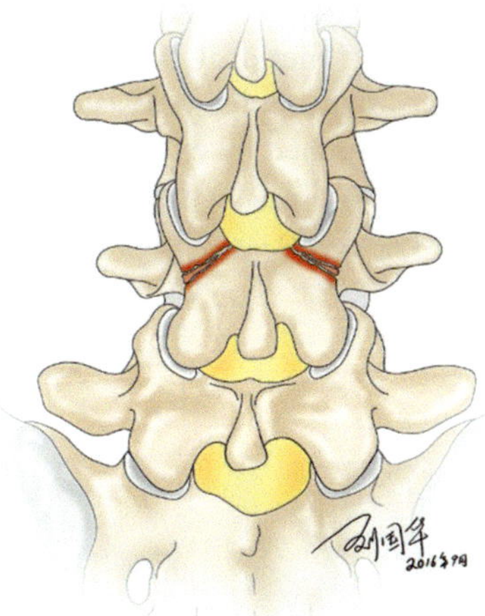

Fig. 14.4 Insert cancellous bone graft. (From W Tian, YJ Liu, D He, et al.: Operative techniques of navigation assisted spine surgery [M], 2017)

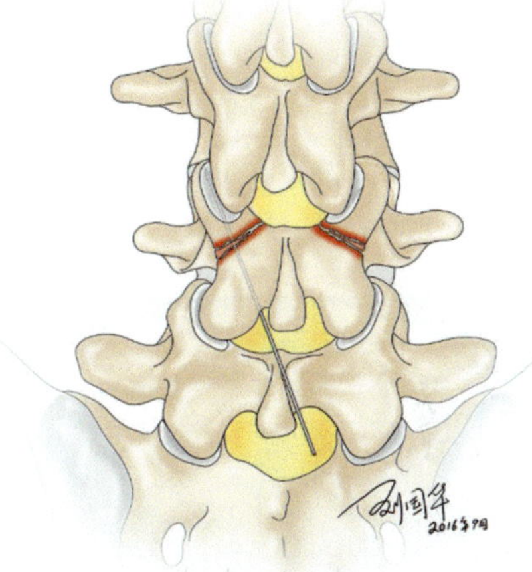

Fig. 14.5 Drill the hole. (From W Tian, YJ Liu, D He, et al.: Operative techniques of navigation assisted spine surgery [M], 2017)

5. Measure the length of the trajectory, usually 40.0–50.0 mm approximately. Create a sliding hole with a 3.5 mm drill. A lag screw is then inserted. Simultaneously, assisted compression may be applied by extension of the lumbar bridge or by pressing the spinous processes together (Fig. 14.6).

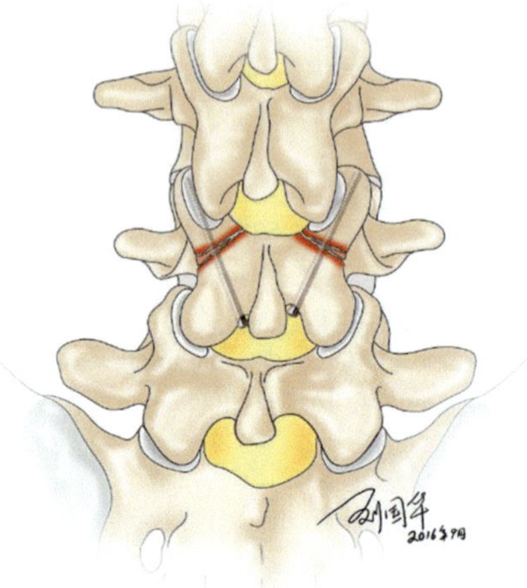

Fig. 14.6 Insert the screw. (From W Tian, YJ Liu, D He, et al.: Operative techniques of navigation assisted spine surgery [M], 2017)

6. Confirm the screws by fluoroscopy. Abrade the cortical surface of lateral portion of lamina and par interarticularis down to the trabecula. Place the fragmented bone graft on the dorsal side of the isthmus (Fig. 14.7a, b).

5 Robot-Assisted Minimally Invasive Procedure

The surgical procedure involved is detailed below:

1. GA, the patient was put on a carbon operating table in prone position. Following localization and marking of the spinous process of the proximal adjacent level, disinfection and draping are performed. A 0.5 cm longitudinal incision is made along the marked spinous process to be subsequently exposed. The patient tracker is placed on the spinous process.
2. Install the designator on the robotic arm. Ensure that the responsible and adjacent levels and robotic designator can all be shown in a single projection. Start automatic continuous scan at 190° using the ISO-3D C-arm connected with the robotic system. Next,

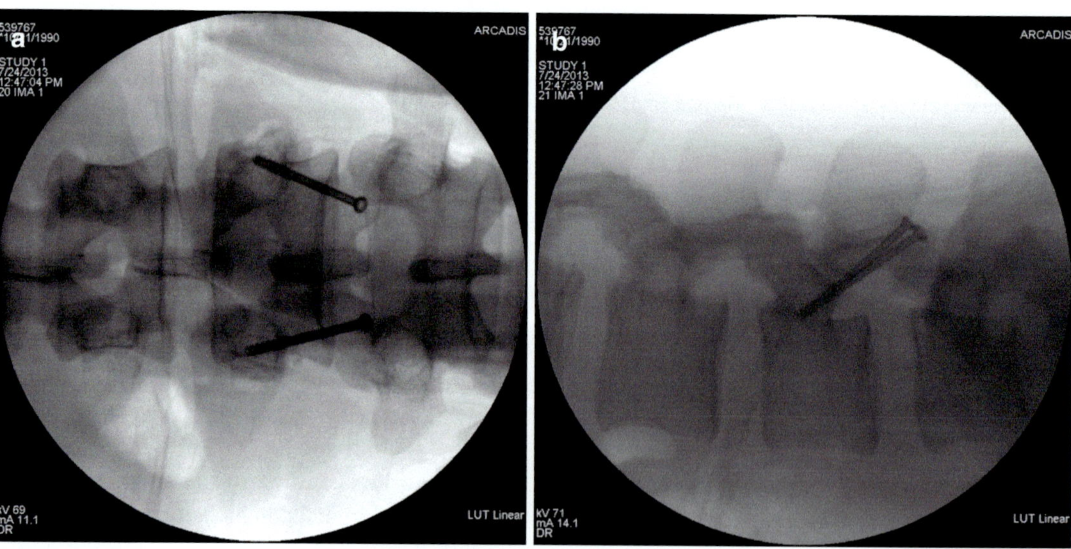

Fig. 14.7 (a, b) Fluoroscopy to confirm the position of screws

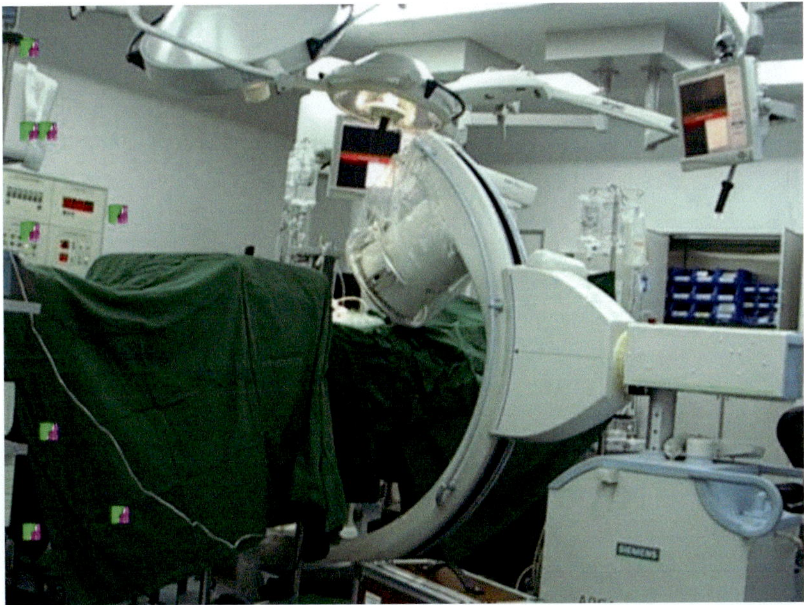

Fig. 14.8 Intraoperative 3D C-arm scanning

automatic registration is completed by the system (Fig. 14.8).

3. Surgeons now can plan the screw trajectory and length of one side using the planning module. The screw should go through the central part of isthmus and be perpendicular to the fracture line. Changes can be made to the designator with a conductor. Operate the robotic arm to the planned trajectory. During the movement of the robotic arm, the real-time accuracy of the orientation will be demonstrated, and the trace of the screw placement will be detected when accuracy less than 0.5 mm (Fig. 14.9).
4. Insert the guide sleeve into the conductor. Make a 2-cm transverse incision and approach according to the contact position of the skin and sleeve. Insert the guiding sleeve further to the cortex of entry point. Dilators should be used if necessary. A guide pin is then inserted along the sleeve. After the pin position is confirmed by fluoroscopy, the robotic arm can now be removed manually (Fig. 14.10).
5. Repeat the planning and subsequent procedure on the contralateral side. Another guide pin is then inserted through the same incision. Confirm the guide pins position by fluoroscopy (Fig. 14.11).
6. Locate the right posterior superior iliac spine (PSIS) by palpation or robotic assistance. Insert a guide pin, dilators, and minimally invasive working sleeve to expose the PSIS. Harvest an adequate amount of cancellous bone by osteotome and curette.
7. Plan two vertical virtual screws pointing at the fracture lines of spondylolysis to ensure their surface projection. Operate the robot twice to guide bilateral incisions. One 1.5-cm incision is sufficient to allow exposure of isthmus on one side. Debride the fibrocartilage and sclerotic bone in the gaps. Implant the cancellous bone graft into the gap.
8. Create a sliding hole with a 3.5-mm drill. Insert one cannulated lag screw onto each side along the guide pin through distal incision. Confirm the placement of the screws by fluoroscopy. Return to the proximal incisions and expose the cancellous bone at the lateral lamina and dorsal isthmus. Place extra bone graft here (Fig. 14.12).
9. Confirm the position of the screws. Close the three transverse incisions and one longitudinal incision and complete the procedure.

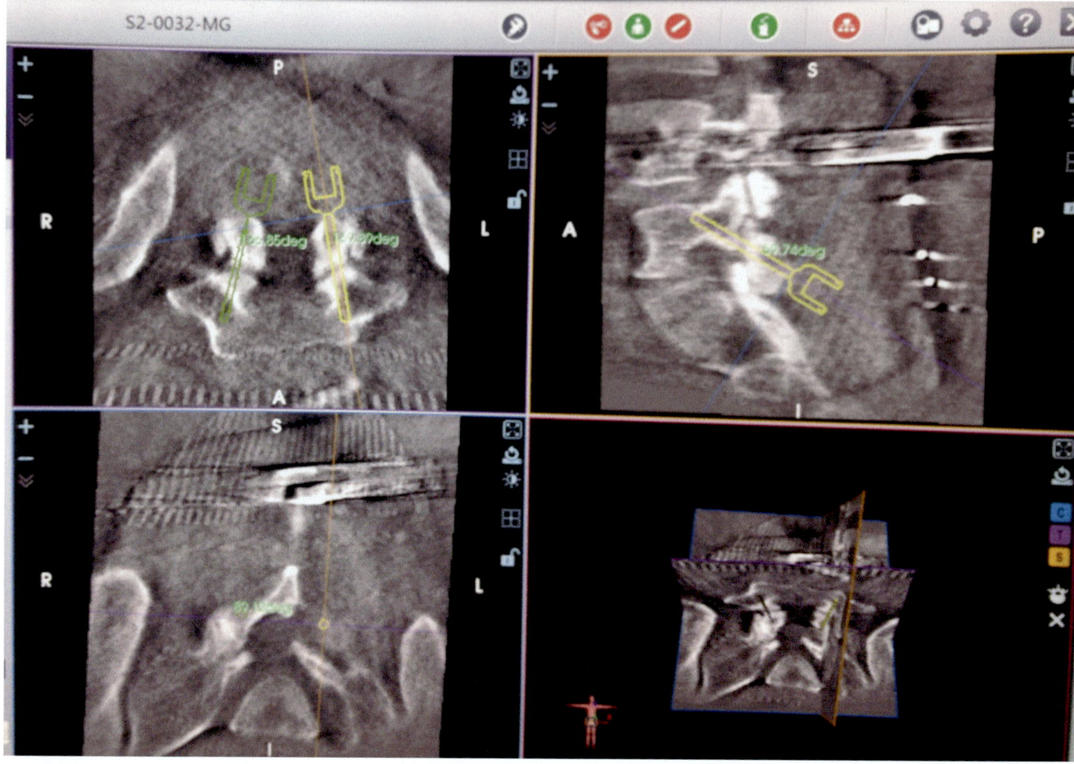

Fig. 14.9 Intraoperative planning

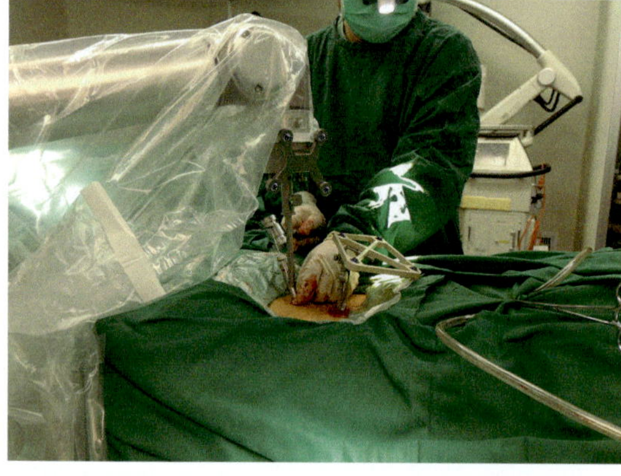

Fig. 14.10 Insert the guide pin through guide sleeve

6 Tips

1. The patient tracker should be fixed on the spinous process firmly.
2. Before the guide pin is inserted into the lamina, a burr can be used to make a hole in the entry point to prevent the sliding of the guide pin.
3. The fibrocartilage and sclerotic bone in the gaps should be removed completely for bone union, and the soft tissue beside the gaps should be retained as much as possible for to improve blood supply.

7 Case

A 30-year-old male complained about repetitive low back pain for 5 years and pain in the right buttock and thigh for 6 months. The symptom aggravated after weight-bearing, walking, or extending the waist with failed conservative treatment. Physical examination demonstrated low back tenderness and painful extension of the lumbar spine. Other signs were all negative bilaterally (SLR, FNST, Bonnet, Kemp).

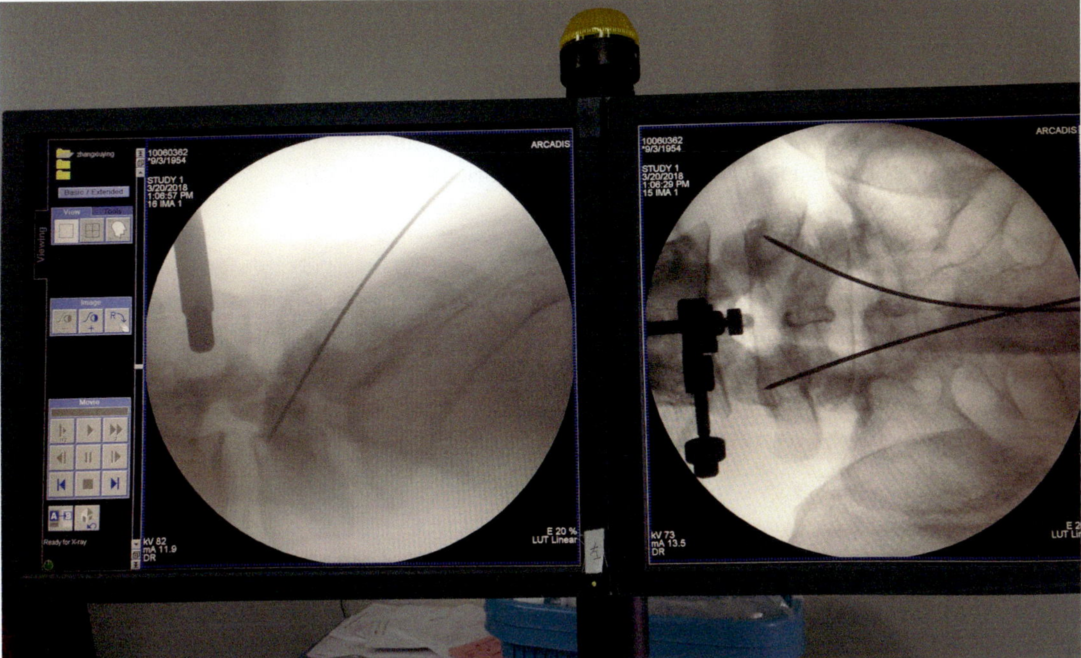

Fig. 14.11 Confirm positions of guide pins

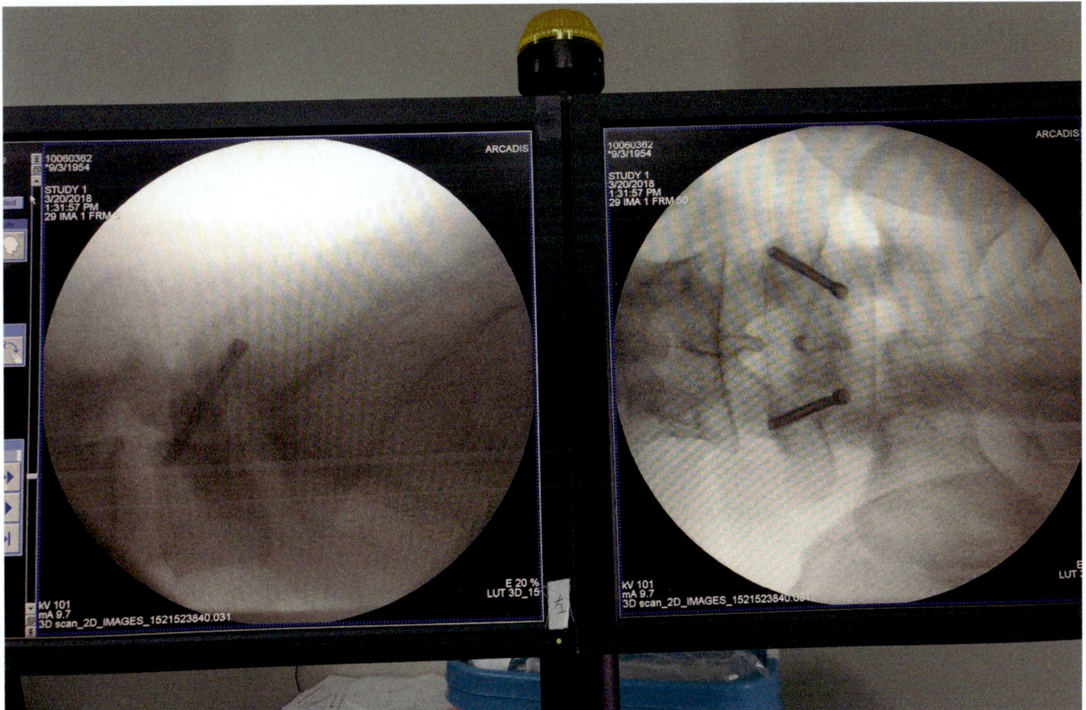

Fig. 14.12 Confirm positions of lag screws

X-rays (AP and lateral views) and MRI showed no obvious degeneration or instability of lumbar spine (Figs. 14.13–14.15). Bilateral oblique views and CT showed bilateral spondylolysis of L5 (Figs. 14.16–14.18).

Robot-assisted translaminar lag screw fixation was performed under general anesthesia, and following the surgical steps illustrated above, bone graft was finished after the gap debridement, and the two lag screws were inserted. Postoperative X-rays and CT images showed good positions of screws (Figs. 14.19–14.22).

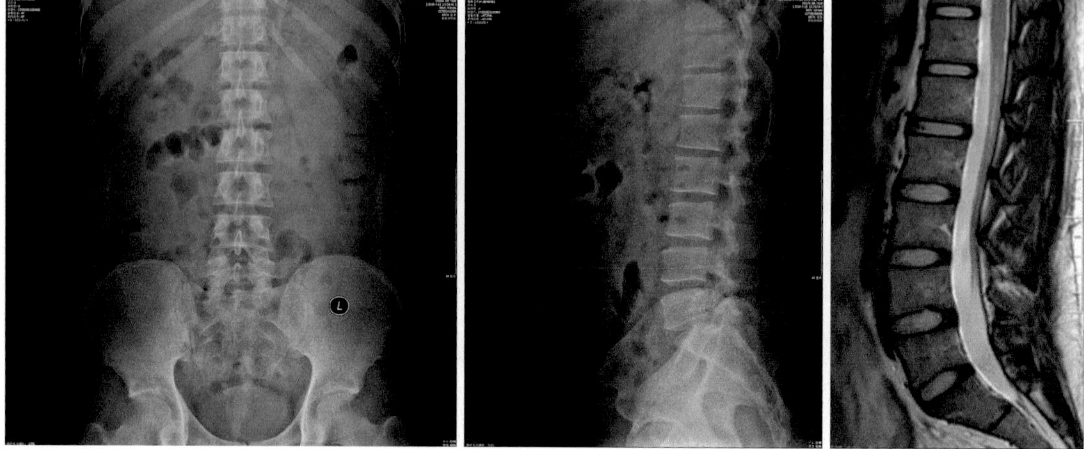

Figs. 14.13–14.15 Preoperative PA and lateral views and sagittal MRI image

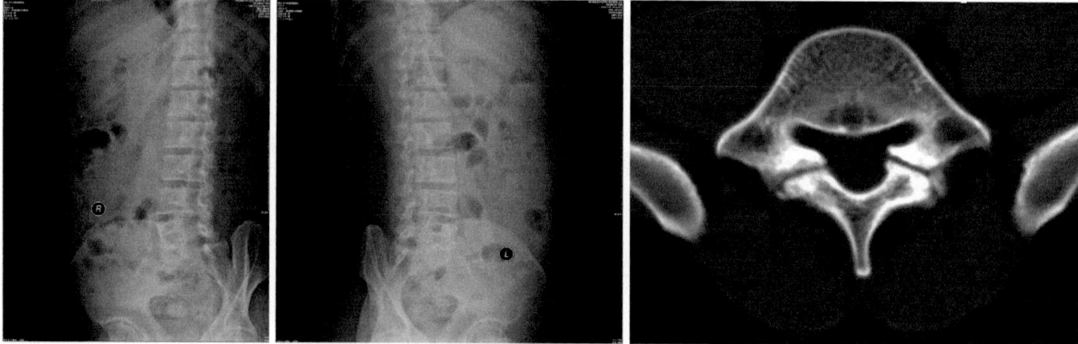

Figs. 14.16–14.18 Preoperative oblique views and axial CT image

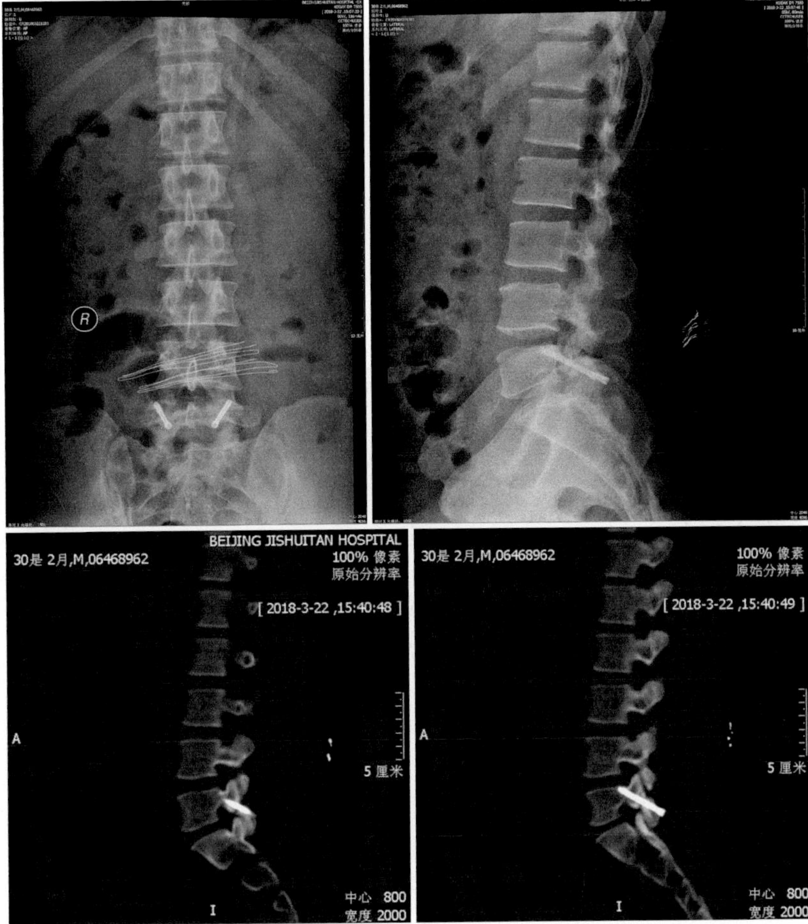

Figs. 14.19–14.22 Post-operative PA and lateral views and sagittal CT image

References

Buck JE. Direct repair of the defect in spondylolisthesis. J Bone Joint Surg Br. 1970;52:432–7.

Dai LY, Jia LS, Yuan W, et al. Direct repair of defect in lumbar spondylolysis and mild isthmic spondylolisthesis by bone grafting, with or without facet joint fusion. Eur Spine J. 2001;10:78–83.

Johnson GV, Thompson AG. The Scott wiring technique for direct repair of lumbar spondylolysis. J Bone Joint Surg Br. 1992;74(3):426–30.

Szypryt EP, Twining P, Mulholland RC, et al. The prevalence of disc degeneration associated with neural arch defects of the lumbar spine assessed by magnetic resonance imaging. Spine. 1989;14(9):977–81.

Trout AT, Sharp SE, Anton CG, et al. Spondylolysis and beyond: value of SPECT/CT in evaluation of low back pain in children and young adults. Radiographics. 2015;35(3):819–34.

Robot-Assisted Percutaneous Transforaminal Endoscopy Discectomy (PTED)

15

Yonggang Xing, Jile Jiang, and Wei Tian

Abstract

Percutaneous transforaminal endoscopy discectomy is a minimally invasive method to treat spinal degenerative disease. On the one hand, it allows direct nerve root decompression under endoscopy through intervertebral foramen. However, it needs a series of intraoperative fluoroscopy to achieve satisfied cannulate position. On the other hand, robot-assisted surgery could improve accuracy of cannulate place, reduce trauma brought by insertion error, and ensure a perfect position for decompression. Robot-assisted endoscopy discectomy also could avoid repeated intraoperative fluoroscopy, reducing radiation exposure of both patients and surgeons. It is recommended in cases with difficult cannulate placement or anatomy variations.

Keywords

Percutaneous transforaminal endoscopy discectomy · Robot-assisted surgery · Minimally invasive surgery · Lumbar disk herniation · Lumbar spinal canal stenosis

Y. Xing · J. Jiang · W. Tian (✉)
Department of Spine Surgery, Beijing Jishuitan Hospital, Fourth Clinical Hospital of Peking University, Beijing, China
e-mail: xingyonggang@vip.163.com; tianweijst@vip.163.com

1 Introduction

In the fourth century BC, ancient Greek Hippocrates described sciatica. Until the 1930s, American doctors Mixter and Barr realized that this disease was caused by "lumbar disk rupture" and could be treated by surgery (Mixter and Barr 1934). Since then, a new era of surgical treatment of lumbar disk herniation has begun. At that time, the "large open" operation of laminectomy or semi-laminar resection was widely used. In the 1970s, authors such as McCulloch reported the use of surgical microscopy for micro-discectomy, which gradually became a gold-standard treatment for lumbar disk herniation (Kahanovitz et al. 1989; Maroon and Abla 1986; McCulloch 1989).

With the continuous advancement of spine surgery technology, minimal surgical trauma, maintaining the integrity and stability of the spine structure, and reducing postoperative complications are the main research directions for the treatment of spinal diseases. In the second half of the last century, the intervertebral foramen approach based on discography was gradually formed. In 1990, Kambin described the concept of the "intervertebral foramen safety triangle" (Fig. 15.1) which provides a theoretical basis for the safety of endoscopic surgery, including the exiting root as the outside boundary, the upper edge of the lower vertebral body as the lower boundary, and the dura mater and the traversing

W. Tian (ed.), *Navigation Assisted Robotics in Spine and Trauma Surgery*,
https://doi.org/10.1007/978-981-15-1846-1_15

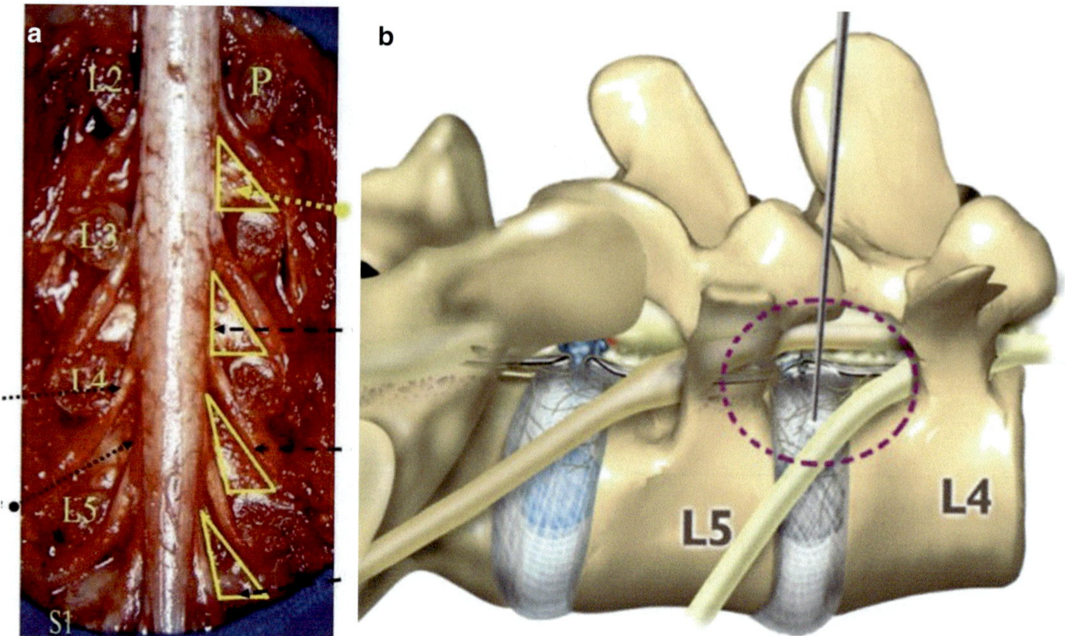

Fig. 15.1 (**a**, **b**) Kambin triangle

root as another boundary (Kambin and Zhou 1996). With the development of surgical endoscopic technology, Attoney Yeung invented the three-generation Yeung multichannel endoscope spine system, which includes operative working channel for insertion of tools, multichannel irrigation, and a cannula system (Yeung 2007; Yeung and Gore 2001). In 2005, Hoogland developed the Thomas Hoogland Endoscopic Spinal System (THESSYS) with a further distance from the midline and easier access to the spinal canal (Hoogland 2003).

The YESS technique emphasizes the entry of the Kambin triangle into the intervertebral disk and the internal excision of the intervertebral tissue first (inside–out). Hoogland emphasizes for foramino-plasty by special designed bone drill, so that working catheter can be placed into spinal canal. The disc tissue or free nucleus pulpopsus fragments can be removed under direct version. This is named as "outside-in technique", the direction of remove is from the outer disk to the inner disk. In 2005, Ruetten proposed a far-lateral approach, similar to the YESS technique, but the entry point was extremely lateral, and this technique was more accessible to the ventral or even contralateral side of the dura mater (Ruetten et al. 2005a). Figure 15.2 shows the different puncture methods for the three approaches. There were a lot of arguments about several approaches in the early days, and also many modified technologies emerged in recent years, and they all can be recognized as PELD (percutaneous endoscopic lateral discectomy) technology or PTED technology (percutaneous transforaminal endoscopic discectomy). In fact, each of them has its only limitation and advantages. Surgeons

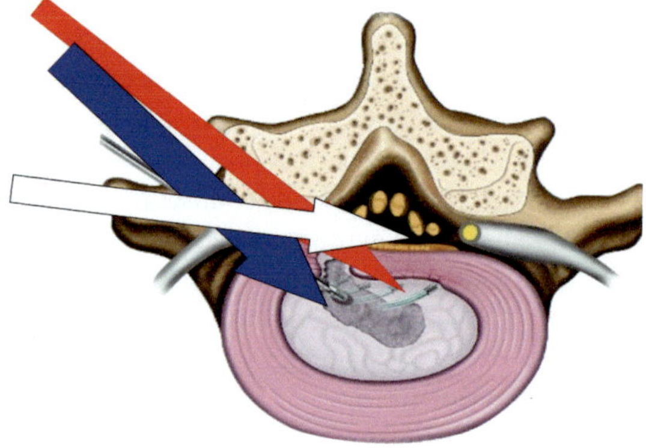

Fig. 15.2 The blue arrow stands for YESS approach, the red one is for THESSYS approach, and the white one is for far-lateral approach

should use the most familiar and appropriate approach for each patient; the details of the surgery will be explained in the following section.

2 Indications

In principle, the indications for PTED are the same as those for open microdissection, mainly for the patients with failure of conservative treatment of lumbar disk herniation. Including central and posterolateral herniation. The YESS approach is best indicated for contained posterolateral herniation, because it could remove the herniation from the inside. For patients with prolapse caudally or cranially, or patients with articular facet hypertrophy, the THESSYS approach is better indicated; the foraminoplasty allows direct visualization and removal of disk fragments. For patients with central disk herniation, the far lateral approach could achieve adequate decompression because it is more transverse in coronal plane compared with other two methods.

Patients with disk herniation or patients with adjacent segmental disk herniation are very suitable for PTED, because the surgical scar from posterior approach will significantly increase difficulties for another posterior approach surgery. However, it had minimal effect on oblique anterior approach, thus making PTED a better choice.

Previously, calcification of herniated disk is a relative contraindication, because there are limited sights with restricted operation field under endoscopy, and the bony structure cannot be removed completely. And also due to size of endoscopic forceps, it is very difficult to separate osteophyte from the bone. Nowadays, with improvement of instrumentation and introduction of endoscopic burr, osteophyte is no longer a barrier of PTED.

The indication also includes specific types of lumbar spinal stenosis, intervertebral foramen stenosis, and lateral recess entrance stenosis. Although we can deal with osteophyte in intervertebral foramen and lateral recess entrance due to the introduction of endoscopic bur, it is still difficult to fully remove hypertrophied ligament flavum around the nerve root. Moreover, because the pathology of spinal stenosis is due to hypermobility and instability, which brings hypertrophied ligament flavum and osteophyte, only removal there compression sites without stop hypermobility and instability may only bring temporary symptom relieve. The long-term results of PTED in the treatment of spinal stenosis remains controversial.

3 Contraindications for PTED Surgery

Mainly, it can be divided by two methods. One is due to limitation of the procedure itself. The PTED could not provide fusion, so it is not indicated for patients combined with lumbar instability, unless combined with fusion surgery, either open or endoscopic.

Another contraindication is due to limitation of instrumentation, take lumbar disk herniation with ossification, for example; it is regarded as contraindication previously, and now due to improvement of endoscopic burr, it has become a relative indication. However, for patients with lateral recess stenosis or central canal stenosis, PTED still could not achieve adequate decompression alone.

4 Advantages of Robot-Assisted Surgery

There are two difficult steps that restricted its wide clinical use. One is endoscopic maneuver, which needs massive training to achieve eye-hand coordination. Another problem is accurate placement of work cannula into the proper position. There are two reasons why cannula position is so important. One is due to the limited endoscopic view, where the range of decompression relies on the position of endoscopy. The other one is due to the Kambin triangle; abundant nerves and vessels around intervertebral foramen require precise acupuncture to avoid associated injury. Previously, surgeons need series of intraoperative fluoroscopy and lots of time to identify position of cannula, especially for new learners. Under the guidance of robot, now we can set up the working cannula precisely, quickly, and safely for endoscopy. Furthermore, we can design different approaches based on direction of herniation and morphology of intervertebral foramen, to achieve the most accurate surgical plan for each patient.

5 Surgical Procedures

1. Position

   Between the lateral and prone position, we are more familiar with the lateral position (the following operation takes the Maxmore system commonly used in our hospital as an example).
2. Mark the target level with a G-arm and a K-wire. As shown in Fig. 15.3b, for the anteroposterior X-ray, the connection between the tip of the superior articular process (SAP) and the lower vertebral endplate center, for the lateral position, has different angles, generally speaking, L5/S1 30°–40°, L4/L5 and L3/L4 20°–25° (Fig. 15.3a). Because intervertebral foramen surgery is a minimally invasive procedure, it can be navigated and positioned in vitro through surface markers. After attaching the body surface marker, registration is performed by C-arm scanning (Fig. 15.4).
3. Select the entry point and direction under the guidance of the robot, and choose YYS, THYSSES, or far outside according to the surgical approach (Fig. 15.5). Targeted skin and lumbosacral fascia was infiltrated with 2 ml 1% lidocaine, and the 18-G needle was advanced under direction of robot until SAP, with another injection of 2 ml lidocaine (can be injected at different sites around SAP to achieve satisfied anesthesia). Incise the skin and fascia after guide wire.
4. Insert the TomShidi needle sleeve along the guide wire, remove the guide wire, and replace

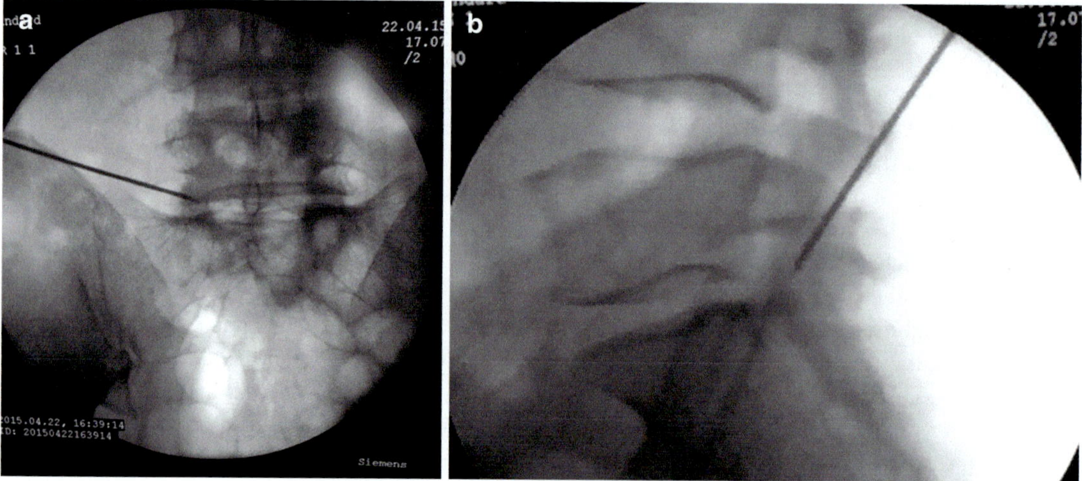

Fig. 15.3 (**a**, **b**) Identify entry point and acupuncture

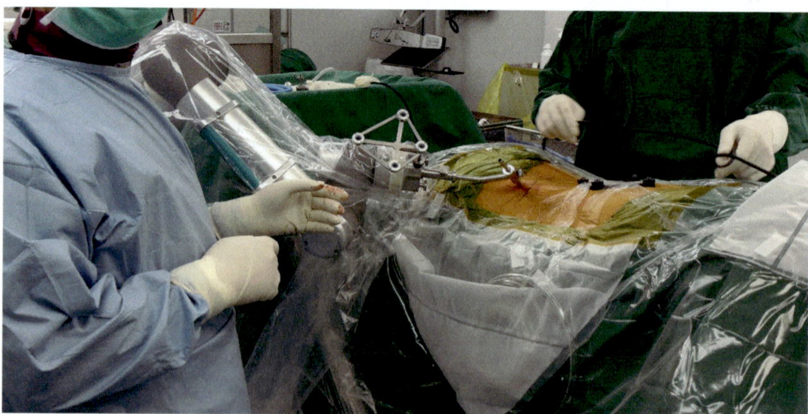

Fig. 15.4 After adhesion of surface marker, we register through C-arm scan, and put cannula under robot guidance

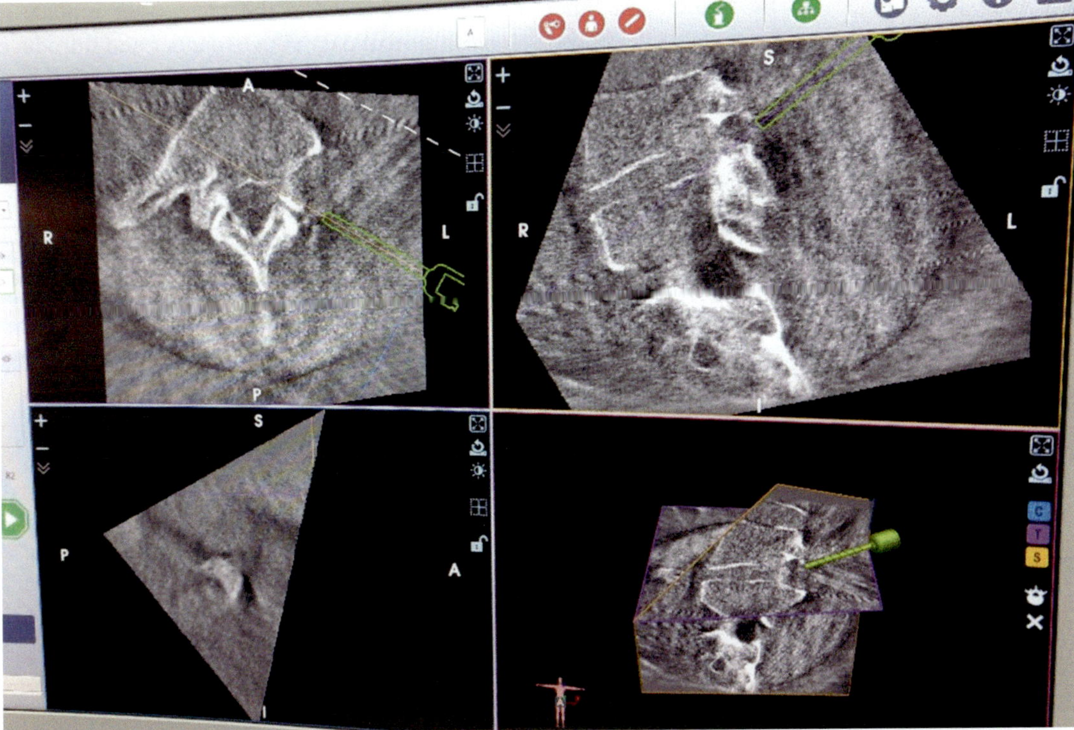

Fig. 15.5 Surgical plan intraoperatively

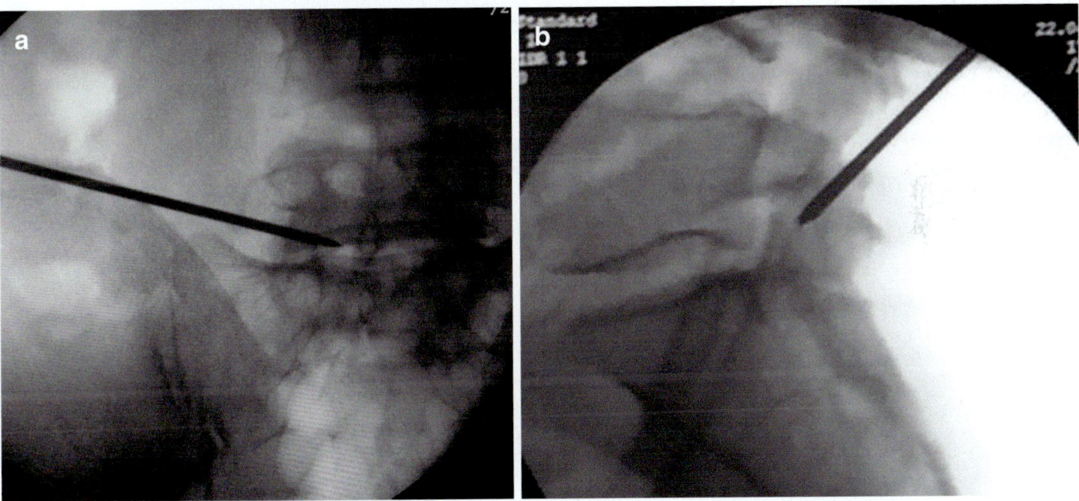

Fig. 15.6 (**a**, **b**) TomShidi needle

it with a sharp Tom needle. Start from SAF and advance it into the intervertebral foramen according to direction planned before the operation. Change to a blunt Tom needle when the feeling of breakthrough came out, or when the tip of the needle crosses inter-pedicle line. Continue tapping the needle into the front of the spinal canal and approach the protruding disk. At this point, replace the Tom needle with a guide wire (Fig. 15.6).

5. Under the guidance of the guide wire, the 4–8 mm bone drill is used to expand the intervertebral foramen. It is necessary to pay attention to the direction of the bone drill along the guide wire to avoid bending or breaking. It is recommended to monitor the position of the bone drill with X-ray closely, try to avoid sharp instrumentation into spinal canal (Fig. 15.7).
6. After withdrawing the bone drill, replace it with a secondary skin expander and introduce the working sleeve so that the tip of the sleeve approaches the level of the protruding disk (Fig. 15.8).
7. Endoscope is placed and endoscopic view is focused. Then it is ready to watch the operation from the monitor. The nucleus pulposus clamp is used to remove the loose debris; try to

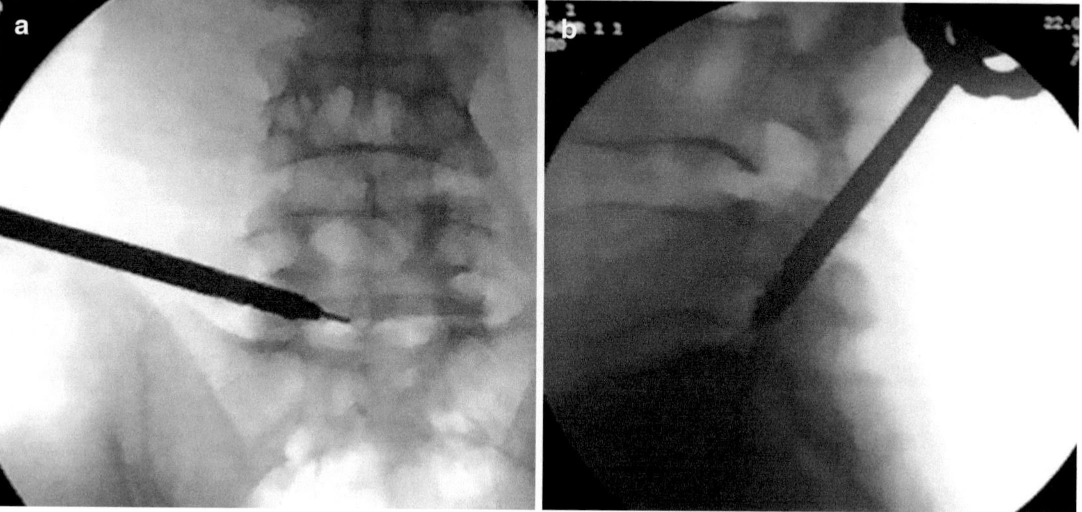

Fig. 15.7 (**a**, **b**) Foraminoplasty with 4–8 mm bone drill

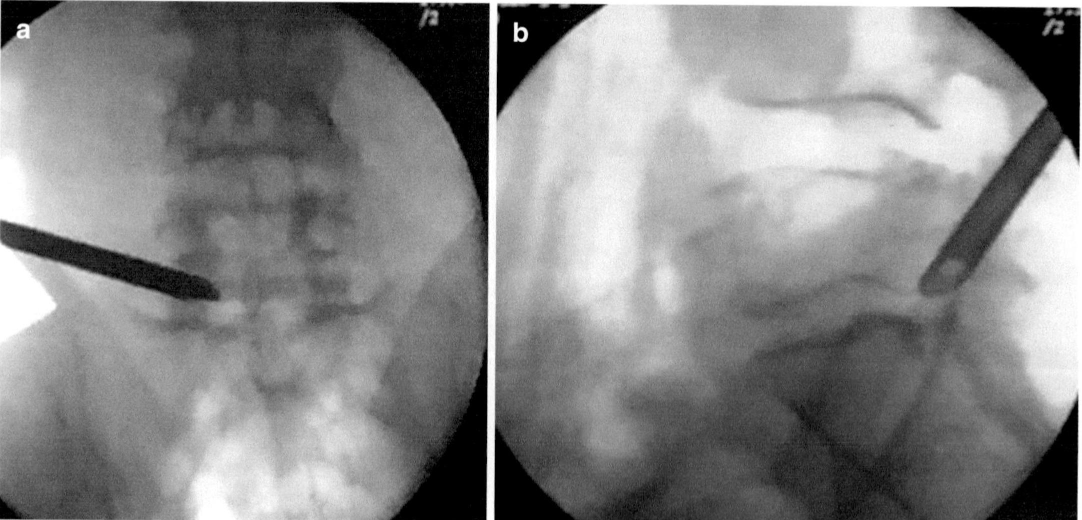

Fig. 15.8 (**a**, **b**) Position of working cannula

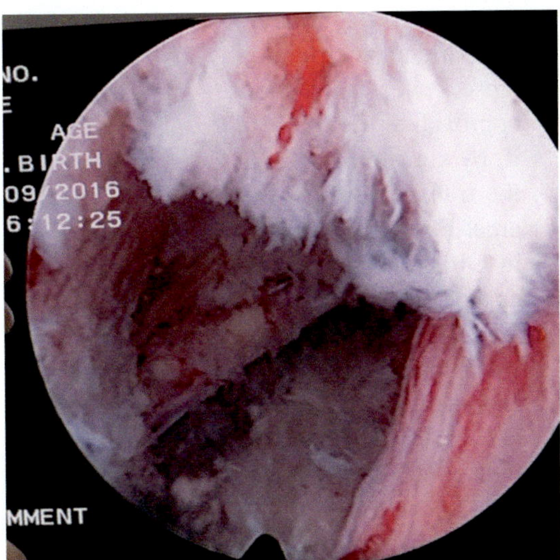

Fig. 15.9 After decompression, the nerve falls down to the view. We can see the traversing nerve root in the upper left, exiting nerve root in the lower right, and Kambin triangle between them

identify the ligamentum flavum, articular process, and intervertebral disk tissue with the help of probe or bipolar radiofrequency probe. At this time, the nerve root is often invisible, and we need to remove the prominent nucleus pulposus tissue patiently and slowly. When the nerve roots and dura mater tissues fall into the endoscopic view (Fig. 15.9), the nerve fluctuations can often be watched during surgery. And when the volume of extracted nucleus pulposus tissue is consistent with size estimated based on MRI scanning preoperatively, the decompression is sufficient. Under local anesthesia, you can ask the patient whether the symptoms are relieved. Patients were encouraged to ambulate 2 h after the operation, but for patients under general anesthesia, we recommended ambulation the next day. There is no need of prophylactic antibiotic or corticoid usage after operation.

6 Complications

Yeung AT summarized nearly a thousand cases of PTED surgery, the overall incidence of surgical complications was 3.5%, and with the accumulation of surgical experience, the incidence rate fell to less than 1% (Yeung 2007). Common surgical complications include (1) dural tears due to puncture tongs or rough operation under the endoscopy. Generally, no special treatment is required in these situations. Postoperative clots can act as a blockage. (2) Nerve root injury. This complication is not likely to occur under local anesthesia. If the patient complains of nerve pain during surgery, the surgeon should stop immediately. If the pain persists, when the adjustment is still impossible, the laminectomy from posterior approach should be kept in mind (3). The abnormality sensation of the exiting nerve root-dominating area has an incidence rate of 5–15%: this is a complication due to the approach. It occurs mostly within a few days after surgery and could resolve spontaneously. It is generally considered to be related to impingement between intraoperative working sleeve and dorsal root ganglion of the nerve root. Local cortisol injection can be considered as a choice (4). Head and neck pain includes severe pain in the head and neck, even muscle pain in extremities. Very few patients had this problem, and it is considered related to overperfusion of intraoperative irrigation fluid. Sedation, oxygen inhalation, avoiding excessive perfusion water pressure, or long-term operation time are helpful for these kinds of patients (5). In addition, there are some rare complications including retroperitoneal hematoma after surgery, intestinal infection, intestinal tube injury, among others, that had been reported (6). Postoperative intervertebral disk recurrence is similar to the incidence of conventional fenestration discectomy (5–11%).

In order to avoid unnecessary risks during surgery, the surgeon must be cautious when dealing with the following symptoms: (1) Patient with local anesthesia has unexpected waist and leg discomfort; at this time, surgeons should carefully adjust the puncture and check under fluoroscopy. (2) When patients present with head and neck pain and abdominal pain, surgeons should first stop the operation, looking for any abnormality, and if necessary, giving up surgery is also an option.

7 Recommendations

1. Anesthesia

   Most surgeons prefer topical 1% lidocaine infiltration anesthesia on the basis of intravenous sedation, but more and more surgeons are willing to give general anesthesia. The advantage of local anesthesia is that the patient can give feedback to the surgeon in time, which plays the role of nerve monitoring, but it is difficult to avoid pain and nervous during procedure around nerve root in the operation, and the patient often cannot tolerate the same posture for a long time. Therefore, for patients who are difficult to cooperate (such as younger patients), or patients with more difficult surgery and longer estimation time, we prefer general anesthesia. The risk of nerve root damage is the major concern for many doctors; if you strictly follow the standard puncture path and avoid sharp instruments entering the spinal canal, you can basically avoid nerve damage during operation.
2. Patient position placement: prone or lateral decubitus, mainly depending on the habits of the surgeon. For doctors with abundant open surgery experience, the prone position is more familiar in anatomy, and the patient's position is more stable. However, lateral position also has advantages: (1) lateral position is more conducive to anesthesia management; (2) if the operation time is long, the lateral position is more tolerable than the prone position, and the prone position is responsible for restricted respiratory function of patients, especially elderly patients; (3) the lateral side due to the bending of the operating bed, making intervertebral foramen bigger, thus makes the puncture and catheterization easier; (4) the lateral position is safer for the abdominal organs and is easy for straight leg elevation test and femoral nerve traction test.
3. Approach selection: For L5/S1, especially for patients with cranially or caudally prolapse, we can choose the THESSYS approach or the BEIS approach derived from it, by cutting the articular process and even the transverse process to achieve the target area. For compression from the ventral side in L4/L5 or L3/L4 level, the extreme lateral approach can be used to avoid damage to the facet joint. For the intervertebral disk herniation with higher level, it is often safer to enter the disk through YESS approach because the peritoneal structure such as the kidney is avoided in the puncture path otherwise. However, if the disk is prolapsed downward or combined with compression from the dorsal side, the THESSYS approach is the best choice, because it is required to cut the superior articular process to expose the dorsal side of the nerve root for decompression.
4. How to judge the decompression is sufficient: a major difficulty in the operation of endoscopy is to determine whether the decompression is sufficient. In the local anesthesia, it can be verified by asking the patient, but this subjective experience is often not very accurate, as there may still be residual disk tissue fragments, resulting in short-term recurrence after surgery. The main basis for our judgment of the end point includes the following points: (1) nerve root fluctuates with the heartbeat beat. (2) The volume of protruding tissue is matched with the size estimated based on MRI scan. (3) The nerves are free to slide intraoperatively during straight leg elevation test (lateral position) or femoral nerve traction test (positive lateral position). (4) Intraoperative probe showed that there are no compression under the nerve from head to tail.

8 Typical Case

Female, 33 years old, left lower limb pain for 3 months, worsened in recent 1 week.

Figure 15.10 showed there was a lumbar disk herniation in L5/S1 level, protruded to the left side. There is significant degeneration change in L4/L5 level, but no obvious disk herniation.

CT images in Fig. 15.11 demonstrated that L5/S1 lumbar disk protrusion to the posterior lateral side, without calcification.

Patient received a robot-assisted percutaneous transforaminal endoscopy discectomy (Figs. 15.12, 15.13, 15.14, 15.15, 15.16, and 15.17). Compression under the nerve root was removed after the surgery. There was reduced nerve tension and dilation of

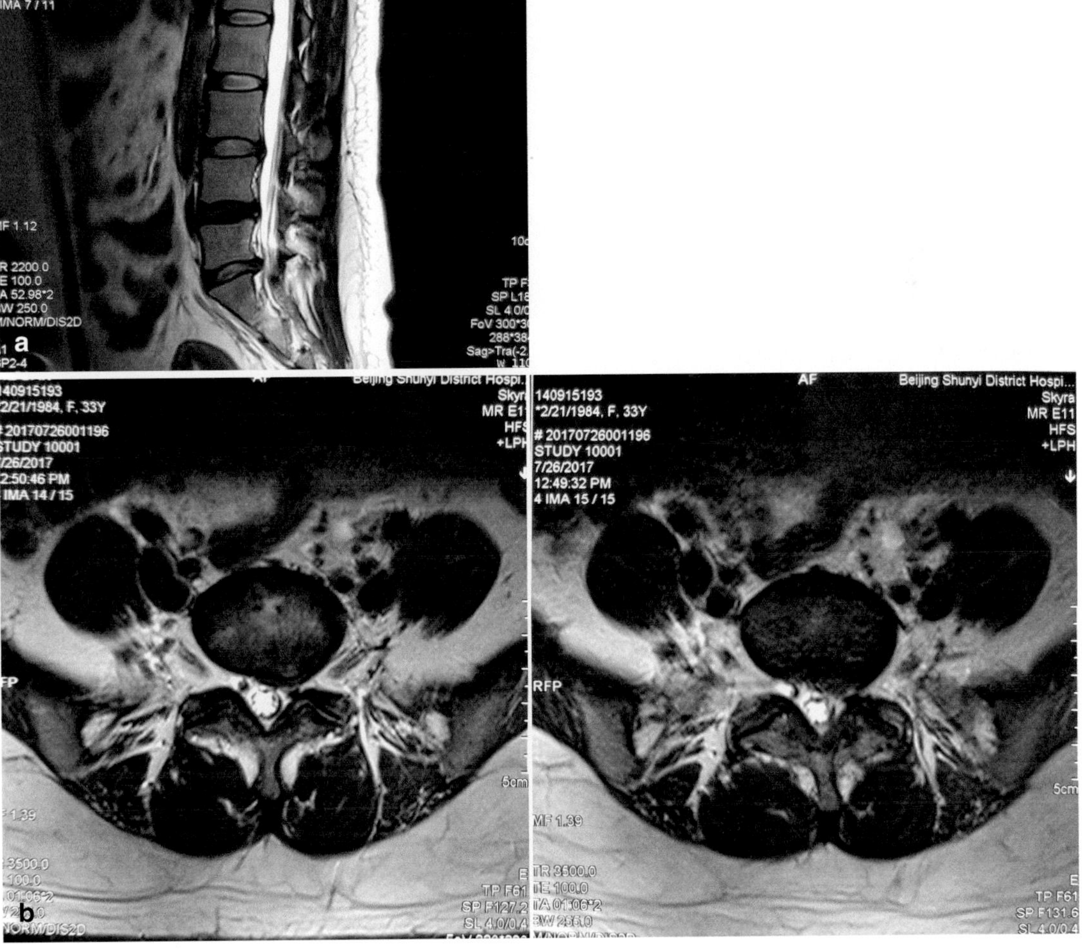

Fig. 15.10 (**a**, **b**) MRI images of the patient

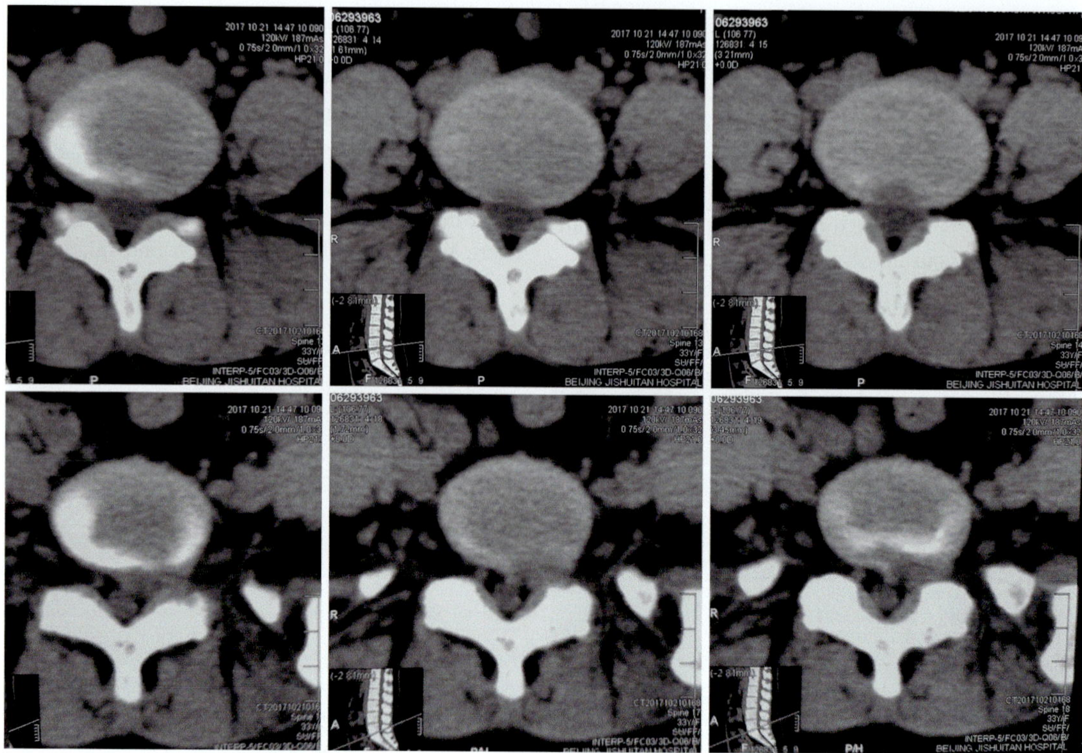

Fig. 15.11 CT images of the patient

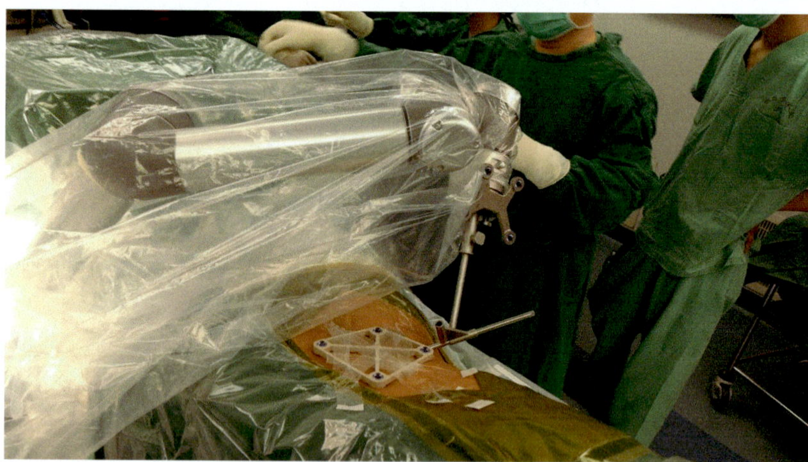

Fig. 15.12 The system setup for the patient

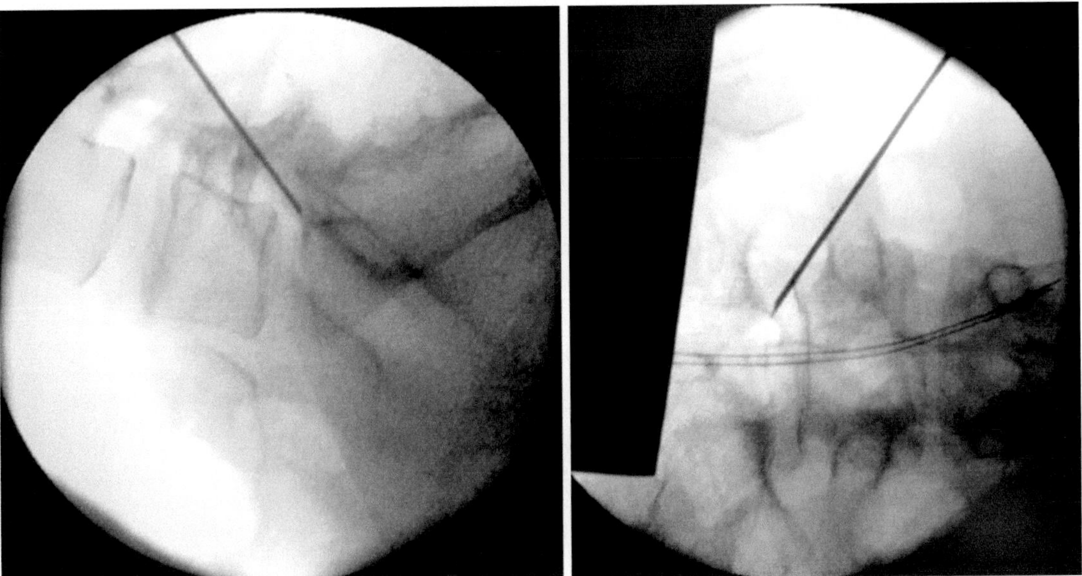

Fig. 15.13 Acupuncture needle under guidance of robot

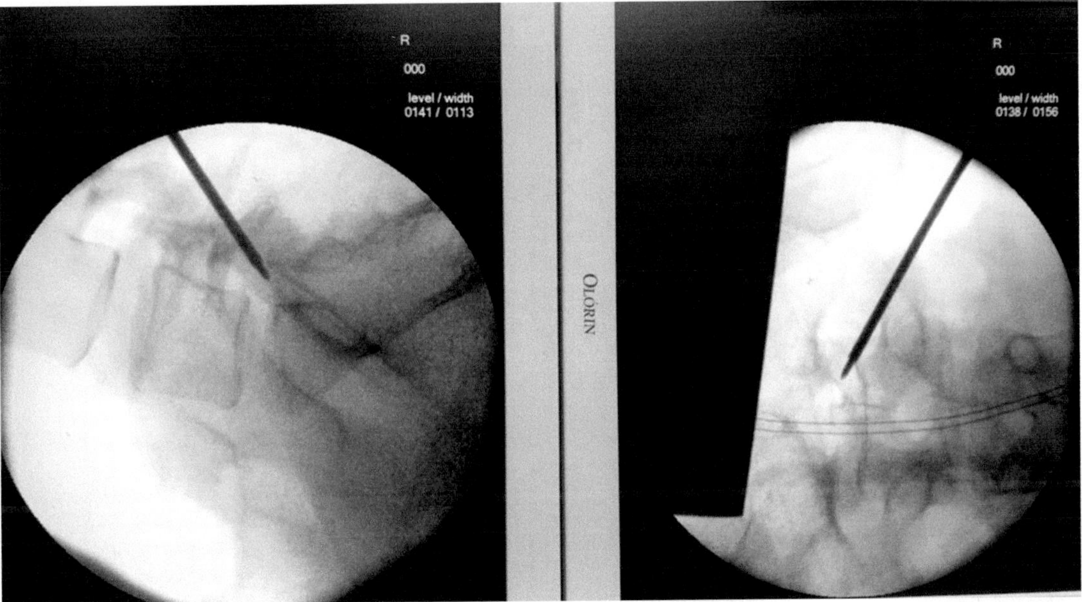

Fig. 15.14 TomShidi needle for final adjustment

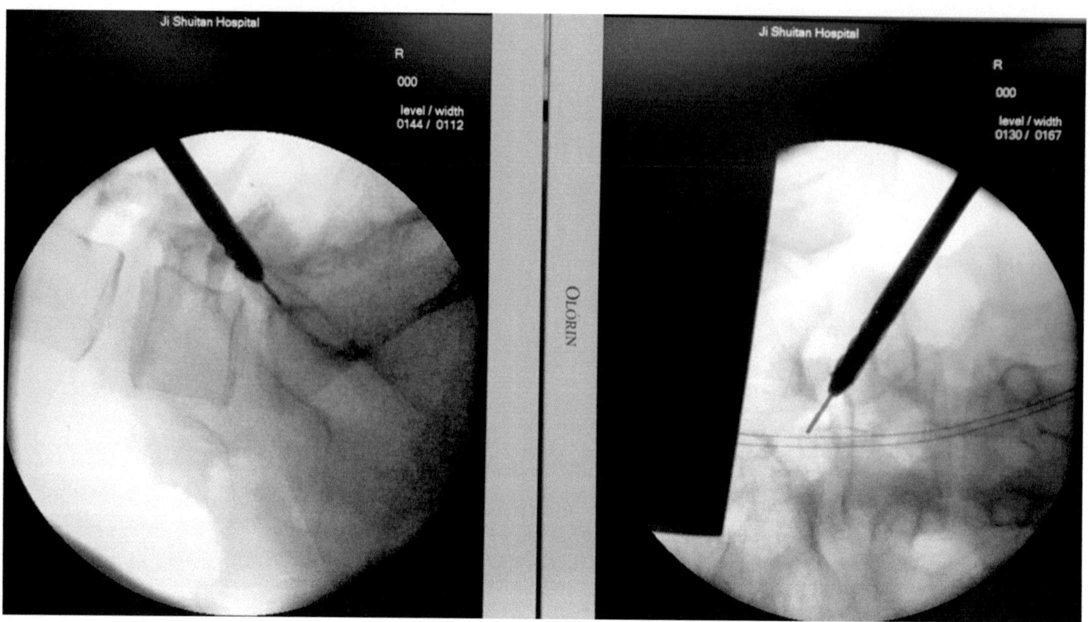

Fig. 15.15 Foraminoplasty with 4–8 mm bone drill

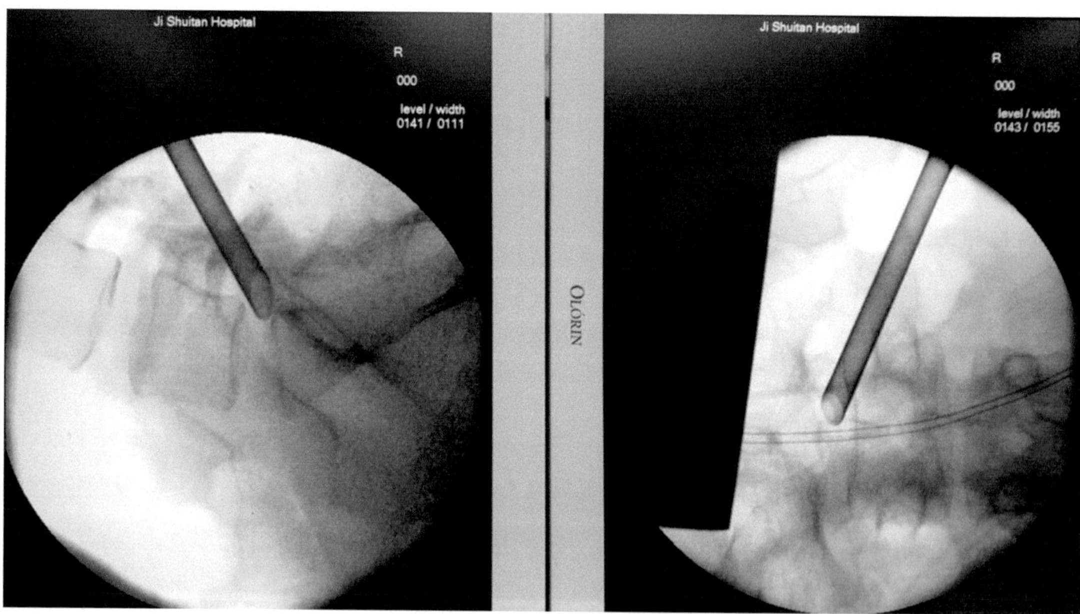

Fig. 15.16 Position of cannula for further endoscopic operation

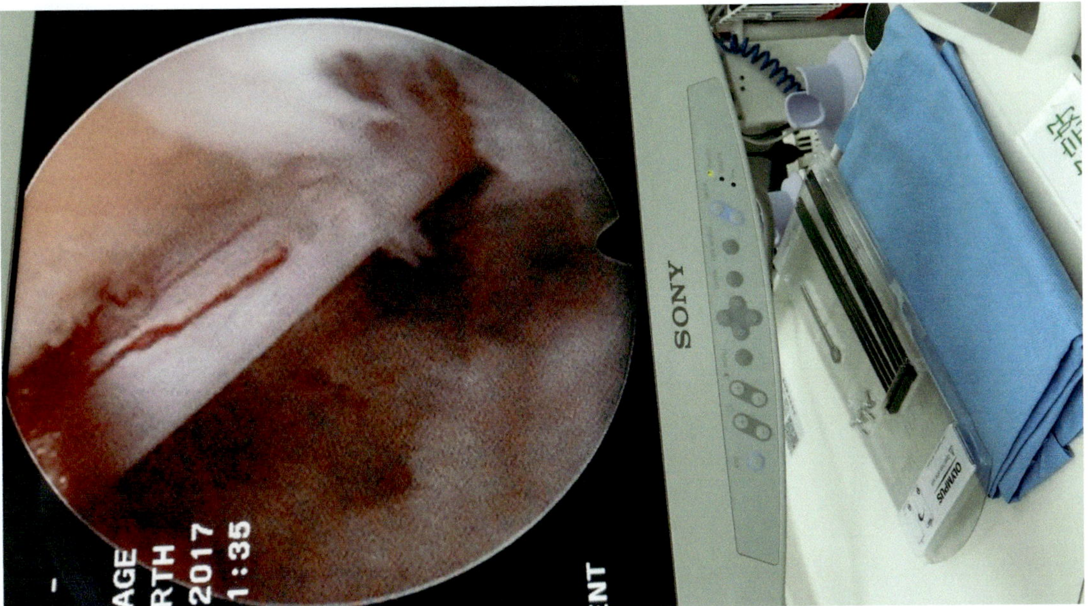

Fig. 15.17 Compression of the herniated disk was removed

surface vessels. The straight leg raise test showed a smooth movement of nerve root, indicating endpoint of decompression.

References

Hoogland T. Transforaminal endoscopic discectomy with foraminoplasty for lumbar disc herniation. Surg Tech Orthop Traumatol. 2003;40:55–120.

Kahanovitz N, Viola K, Mcolloch J. Limited surgical discectomy and microdiscectomy: a clinical comparison. Spine. 1989;14:79.

Kambin P, Zhou L. History and current status of percutaneous arthroscopic disc surgery. Spine. 1996;21:57–61.

Maroon JC, Abla A. Microlumbar discectomy. Clin Neurosurg. 1986;33:407.

McCulloch JA. Principles of microsurgery for lumbar disc diseases. New York: Raven Press; 1989.

Mixter WJL, Barr JS. Rupture of the intervertebral disc with involvement of spinal canal. N Engl J Med. 1934;211:210.

Ruetten S, Komp M, Godolias G. An extreme lateral access for the surgery of lumbar disc herniations inside the spinal canal using the full-endoscopic uniportal transforaminal approach-technique and prospective results of 463 patients. Spine (Phila Pa 1976). 2005a;30:2570–8.

Yeung AT. The evolution and advancement of endoscopic foraminal surgery: one surgeon's experience incorporating adjunctive technologies. SAS J. 2007;1:108–17.

Yeung AT, Gore SR. Evolving methodology in treating discogenic back pain by selective endoscopic discectomy (SED) and thermal annuloplasty. J Minimally Invasive Spinal Tech. 2001;1:8–16.

16 Cortical Bone Trajectory for Lumbar Pedicle Screws Placement

Qiang Yuan, Nan Li, Jie Yu, and Wei Tian

Abstract

There have been a number of reports of alternative screw trajectories aimed at enhancing screw purchase with higher-density bone regions. The cortical bone trajectory (CBT) is laterally directed in the transverse plane and caudo-cephalad in the sagittal plane. This technique has been advocated because it is minimally invasive and reduces neurovascular injuries. However, the CBT technique do have several drawbacks when compared with the traditional pedicle screw approach. The use of navigation and robot-assisted surgery can both increase the accuracy of CBT screw placement.

Keywords

Cortical bone trajectory · Medio–lateral–superior trajectory · Pedicle screw · Robot-assisted surgery · Minimally invasive

Q. Yuan (✉) · N. Li · J. Yu · W. Tian
Department of Spine Surgery, Beijing Jishuitan Hospital, Fourth Clinical Hospital of Peking University, Beijing, China
e-mail: yuanqiang@jsthospital.org; tianweijst@vip.163.com

1 Previous Studies and Development

Santoni et al. first introduced the concept of CBT (Santoni et al. 2009). Previously, some surgeons had designed alternative screw trajectories that did not go through the pedicle anatomical axis. In 1976 and 1992, Roy-Camille et al. described an alternative screw trajectory that crossed the pedicle axis vertically. The vertical screw contacted more cortical bone at its end, which contributed to the biomechanical characteristics of pullout strength and stability.

The "medio–latero–superior trajectory" (MLST) that came to be known as the CBT was initially used in screw fixation of single-level thoracolumbar burst fractures. The application of the CBT approach in clinical practice has been reported for over 10 years, which all included satisfactory outcomes, with no occurrences of neurological injury or screw instrumentation failure. These early studies laid the foundation for the deeper research for alternative pedicle screw trajectories.

2 Advantages and Disadvantages

The novel CBT technique has several advantages over the traditional pedicle screw trajectory approaches.

W. Tian (ed.), *Navigation Assisted Robotics in Spine and Trauma Surgery*,
https://doi.org/10.1007/978-981-15-1846-1_16

1. The novel CBT technique has the advantages of less blooding, less invasive, and faster postoperative recovery. The CBT insertion point is located medial on the pars interarticularis, which means smaller initial incisions and less soft tissue retraction and injury compared with the traditional approach. Minimal invasive means less intraoperative blood loss and postoperative pain for patients.
2. The novel CBT technique has a lower risk of neurovascular injury compared with the traditional pedicle screw trajectory. The CBT is laterally directed in the transverse plane and caudo-cephalad in the sagittal plane, and the screw follows a path away from the anterior vascular structures and the medial branch nerves arising from lumbar spinal nerve, which is susceptible to injury by traditional pedicle screw path.
3. The novel CBT technique is more suitable for obese patients. The exposure and access to the surgical site are challenging in obese patients, while the more minimally invasive CBT approach seemed to conquer this problem.

There still remain several drawbacks and complications in the CBT technique.

1. An inappropriate diameter of cortical screws may lead to the risk of pedicle fractures, and an incorrect depth of screw penetration can also increase the risk of the upper nerve root injury. These potential negative consequences cautioned surgeons about the relationship between the cortical screw and the anatomical pedicle size both pre- and intraoperatively.
2. The CBT technique does not apply to the patients with partially or fully destructed articular joints, since the landmarks for the CBT insertion point may no longer be available. Iwatsuki et al. proposed the isthmus-guided CBT approach to deal with this problem.
3. Failure of the pedicle screws to line up in the sagittal plane may increase the challenge and difficulty of rod placement.
4. Intraoperative imaging is necessary in the CBT approach; thus, there are potentially increased radiation exposure and longer operation times in CBT procedures, particularly for surgeons not familiar with this new technique.

Keorochana et al. (2017) searched eight studies (seven studies were cohort studies, one study was randomized control trial), and there was no significant difference in clinical outcomes between the CBT technique and traditional pedicle approach, including JOA, ODI, VAS (back and leg), and intraoperative complication and fusion rates in posterior lumbar fixation. There was an interesting result that patients in the CBT group had significantly lower postoperative complications of approximately 50% compared with the traditional pedicle group. Postoperative complications included wound problems (infection or hematoma) that could be associated with the wider and longer dissection required for PS fixation, and other problems (loss of reduction, implant migration, ASD, and osteolysis) could be associated with facet violation from the PS fixation. Pedicle screw has been widely used in fusion surgery of the lumbar spine because of its biomechanical characteristics, and PS still has the risk of facet violation and intraoperative injury to the intraspinal structure (dura mater and spinal nerve root). Thus, the CBT technique was invented in lumber fusion surgery and reduces the risk of that postoperative complications.

3 Indications

1. Posterior fixation in single segmental degenerative and traumatic cases.
2. Decompressive laminectomy and transforaminal lumber interbody fusion requiring instrumentation.

3. Obese patients who require smaller incision and less soft tissue injury.
4. Patients with osteopenia or osteoporosis requiring instrumentation.

4 Contraindications

Relative contraindications include (1) posterior fixation in multilevel scoliosis, (2) narrow or medialized pars, and (3) congenitally small pedicles.

Absolute contraindications include (1) congenital pars defects and lack of cortical bone at the pars.

Several shortcomings still exist in the CBT approach. First, CBT screws are generally used in single segmental degenerative and traumatic cases, whereas pedicle screws are already used in multiple levels lumber diseases. However, the CBT technique is suitable for patients with osteoporosis. The unique CBT enhanced screw purchase due to maximum contact of the screw with higher-density bone regions. This would reduce the risk of pedicle screw loosening in patients with osteoporosis. A cadaveric biomechanical study revealed that the screw surrounding bone ROIs in CBT fixation displays much more than that of the traditional fixation. Differences are statistically significant, and the mean maximum torque of the CBT screws was 1.7–2.3 times higher than that of the traditional screws. There is no significant difference between the mean CT measurements in CBT screws and traditional screws. It is mainly due to the depth of cortical bone in vertebral pedicle and the lack of bone mass in vertebral plate. In these patients, because of the disadvantages of CBT mechanical property, there is no significant advantage between the two screws.

Oshino et al. (2015) conducted a biomechanical research in biomechanical properties of functional spine units. In this study, 20 lumbar spine (L5–L6) specimens from a 3-year-old male deer cadaver were assigned to two groups: the mean ROM in the bend and rotation tests and the mean rate of relative change of ROM in both the bend and rotation tests were compared between the CBT and PS groups. There were no significant differences between the mean ROMs and the mean rate of relative change of ROMs in both the bend and rotation tests between the two approaches.

5 Surgical Procedures and Illustrations (Tradition and Navigation, Robotic Methods)

Freehand screw placement:

1. Anesthesia: After general anesthesia, the patient was placed prone on the carbon bed chest pad, and the abdomen was vacated.
2. Exposure: After the surgical segment marker needle was positioned, it was routinely disinfected and spread. The midline incision of the lumbar posterior segment was performed. The layers were exposed to the spinous process. The paravertebral muscles on both sides of the spinous process were dissected beneath the subperiosteal, revealing the lateral lamina and the medial border structure of the articular process.
3. Drilling: After the exposure is complete, the initial starting point is identified at media and caudal 2 mm laminar point of superior articular process. Using a diamond drill, we make the initial hole. Into the direction of the screw, the coronal position tilts 5° to 15° medial–lateral, and the sagittal position is 30° to −10° caudo-cranial. After the screw passage with the opener, the surgeon advances the pedicle probe to the walls and the bottom. After investigating the integrities of the walls, place the marking needles. After the perspective position is good, use the taper cone channels to explore the four walls and bottom again and measure the length of the required screws.
4. Screw placement: Into the screw (selection of anterior segment cancellous bone thread, posterior cortical bone thread, universal screw).

Screw diameter generally chooses 4.5 mm (3.5–5.0 mm), and screw length 40 mm is better (35 mm is enough for stability). Screw head is close to the cortex of the vertebral body wall through the pedicle. The non-self-tapping nail for the round head may pass through the cortex, and the self-tapping nail for the pointed head should not pass through the cortex.

Placement of CBT screws based on 3D navigation system:

1. Anesthesia, posture, surgical preparation, and incision with the freehand screw placement.
2. Revealing:When revealing, the upper facet joint is not necessary (such as L4/L5 interbody fusion surgery; L3/L4 facet joints do not have to be revealed, only L4 lamina and isthmus need to be revealed); hence, for the navigation tracer placement, one spinous process is less revealed compared with the insertion of pedicle screws.
3. Drilling:After the exposure, a reasonable point of entry is found using the nose cone of the navigation system. After the cortex and some channels are drilled out with a sharp diamond, the entire screw channel is prepared using a navigation opener.
4. Screw placement:The length of the screw can be measured accurately to reach the cortex of the vertebral body based on the 3D navigation system.

Robot-assisted placement of CBT screws:

1. Preparation: Surgical preparation is basically the same as navigation-assisted surgery.
2. Tracer placement: Due to the fact that the size of the passive tracer for robotic surgery is larger than that of navigation, it is recommended to place the tracer on the superior spinous process.
3. Revealing: Revealing part is the same as the navigation surgery.
4. Image acquisition: After the image acquisition, the entry point, screw direction, the diameter, and length of each CBT screw are planned by the surgeon.
5. K-wires placement: The placement of each CBT screw is started based on the standard robot system. After the operation channel has been placed, the diamond must be used drilling at the entry point instead of drilling directly with the tip of the Kirschner wire. Since the lamina cortex on the medial side of the isthmus is stiff and sloped, the point of entry of the drill after grooving is perpendicular to the direction of the Kirschner wire, preventing the Kirschner wire from shifting to varying degrees. Poor handling of the entry point often causes the Kirschner wire to deflect outward and upward.
6. Screw placement: After all K-wires have been placed, the surgeon advances the position of the screws with the use of AP and lateral images, and then insert the taps and screws.

On the one hand, regardless of the manner in which the CBT screw is placed, special care must be taken when performing decompression surgery, especially interbody fusion cage placement, since the CBT screw entry point is close to the upper edge of the next gap. The screw will affect the sight when performing decompression. On the other hand, the expansion of the decompression will affect the bone mass in the cortex of the screw. For a 4.5 mm screw selection, the operating guide requires that the decompression edge is 3 mm away from the screw. During decompression surgery including TLIF, PLIT, or MIDLIF, the surgeon drills the screws in advance according to the standard entry point to complete the screw channel. After sufficient decompression, the surgeon inserts the screws. Since the inner part of the screw is tapered, it is not necessary to fully screw, while approximately 1/2 or 2/3 is appropriate. If there is a navigation or robot assistance, observe the position of the lamina first corresponding to the upper edge of the disk before selecting a reasonable entry point. Leave 3 mm space and then plan the entry point and screw passage.

Isthmus spondylolisthesis: In the case of isthmus spondylolisthesis requiring surgery, the issue of whether CBT screws can be fixed and resettling requires the specific analysis of the bone shape of the isthmus fissure.

6 Surgical Points

Matsukawa et al. (2013) performed 3D reconstruction of CT images of lumbar spine in 100 adult patients and analyzed screw diameters, lengths, and screw penetration angles of CBT screw fixation techniques. The study pointed out that the CBT screw entry point is located at the intersection of the top line of the upper articular process with the 1 mm below the lower edge of the transverse process. The screw diameter gradually increases from L1 (6.2 mm ± 1.1 mm) to L5 (8.4 mm ± 1.4 mm); the L3 and L4 screw lengths are the longest, from L1 to L5 are (36.8 ± 3.2) mm, (38.2 ± 3.0) mm, respectively, (39.3 ± 3.3) mm, (39.8 ± 3.5) mm, and (38.3 ± 3.9) mm; there is no significant difference in screw head inclination, roll angle from L1 to L5, and the head inclination is (26.2 ± 4.5)°, (25.5 ± 4.5)°, (26.2 ± 4.9)°, (26.0 ± 4.4)°, and (25.8 ± 4.8)°, roll angles (8.6 ± 2.3)°, (8.5 ± 2.4)°, (9.1 ± 2.4)°, (9.1 ± 2.3)°, and (8.8 ± 2.1)°. After 3D reconstruction of the CT image, the authors also found that in the lumbar segment, the CBT screw's entry point on the left side is always at the 5 o'clock position of the pedicle isthmus contour and the right side corresponds to the 7 o'clock direction (Fig. 16.1). Based on this finding, they proposed another CBT entry point positioning method: the lumbar AP image was taken during the operation. For the left pedicle, the entry point was at 5 o'clock in the pedicle isthmus, and the right pedicle was corresponding to the 7 o'clock direction; the screw direction is on the left side to the 11–12 o'clock direction, and the right-pointing position is not interfered with the articular process position, and it is still applicable when the facet joint is displaced and destroyed. This method can reduce the anatomic exposure area.

Iwatsuki et al. (2014) designed another CBT screw positioning method: Inserting the screw at a point 3 mm medial to the lateral margin of the isthmus, with the superior margin of the intervertebral foramen as imaged by lateral fluoroscopy serving as the reference point for insertion on the craniocaudal axis. The modified CBT technique is not superior to the original CBT method in the following aspects because the screws used are shorter and their insertion points closer to the cranial side than with the original CBT technique. The pullout force is slightly lower than the original CBT technique, but it can reduce the possibility of screws entering the intervertebral foramen and the spinal canal and injuring the nerves.

Initially, CBT screw fixation was only used for lumbar fixation. Matsukawa et al. 2014 studied the thoracic CBT screw fixation technique. From T9 to T12, the vertical coronal plane enters the screw obliquely upward, and the entry point is located near the lowest point along the lower edge of the upper articular process 2/3. All morphometric parameters of thoracic CBT increased from T9 to T12 (the mean diameter: from 5.8 mm at T9 to 8.5 mm at T12; the length: from 29.7 mm at T9 to 32.0 mm at T12; and the cephalad angle: from 21.4° at T9 to 27.6° at T12). The mean maximum insertional torque of CBT screws and traditional screws were 1.02 ± 0.25 and 0.66 ± 0.15 Nm, respectively. The new technique demonstrated average 53.8% higher torque than the traditional technique ($P < 0.01$).

The scholar Matsukawa et al. 2017 also extended the application scope of CBT screw fixation to the lumbosacral region, based on the CT scans of 50 adults studied for morphometric measurement of the new trajectory. The entry point was supposed to be the junction of the center of the superior articular process of S-1 and approximately 3 mm inferior to the most inferior border of the inferior articular process of L-5. The mean cephalad angle in these 50 patients was 30.7° ± 5.1°. The direction was straightforward in the axial plane without convergence, angulated cranially in the sagittal plane penetrating the middle of the sacral endplate. The new technique demonstrated an average of 141% higher insertional torque than the traditional monocortical technique.

The use of navigation can increase the accuracy of CBT screw placement. In a retrospective study of Snyder et al. (Snyder et al. 2016), it was found that there were no shifts in the placement of CBT screws in 69 patients using navigation aids. Other documents (Yson et al. 2013; Sipos et al. 1996; Youkilis et al. 2001) also show that navigation guidance can significantly improve the accuracy of screw placement.

7 Typical Cases (Figs. 16.1–16.18)

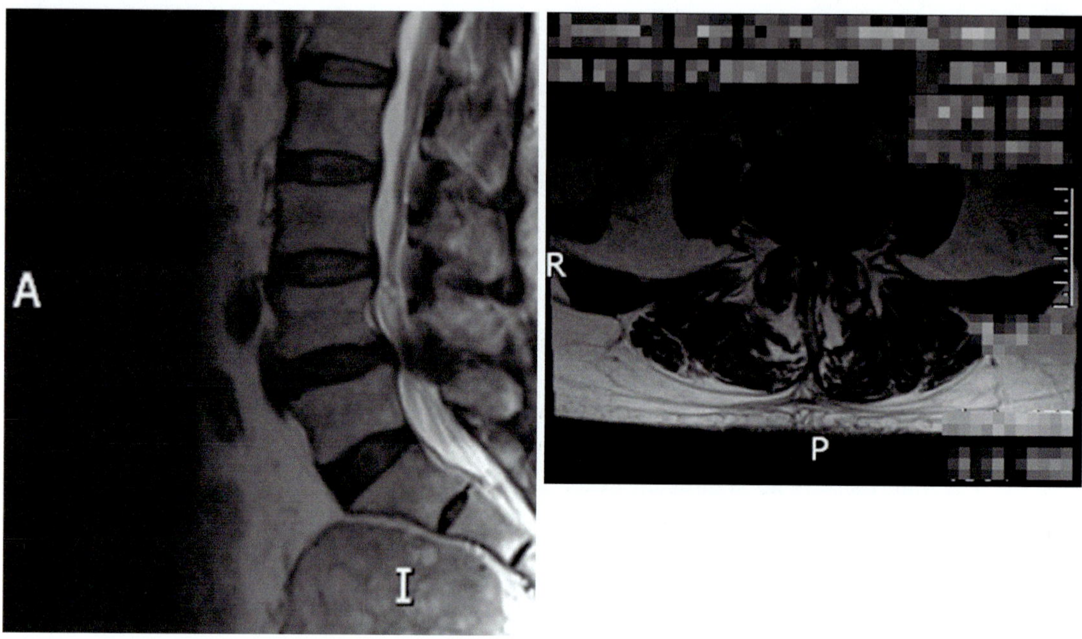

Fig. 16.1 and 16.2 Age 61, female, preoperative diagnosis: lumbar spondylolisthesis (L4/L5). Preoperative MRI shows segmental spondylolisthesis with stenosis in L4/L5

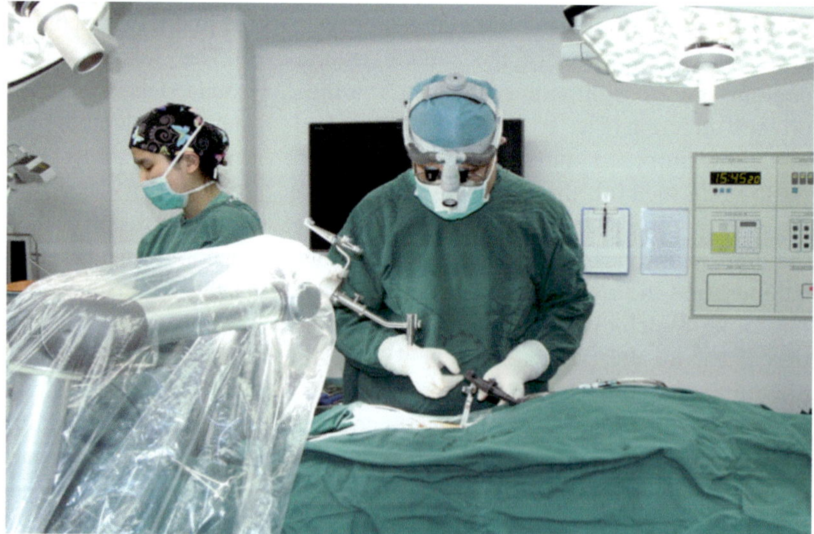

Fig. 16.3 The surgery is robot-assisted. The surgeon placed the tracer and adjusted the robotic arm

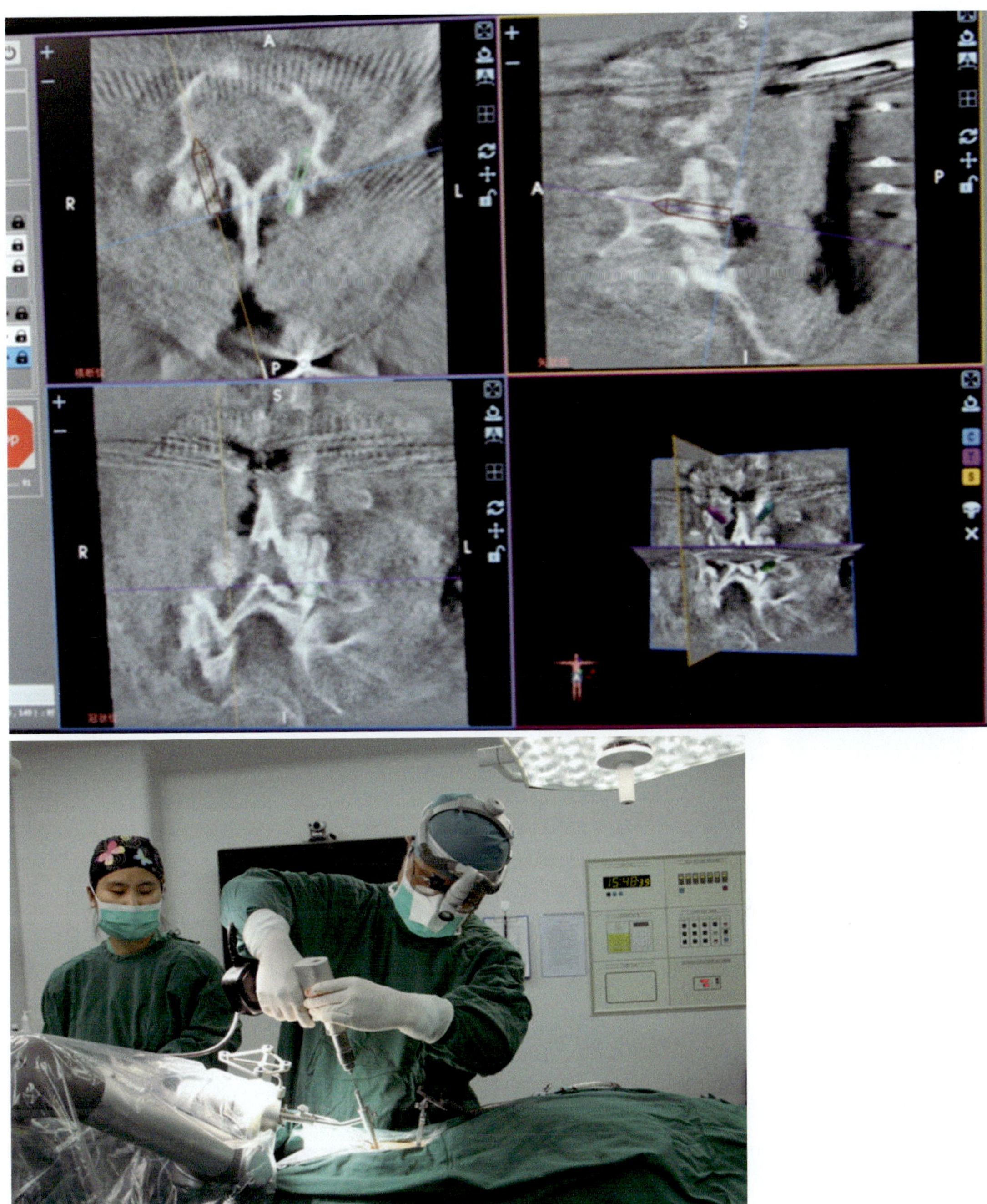

Fig. 16.4 and 16.5 CBT screw planning during surgery indicating probe needle placement guided by a robotic arm

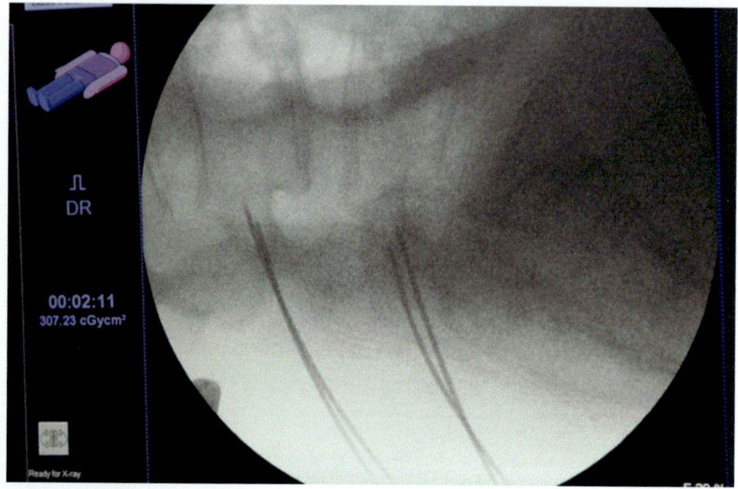

Fig. 16.6 After all guide needles are inserted, the fluoroscopy-image confirmation position is good

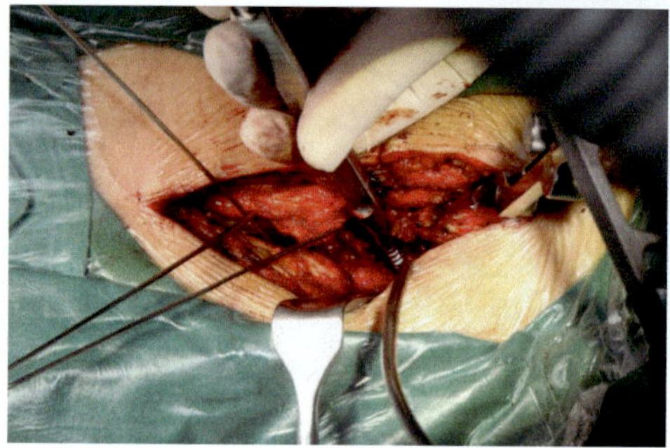

Fig. 16.7 Measurement of the length of each CDT screw

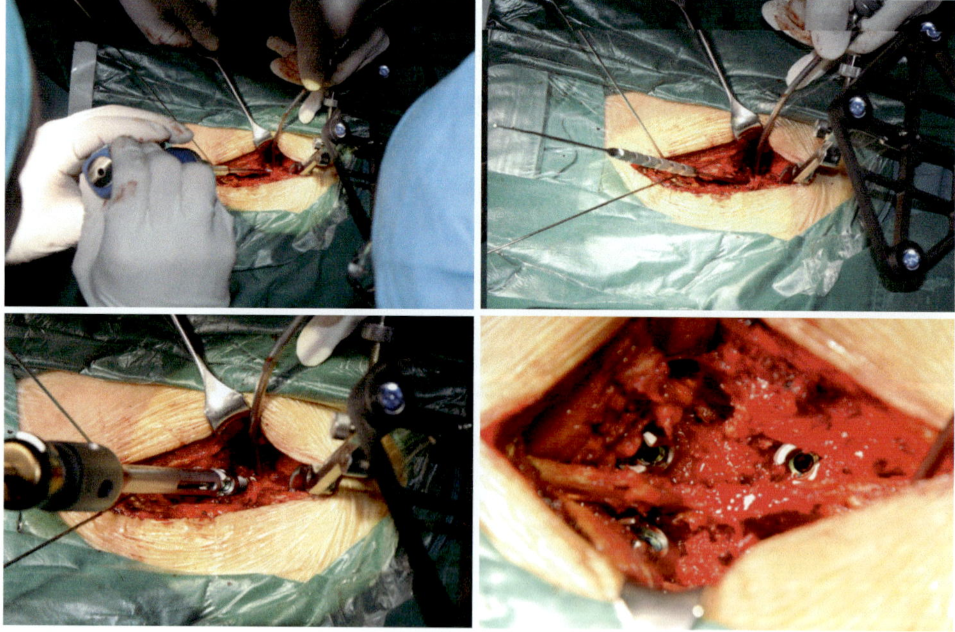

Fig. 16.8–16.11 Tap to make channel for CBT screw, probe the four walls and the bottom of the screw, and confirm that the four walls are complete (the bottom may have just broken), screw down CBT screws, screw down completely

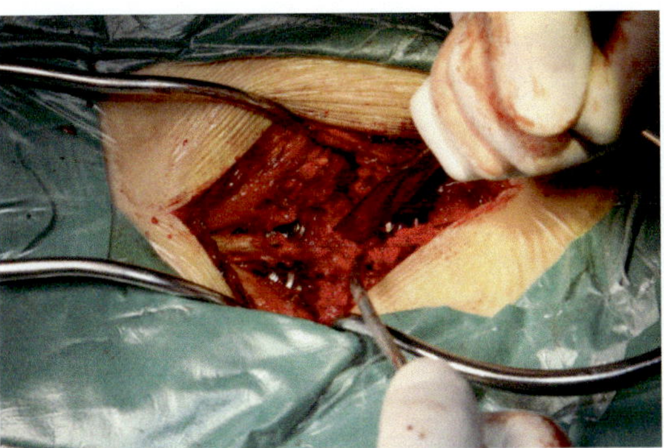

Fig. 16.12 Performing decompression and lumber interbody fusion procedure

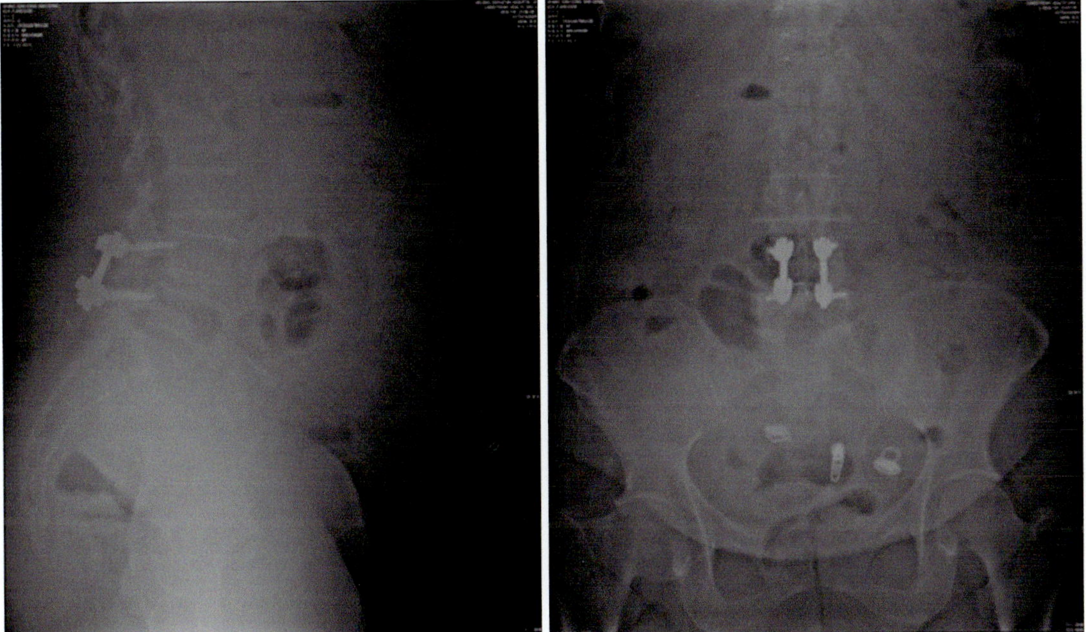

Fig. 16.13 and 16.14 The X-ray on the posterolateral position shows that the CBT screw is in a good position, the spondylolisthesis is completely reset, and the position of the interbody fusion cage is satisfactory

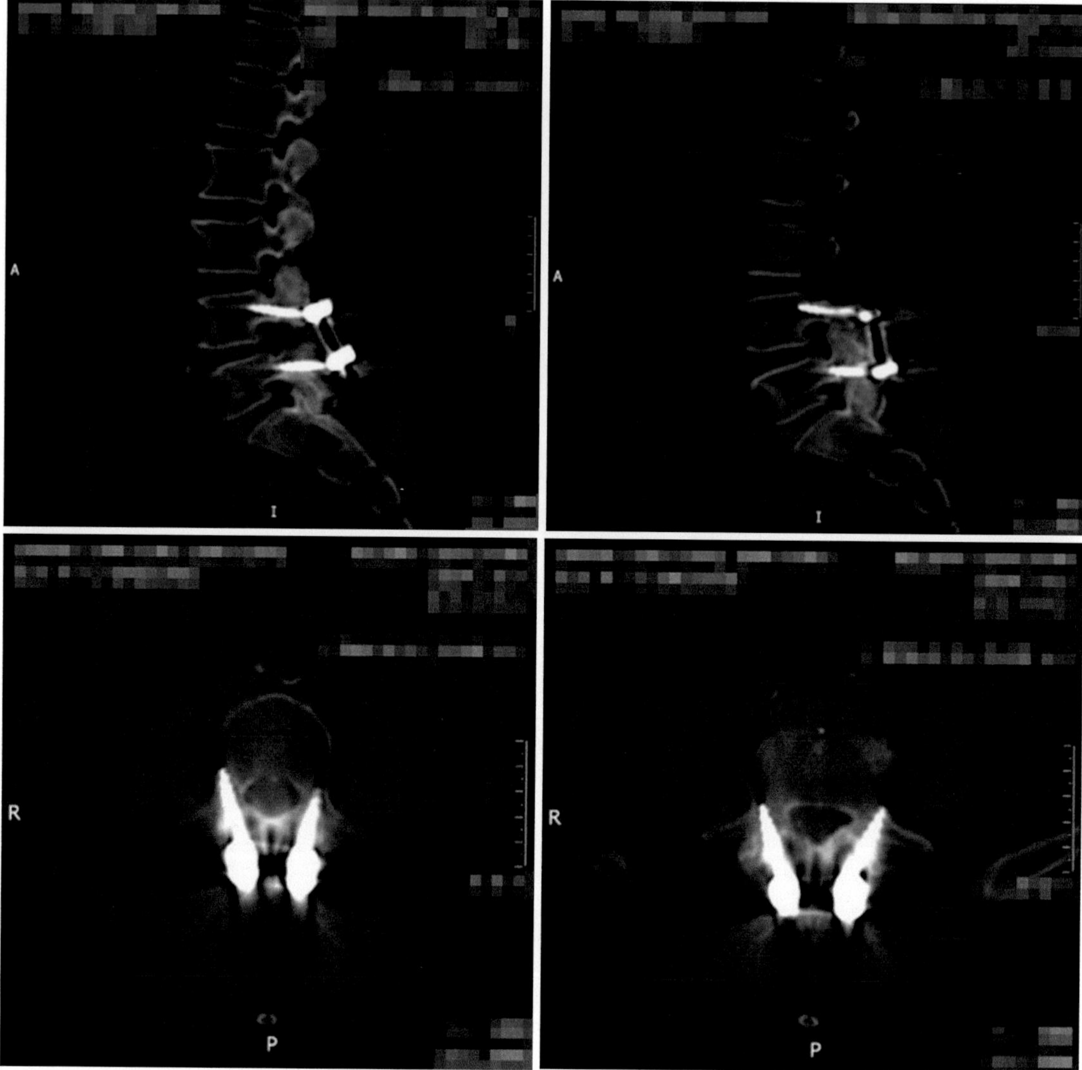

Fig. 16.15–16.18 Postoperative CT shows good position of CBT screws

References

Iwatsuki K, Yoshimine T, Ohnishi Y, et al. Isthmus-guided cortical bone trajectory for pedicle screw insertion. Orthop Surg. 2014;6(3):244–8. https://doi.org/10.1111/os.12122.

Keorochana G, Pairuchvej S, et al. Comparative outcomes of cortical screw trajectory fixation and pedicle screw fixation in lumbar spinal fusion: systematic review and meta-analysis. World Neurosurg. 2017;102:340–9.

Matsukawa K, Yato Y, Nemoto O, et al. Morphometric measurement of cortical bone trajectory for lumbar pedicle screw insertion using computed tomography. J Spinal Disord Tech. 2013;26(6):E248–53.

Matsukawa K, Yato Y, Kato T, et al. Cortical bone trajectory for lumbosacral fixation: penetrating S-1 endplate screw technique: technical note. J Neurosurg Spine. 2014;21(2):203–9. https://doi.org/10.3171/2014.3.SPINE13665.

Matsukawa K, Yato Y, Hynes RA, et al. Cortical bone trajectory for thoracic pedicle screws: a technical note. J Spinal Disord Tech. 2017;30(5):E497–504.

Oshino H, Sakakibara T, et al. A biomechanical comparison between cortical bone trajectory fixation and pedicle screw fixation. J Orthop Surg Res. 2015;10:125.

Roy-Camille R. Posterior screw plate fixation in thoracolumbar injuries. Instr Course Lect. 1992;41:157–63.

Roy-Camille R, Saillant G, Berteaux D, Salgado V. Osteosynthesis of thoraco-lumbar spine fractures with metal plates screwed through the vertebral pedicles. Reconstr Surg Traumatol. 1976;15:2–16.

Santoni BG, Hynes RA, McGilvray KC, et al. Cortical bone trajectory for lumbar pedicle screws. Spine J. 2009;9:366–73.

Sipos EP, Tebo SA, Zinreich SJ, Long DM, Brem H. In vivo accuracy testing and clinical experience with the ISG viewing wand. Neurosurgery. 1996;39:194–202.

Snyder LA, Martinez-Del-Campo E, Neal MT, Zaidi HA, Awad AW, Bina R, et al. Lumbar spinal fixation with cortical bone trajectory pedicle screws in 79 patients with degenerative disease: perioperative outcomes and complications. World Neurosurg. 2016;88:205–13.

Youkilis AS, Quint DJ, McGillicuddy JE, Papadopoulos SM. Stereotactic navigation for placement of pedicle screws in the thoracic spine. Neurosurgery. 2001;48:771–8.

Yson SC, Sembrano JN, Sanders PC, Santos ER, Ledonio CG, Polly DW Jr, et al. Comparison of cranial facet joint violation rates between open and percutaneous pedicle screw placement using intraoperative 3-D CT (O-arm) computer navigation. Spine. 2013;38:E251–8.

The Complications of Robot-Assisted Spine Surgery

17

Wei Tian, Xiaohui Tao, and Sai Ma

Abstract

Responding complications of robot-assisted spine surgeries include hardware malposition and other injuries related to the robot-assisted method. Surgeons should pay more attention to the complications with different morbidities and consequences.

Keywords

Robot · Spine surgery · Complication Pedicle screw

Robot-assisted spine surgeries have been performed widely. However, various complications emerge, resulting in clinical consequence. Malposition of the instrumentation and other injuries related to the robot-assisted method are the most important complications.

1. Malposition of the Screw: Although the robot system is delicate theoretically, false position of screw might appear as a result of system or manual deviation, which could damage some vital structures near the pedicle, such as the spinal cord, nerve root, muscle, vessel, and associated internal organs (Wang et al. 2015).

   Pechlivanis et al. reported that 31 patients were used a novel robotic system to complete the posterior percutaneous pedicle screw insertion. A total of 133 pedicle screws were placed, in which there was 1 screw that was categorized to group C (axial plane) and D (longitudinal plane) in the postoperative evaluation (Pechlivanis et al. 2009). In this patient, CT scan showed that the position of this screw was different from the original plan. An accidental slippage of this screw occurred because of the oblique pedicle wall, which might be the most possible reason, and the author tried to modify the fixation tools to prevent the occurrence of slippage.

   Ringel et al. reported that a total of 298 pedicle screws were implanted in 60 patients (group of freehand (FH), 152; group of robot-assisted (RA), 146) (Ringel et al. 2012). About 93% had good positions (A or B) in FH and 85% in RA. There were 7 patients with 10 pedicle screws in RA changing to the FH method, in which the robot-guided drill hole was misplaced away from the correct pedicle trajectory. One patient in FH had a severe radicular pain postoperatively as a result of a misplaced screw, and the author had to perform a second surgery to revise the group E screw.

W. Tian (✉) · X. Tao · S. Ma
Department of Spine Surgery, Beijing Jishuitan Hospital, Fourth Clinical Hospital of Peking University, Beijing, China
e-mail: tianweijst@vip.163.com

W. Tian (ed.), *Navigation Assisted Robotics in Spine and Trauma Surgery*,
https://doi.org/10.1007/978-981-15-1846-1_17

Schatlo et al. reported that a perfect trajectory was observed in 204 screws (83.6%) in the robot group (Schatlo et al. 2014). In three cases, the author found the insert point guided by the robot was not pointing directly on the anatomical center of the pedicle. Thus, a new screw trajectory was made with the lateral fluoroscopy.

Although robot-guided system is a safe and effective tool for placement of pedicle screw in cases of degenerative spine, technical aberration remains, and freehand method with fluoroscopy should be the necessary backup.

The reasons of malposition of instrumentation could be divided into two parts. One is skidding of the cannula. Most entry points for pedicle screws are on the slope of the lateral aspect of the facet joint rather than on the top, especially in cases of degenerative facet joint hypertrophy. Therefore, the slope can get steep giving rise to a lateral skidding of the cannula at the entrance point because cannula is not anchored to the bony entrance firmly. The other reason is disturbance of surrounding tissue. Influence of soft tissue is one of the many reasons for the deflection of the cannula from the planned trajectory. When the muscle was bluntly perforated by the cannula, any muscle bundles could interfere the direction of the cannula. Another reason is the bony block which arises at the S1 level. When the cannula was made in S1, converging screws coming from far lateral might get displaced by the iliac crest, resulting in a more medial trajectory.

2. The misplacement of pedicle screws could result in the secondary complications, which include any crucial organs injury. Clinical complications with the robot-assisted system included hemothorax (Barzilay et al. 2014), CSF leakage, and pulmonary embolism (Urakov et al. 2017). Devito presented reversible neurological complications in 4 of 593 (0.7%) cases with the robot-assisted method for pedicle screw placement (Devito et al. 2010); however, freehand group had higher rates of dural tears (four compared with one) when compared with robot-assisted group (p = 0.142) (Keric et al. 2017). Moreover, Schatlo and Solomiichuk reported radiculopathic nerve root injury in a fluoroscopy-guided procedure, but none in the robot-assisted group (Schatlo et al. 2014; Solomiichuk et al. 2017).

Kantelhardt et al. reported a lower rate of postoperative infection in robot-guided procedures (2.7%) when compared with open non-robotic group (10.7%) (Kantelhardt et al. 2011). Therefore, some of the infection cases were required operative intervention, in which there were 10 cases including 0.6% percutaneous procedures, 12.6% open robotic-guided procedures, and 12.2% open procedures.

Keric et al. noted a higher rate of wound infection in either the open surgery group (20.8%) or the robot-assisted percutaneous group (10.6%) (Keric et al. 2017). One of the open procedures was treated by antibiotics, and surgical intervention were performed in four cases. Meanwhile, in robot-assisted group, three patients were resolved by antibiotics as compared with four whose complications required additional surgery.

References

Barzilay Y, Schroeder JE, Hiller N, Singer G, Hasharoni A, Safran O, et al. Robot-assisted vertebral body augmentation: a radiation reduction tool. Spine. 2014;39(2):153–7.

Devito DP, Kaplan L, Dietl R, Pfeiffer M, Horne D, Silberstein B, et al. Clinical acceptance and accuracy assessment of spinal implants guided with SpineAssist surgical robot: retrospective study. Spine. 2010;35(24):2109–15.

Kantelhardt SR, Martinez R, Baerwinkel S, Burger R, Giese A, Rohde V. Perioperative course and accuracy of screw positioning in conventional, open robotic-guided and percutaneous robotic-guided, pedicle screw placement. Eur Spine J. 2011;20(6):860–8.

Keric N, Eum DJ, Afghanyar F, Rachwal-Czyzewicz I, Renovanz M, Conrad J, et al. Evaluation of surgical strategy of conventional vs. percutaneous robot-assisted spinal trans-pedicular instrumentation in spondylodiscitis. J Robot Surg. 2017;11(1):17–25.

Pechlivanis I, Kiriyanthan G, Engelhardt M, Scholz M, Lucke S, Harders A, et al. Percutaneous placement of pedicle screws in the lumbar spine using a bone mounted miniature robotic system: first experiences and accuracy of screw placement. Spine. 2009;34(4):392–8.

Ringel F, Stuer C, Reinke A, Preuss A, Behr M, Auer F, et al. Accuracy of robot-assisted placement of lumbar and sacral pedicle screws: a prospective randomized comparison to conventional freehand screw implantation. Spine. 2012;37(8):E496–501.

Schatlo B, Molliqaj G, Cuvinciuc V, Kotowski M, Schaller K, Tessitore E. Safety and accuracy of robot-assisted versus fluoroscopy-guided pedicle screw insertion for degenerative diseases of the lumbar spine: a matched cohort comparison. J Neurosurg Spine. 2014;20(6):636–43.

Solomiichuk V, Fleischhammer J, Molliqaj G, Warda J, Alaid A, von Eckardstein K, et al. Robotic versus fluoroscopy-guided pedicle screw insertion for metastatic spinal disease: a matched-cohort comparison. Neurosurg Focus. 2017;42(5):E13.

Urakov TM, Chang KH, Burks SS, Wang MY. Initial academic experience and learning curve with robotic spine instrumentation. Neurosurg Focus. 2017;42(5):E4.

Wang H, Zhou Y, Liu J, Han J, Xiang L. Robot assisted navigated drilling for percutaneous pedicle screw placement: a preliminary animal study. Indian J Orthop. 2015;49(4):452–7.

18

Robot-Assisted Free Vascularized Fibular Grafting for the Treatment of Osteonecrosis of the Femoral Head

Shanlin Chen and Wei Tian

Abstract

Placing the tip of the fibula at the center of the load-bearing region of the femoral head, close to the subchondral plate, is essential for the treatment of osteonecrosis of the femoral head in pre-collapse stage by free vascularized fibular grafting. The orthopedic robot-assisted system could help us to insert the guide pin and place the fibula precisely, thereby allowing the tip of the fibula to be inserted into the optimal anatomical position and maximizing its mechanical efficacy.

Keywords

Surgical robot · Avascular necrosis of femoral head · Free vascularized fibula grafting

Placing the tip of the fibula at the center of the load-bearing region of the femoral head, close to the subchondral plate, is essential for treatment of osteonecrosis of the femoral head (ONFH) in pre-collapse stage by free vascularized fibular grafting. The orthopedic robot-assisted system could help us to insert the guide pin and place the fibula precisely, thereby allowing the tip of the fibula to be inserted into the optimal anatomical position and maximizing its mechanical efficacy.

1 Introduction

There are many surgical procedures that preserve the pre-collapse stage ONFH, with free vascularized fibular grafting (FVFG) being the most common (Yoo et al. 1992; Judet and Gilbert 2001; Edward et al. 2012).

FVFG is a complex treatment for ONFH. Essential aspects of the surgical procedure include thorough curettage of necrotic bone and filling of the cavity with cancellous bone or artificial bone, ensuring that the fibular graft does not penetrate the joint and that anastomosis allows blood flow in the fibular graft. Malizos (Malizos et al. 2004), Della Valle (Gonzalez Della Valle et al. 2005), and Beris (Beris and Soucacos 2001) suggest that placing the tip of the fibula in the optimal position—center of the load-bearing region of the femoral head, as close as possible to the subchondral bone—is the most important compared with the other factors. However, it is not easy to place the fibula in the optimal position in a 3D space, especially using the most common extracapsular technique. The orthopedic robot-assisted system

S. Chen
Department of Hand Surgery, Beijing Jishuitan Hospital, Fourth Clinical Hospital of Peking University, Beijing, China

W. Tian (✉)
Department of Spine Surgery, Beijing Jishuitan Hospital, Fourth Clinical Hospital of Peking University, Beijing, China
e-mail: tianweijst@vip.163.com

W. Tian (ed.), *Navigation Assisted Robotics in Spine and Trauma Surgery*,
https://doi.org/10.1007/978-981-15-1846-1_18

could help us to insert the guide pin and place the fibula precisely, thereby allowing the tip of the fibula to be inserted into the optimal anatomical position and maximizing its mechanical efficacy.

1.1 Indications

1. Hip pain and positive findings for femoral head changes on radiography and magnetic resonance imaging (MRI).
2. Patients younger than 50 years of age, Ficat stage II and early-stage III osteonecrosis, Steinberg stages III and IV, and Marcus stages II, III, and IV.
3. Patients younger than 20 years of age with stage V disease and a good range of motion of the hip are eligible for the procedure.

1.2 Contraindications

1. Age older than 50 years.
2. Hip arthrosis.
3. Bilateral lower-extremity vasculopathy based on either symptomatic claudication or absence of distal pulses.

2 Problems with the Traditional Method and Advantages of Robotic Surgery

FFVG is a complex procedure, and complications are not uncommon. Most surgeons agree with "Precise placement of the bone graft supporting the subchondral plate might be the most important factor in deterring subchondral collapse" (Malizos et al. 2004; Gonzalez Della Valle et al. 2005; Beris and Soucacos 2001).

Thus, the key to fibula grafting for the treatment of ONFH is to place the tip of the fibula at the center of the weight-bearing area. The smaller the angle between the fibular axis and the longitudinal axis of the body, the stronger the supporting effect on the subchondral bone plate. The risks of the surgery are mainly due to operational difficulties, such as operating under traditional fluoroscopy, improper identification of the center of the necrotic area, and manual guide pin insertion impeded by femoral neck anteversion.

With the assistance of an orthopedic robot system, the surgeons can perform surgical planning based on intraoperative 3D images and guide the pin to be accurately positioned, thereby allowing the tip of the fibula to be inserted into the optimal anatomical position and maximizing its mechanical efficacy.

3 Surgical Procedures

1. Anesthesia and positioning. General anesthesia, supine position.
2. The descending branch of the lateral circumflex femoral artery was exposed (Fig. 18.1), and a patient tracer was placed at the medial side of the femur (Fig. 18.2). A 10 cm longitudinal incision was made on the side of the anterolateral part of the thigh to expose the descending branch of the lateral circumflex femoral artery and veins between the vastus lateralis and rectus femoris, free toward the proximal end. The lateral circumflex femoral artery was exposed between the rectus femoris and vastus medialis, and free blood vessels could reach lengths of 10 cm or above. The vastus intermedius was exposed, and blunt

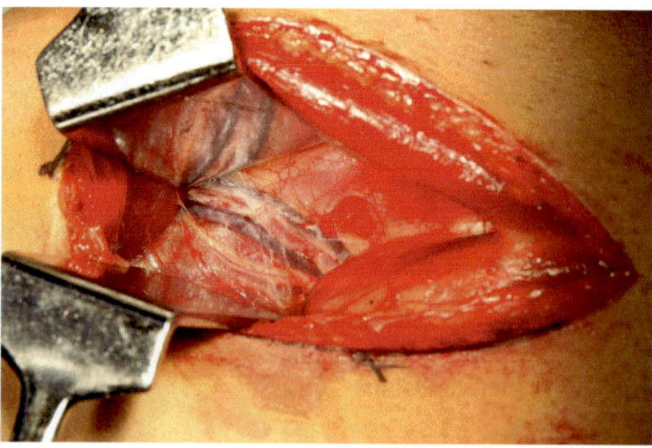

Fig. 18.1 The descending branch of the lateral circumflex femoral artery is exposed between the rectus femoris and vastus medialis, and free blood vessels could reach lengths of 10 cm or above. The branches of the femoral nerve along the course of the vessels should be saved

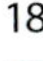

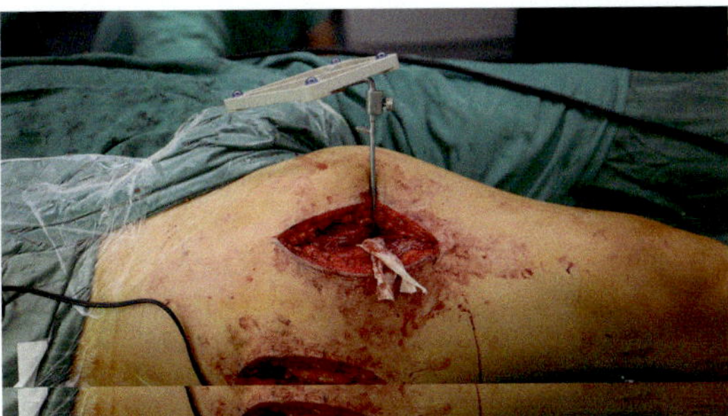

Fig. 18.2 The vastus intermedius is exposed, and the medial femoral cortex is revealed by blunt dissection. A patient tracer was firmly fixed here

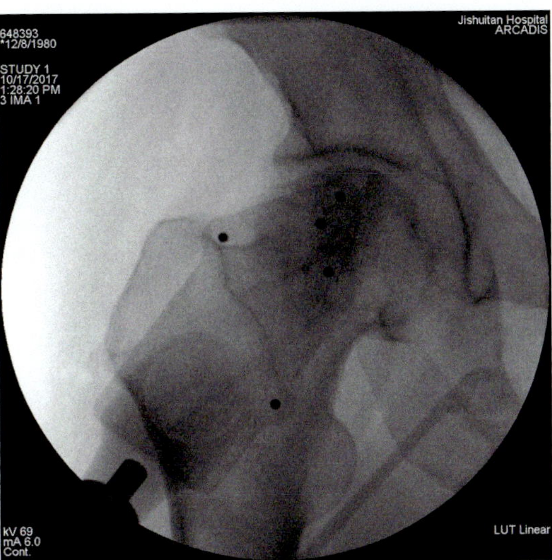

Fig. 18.3 The hip position is confirmed by fluoroscopy after the patient tracer is fixed, requiring that the frontal and lateral hip, femoral neck, and proximal femur were included in the fluoroscopic images, and four markers at least could be seen on the screen

dissection revealed the medial femoral cortex. Patient tracer was firmly fixed before we confirmed the hip position by fluoroscopy, requiring that the frontal and lateral hip, femoral neck, and proximal femur were included in the fluoroscopic images (Fig. 18.3).

3. The robot and scanning system were then registered, and the ARCADIS Orbic 3D system (Siemens Medical Solutions, Germany) was used to scan the hip joint of the patient. The raw 3D data generated from the scan was uploaded on the orthopedic surgical robot workstation. The workstation was used to plan the entry point and target of the guide pin (Fig. 18.4).
4. The workstation controls the robotic arm, guides it to place a sleeve in the optimal position, and inserts and calibrates the sleeve for the guide pin (Fig. 18.5).
5. A guide pin that was threaded at the top with a diameter of 2.8 mm is inserted along the sleeve, and the length of insertion is based on the preoperative plan. An intraoperative CT scan is performed to confirm that the path and the tip position of the guide pin are satisfactory before the robot-assisted part of the surgery is considered complete (Fig. 18.6).
6. A bone window is made around the entry point, and cancellous bone is harvested from the bone window. And then open up a bone tunnel and grind the necrotic area of the femoral head. We may select a cannulated drill with a diameter of 9 mm to open up a bone tunnel along the guide pin. The depth of the tunnel was in accordance with the plan produced by the robot. Using intraoperative fluoroscopy to ensure that the tip of the cannulated drill is placed at the planned target point. A high-speed grinding bur is used to drill the surrounding bone cortex at the entry point and open up a bone window until it is large enough to accommodate the fibula. Cancellous bone around the bone window is chiseled and reserved for later use. The diameter of the bone tunnel is gradually expanded by using a reamer that enlarges in diameter (to a maximum of 14 mm). This step is carried out under fluoroscopy also (Fig. 18.7). By inserting a specially designed scraping knife (up to 30 mm in diameter) that has an enlargeable tip into the necrotic area of the femoral head, we can remove the sclerotic necrotic bone (Fig. 18.8). Finally, the bone knife diameter is reduced to about 20 mm and pulled out while rotating in order to further expand the bone tunnel to make it sufficient to accommodate the fibula.
7. The ipsilateral vascularized fibula is harvested (Fig. 18.9), and the cancellous bone and/or artificial bone is used to fill the cavity after grinding the necrotic area of the bone.

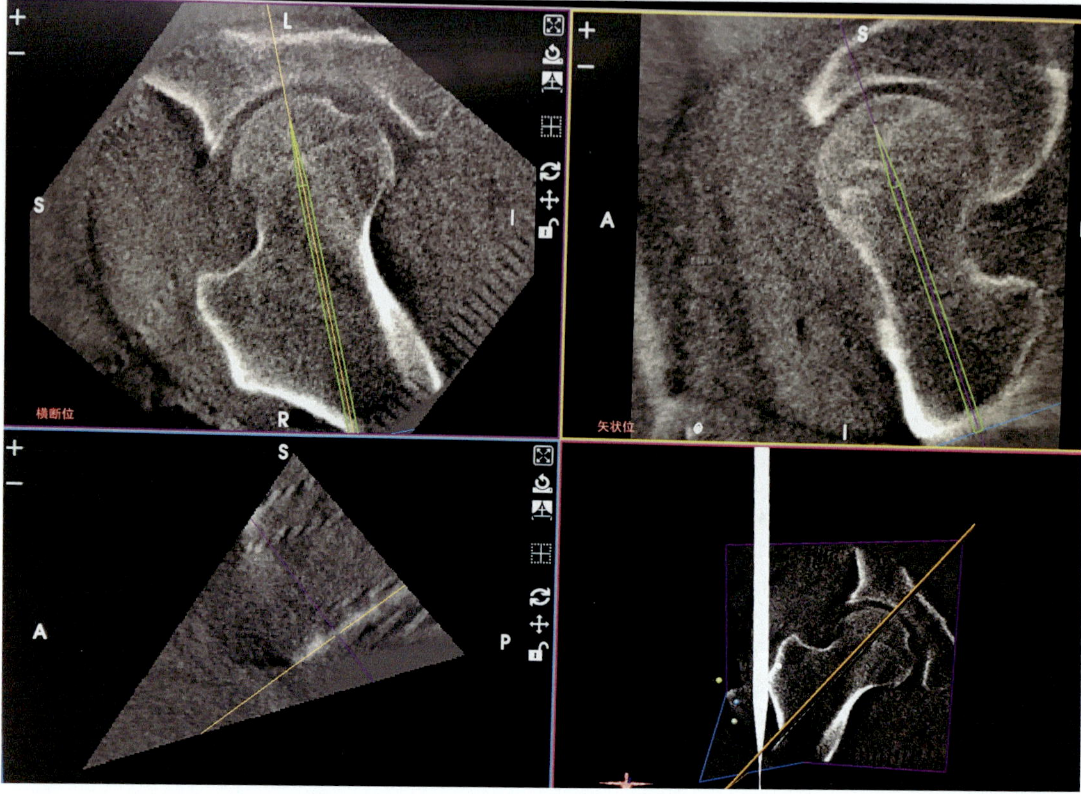

Fig. 18.4 The raw 3D data generated from the scan was uploaded on the orthopedic surgical robot workstation. Doctors could set the implant path of the guide pin based on the newly matched 3D raw image, which included the target (center of the load-bearing region of the femoral head, 4–6 mm from the articular surface), entry point, and length of the required fibula

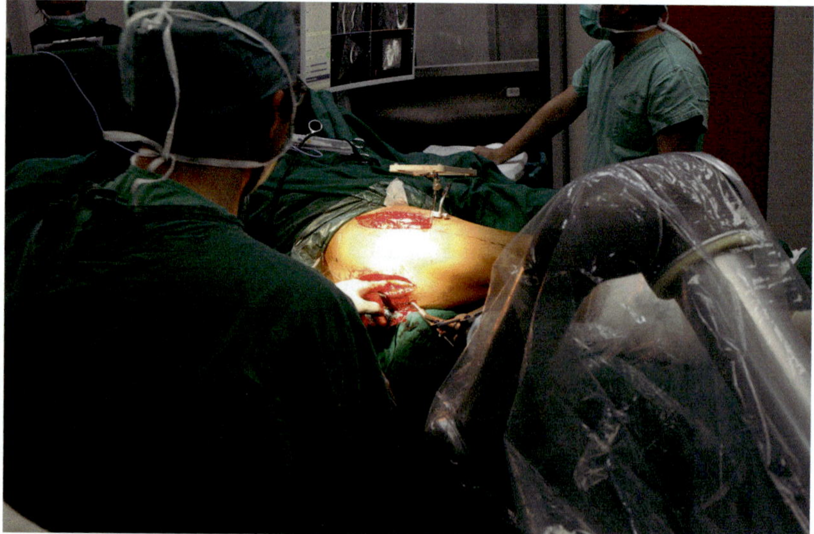

Fig. 18.5 The workstation controls the robotic arm and guides it to place a sleeve in the optimal position. A guide pin that was threaded at the top with a diameter of 2.8 mm is inserted along the sleeve, and the length of insertion is based on the preoperative plan

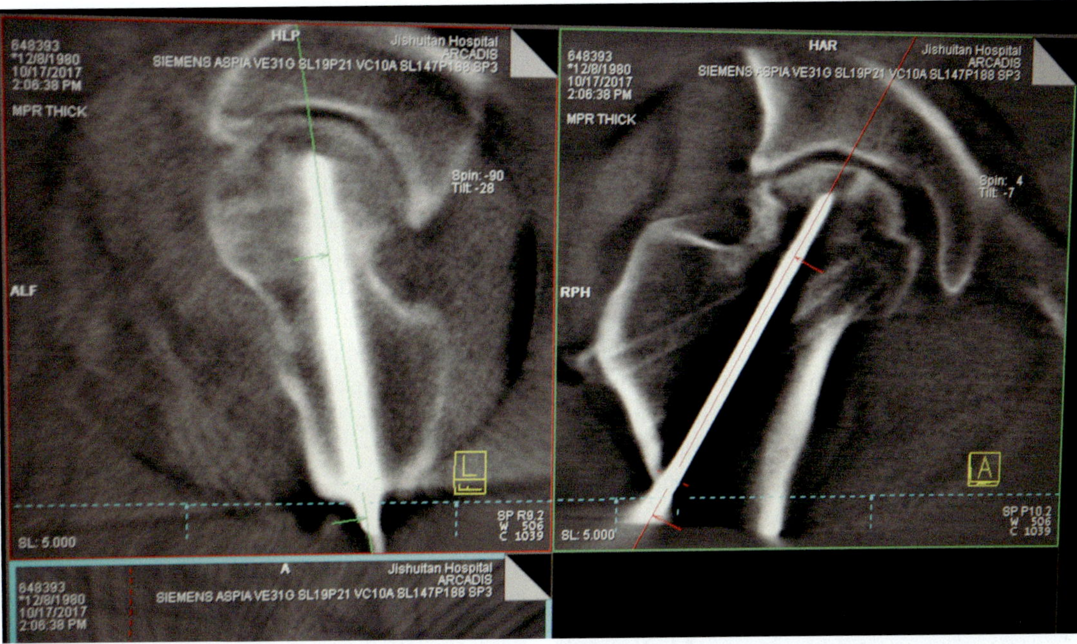

Fig. 18.6 An intraoperative CT scan is performed to confirm that the path and the tip position of the guide pin are satisfactory before the robot-assisted part of the surgery is considered complete

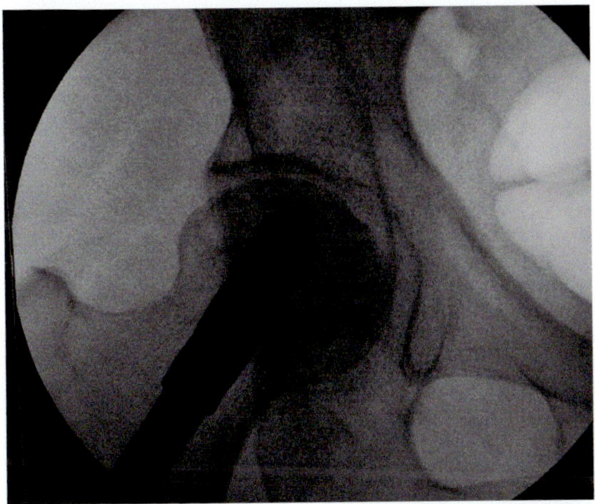

Fig. 18.7 A hollow drill is chosen with a diameter of 10 mm to open up a bone tunnel along the guide pin, and then the tunnel is gradually expanded by using a reamer that enlarges in diameter (to a maximum of 14 mm). This step is carried out under fluoroscopy also

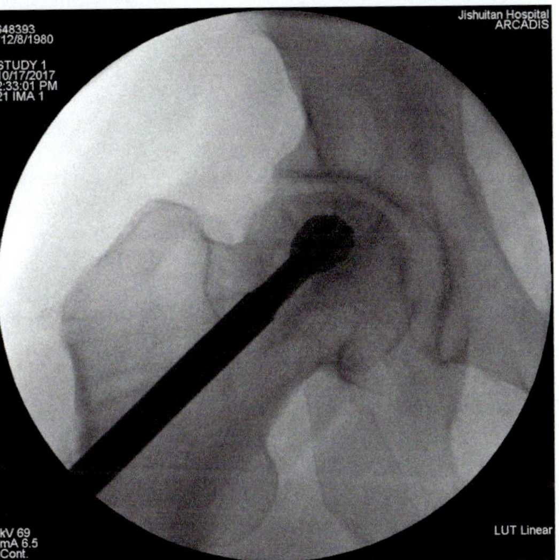

Fig. 18.8 By inserting a specially designed scraping knife (up to 30 mm in diameter) that has an enlargeable tip into the necrotic area of the femoral head, we can remove sclerotic necrotic bone

8. The fibula is inserted into the bone tunnel, and placement was confirmed with the use of fluoroscopy. First, the fibula is trimmed, and 1 cm of periosteum at the distal severed end is elevated toward the proximal end to excavate sclerotic bone and the sharp edge of the severed end. The contralateral periosteum of the vessel pedicle is stripped to reveal the protruding spine. A high-speed bur is used to make the appearance "smooth," making insertion easier. After a trial insertion, depending on the situation, it may be necessary to expand the tunnel entrance and the tunnel itself until the fibula can be successfully inserted. A large amount of saline is used to rinse the surgical area before the cancellous bone and artificial bone are implanted into the lesion area, using a bone grafting instrument for suppression and compaction. The fibula is inserted with caution to protect the fibular vessels. After grafting the fibula, its end is tapped to ensure the distal end would be as close as possible to the subchondral bone. The fibular artery and veins are extracted through the bone channel and reserved. Intraoperative fluoroscopy is used to examine the removal of lesions and bone graft and to confirm the ideal position of the distal end of the fibula (Fig. 18.10).
9. Finally, anastomosis of the vessels is performed (Fig. 18.11).

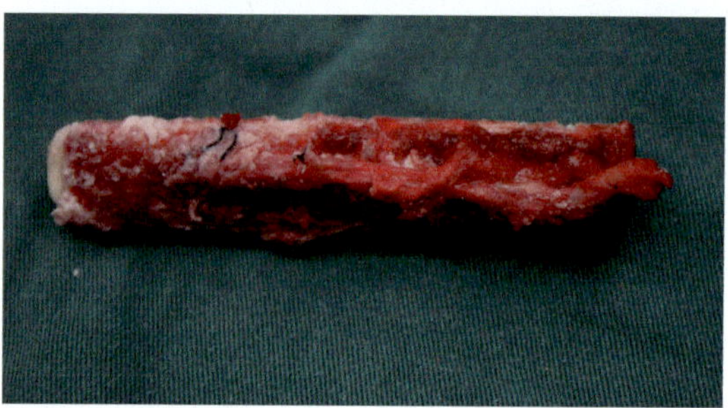

Fig. 18.9 The ipsilateral vascularized fibula is harvested. The length of fibula is in accordance with the requirements of the computerized plan and measurements

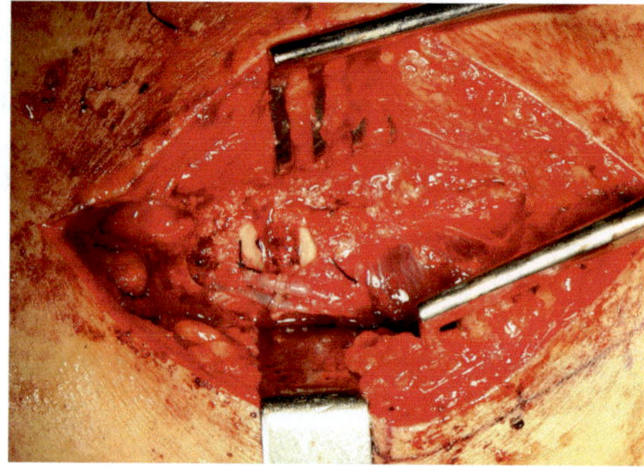

Fig. 18.11 Under a microscope with 9-0 microscopic sutures, the descending branch of the lateral circumflex femoral artery and the fibular artery was separately anastomosed

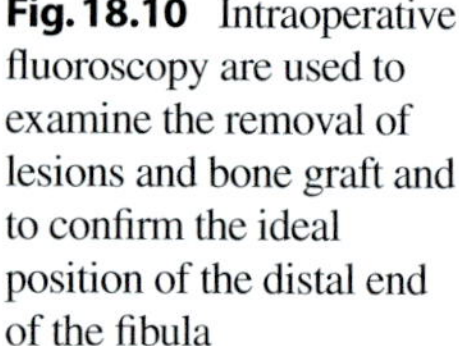

Fig. 18.10 Intraoperative fluoroscopy are used to examine the removal of lesions and bone graft and to confirm the ideal position of the distal end of the fibula

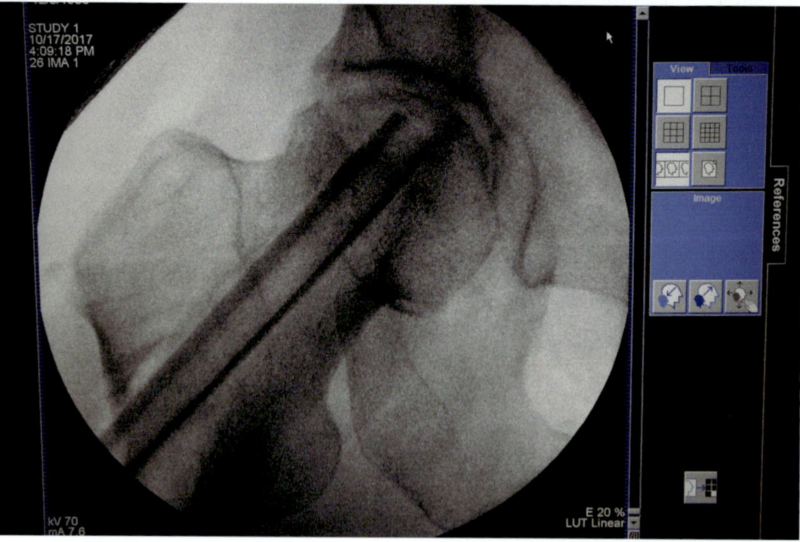

4 Postoperative Treatment

The patients undergo vasodilation, anticoagulant, antispasmodic, and anti-infective treatments for a week, after which a radionuclide scan is performed to examine the blood flow in the free vascularized fibula. Patients rest in bed completely for 2 weeks and are gradually able to sit and stand after that period. Three weeks after surgery, the patients engage in non-weight-bearing functional activities for the hip joint. From the fifth week, they may walk with crutches. The affected limb does not bear weight for 3 months, after which the patients practice walking while-bearing weight. They are able to walk without crutches 6 months after the surgery.

5 Typical Case

A 55-year-old female, with femoral head necrosis in Ficat stage II on the right side (Fig. 18.12).

The planed tunnel accommodates the fibular designed by robot system (Fig. 18.13). Anteroposterior view and lateral view (Fig. 18.14a, b) radiographs of the hip joint 6 months after operation showed the tips of the fibulae were placed at the center of the load-bearing region, 4–6 mm from the articular sur-

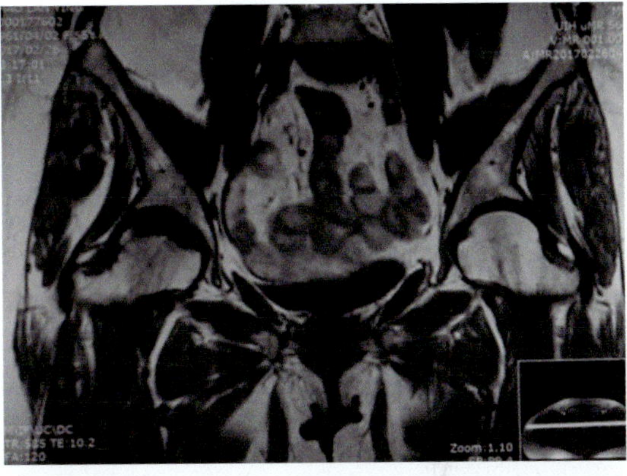

Fig. 18.12 A 55-year-old female, with femoral head necrosis in Ficat stage II on the right side

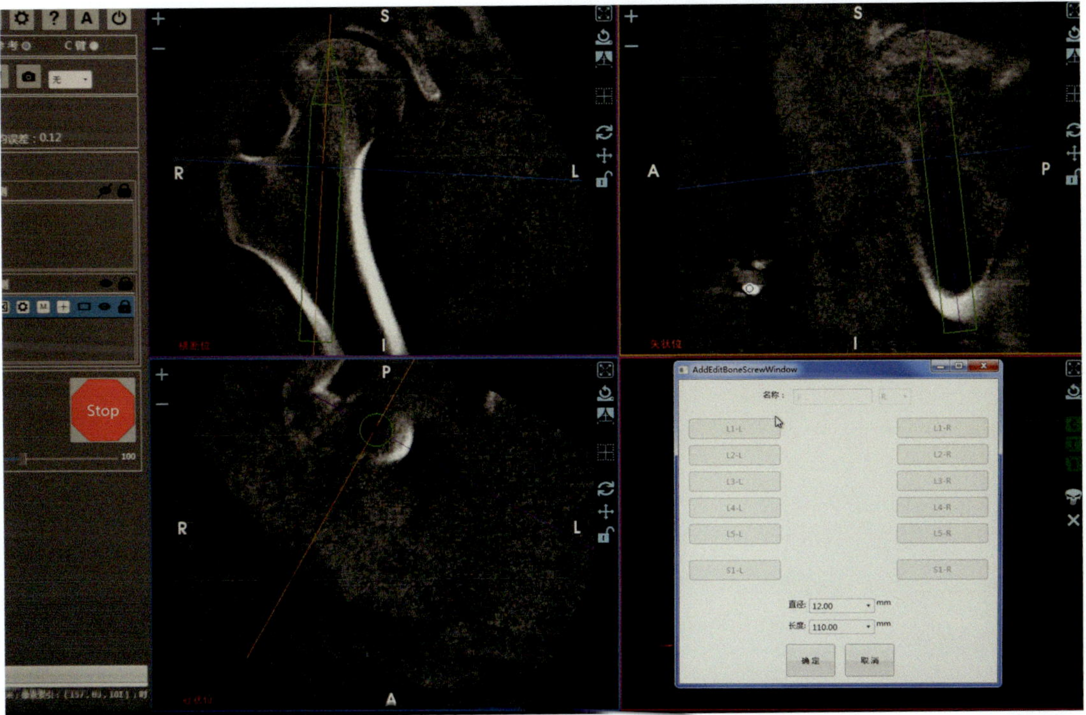

Fig. 18.13 The planed tunnel which accommodate the fibular designed by robot system

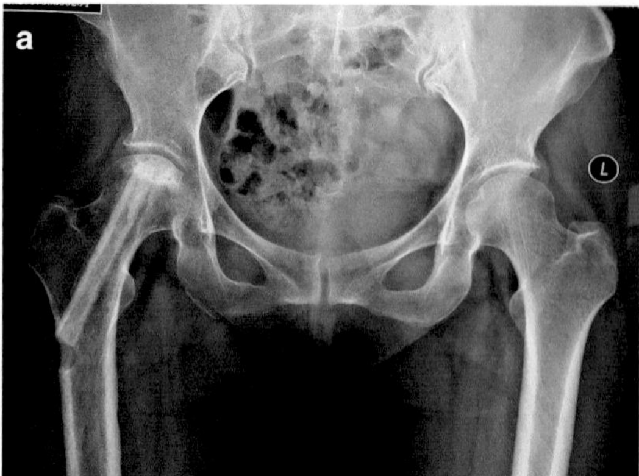

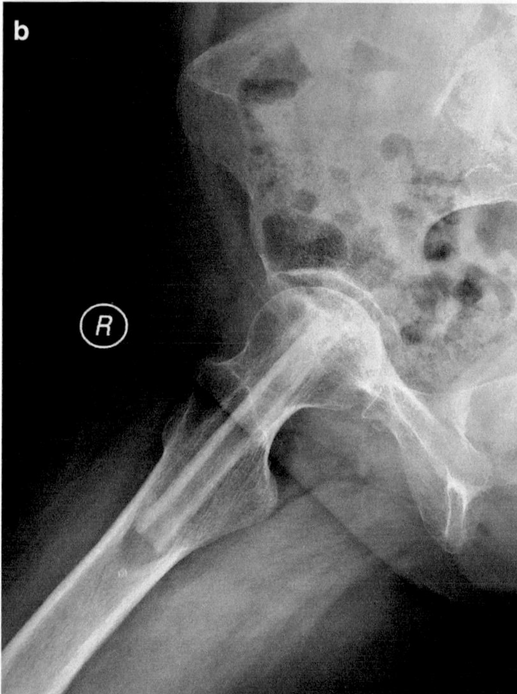

Fig. 18.14 (**a**, **b**) The anteroposterior view and lateral view of 6 months post-op x-rays

face, and did not penetrate the joint. Hip pain disappeared totally and she was satisfied with the final result according to the 2-year follow-up.

References

Beris AE, Soucacos PN. Optimizing free fibular grafting in femoral head osteonecrosis. The Ioannina aiming device. Clin Orthop. 2001;386:64.

Edward WC, Rineer CA, Urbaniak JR, et al. The vascularized fibular graft in precollapse osteonecrosis: is long-term hip preservation possible? Clin Orthop Relat Res. 2012;470(10):2819–26.

Gonzalez Della Valle A, Bates J, Di Carlo E, et al. Failure of free vascularized fibular graft for osteonecrosis of the femoral head: a histopathologic study of 6 cases. J Arthroplast. 2005;20(3):331–6.

Judet H, Gilbert A. Long-term results of free vascularized fibular grafting for femoral head necrosis. Clin Orthop Relat Res. 2001;386:114–9.

Malizos KN, Quarles LD, Dailiana ZH, et al. Analysis of failures after vascularized fibular grafting in femoral head necrosis. Orthop Clin N Am. 2004;35:305–14.

Yoo MC, Chung DW, Hahn CS. Free vascularized fibular grafting for the treatment of osteonecrosis of the femoral head. Clin Orthop Relat Res. 1992;277:128–38.

19 An Overview of Robotic Applications in Traumatic Orthopedics

Xinbao Wu, Yu Wang, Gang Zhu, Junqiang Wang, and Wei Tian

Abstract

This chapter gives an overview of the research status of traumatic orthopedics robot. Also, the application of robot-assisted navigation system in traumatic orthopedics at Beijing Jishuitan Hospital is introduced. There are a lot of researches for traumatic orthopedics robot; however, due to the complexity of the procedures of traumatic orthopedics and the significant individual differences in patients' conditions, the application of these robots in trauma is relatively rare. In traumatic orthopedic surgery, surgical robots generally play two major roles: robotic-assisted screw navigation and robotic-assisted reduction. Some of the navigation robots have been applied in clinical. However, the reduction robots, which are still in the laboratory prototype stage, have not been used clinically.

X. Wu · J. Wang
Trauma Orthopedic, Beijing Jishuitan Hospital, Fourth Clinical Hospital of Peking University, Beijing, China
e-mail: wuxinbao@jst-hosp.com.cn

Y. Wang · G. Zhu
School of Biological Science and Medical Engineering, Beihang University, Beijing, China
e-mail: wangyu@buaa.edu.cn

W. Tian (✉)
Department of Spine Surgery, Beijing Jishuitan Hospital, Fourth Clinical Hospital of Peking University, Beijing, China
e-mail: tianweijst@vip.163.com

Keywords

Robot-assisted navigation system · trauma orthopedic · Robotic-assisted reduction Overview · Clinic application · Research status

1 Research Status and Progress of Robots in Traumatic Orthopedics at Home and Abroad

Due to the complexity of the procedures of traumatic orthopedics and the significant individual differences in patients' conditions, the application of robots in trauma are relatively rare. In traumatic orthopedic surgery, surgical robots generally play two major roles: robotic-assisted reduction and robotic-assisted screw navigation. The former mainly achieves the correct reduction of the displaced bone after fracture, and the latter mainly achieves the accurate positioning of the fixation screw after the reduction.

The robot-assisted reduction technique, also known as reduction robot technique, is mainly to achieve a correct reduction of the displaced bone after fracture. Because the fractured bone is deeply buried under the skin, repeated fluoroscopy and large reduction force are required, which imposes a huge burden on the orthopedists.

W. Tian (ed.), *Navigation Assisted Robotics in Spine and Trauma Surgery*,
https://doi.org/10.1007/978-981-15-1846-1_19

The robot is expected to solve the problem of a large reduction force requirement and insufficient reduction accuracy during the reduction procedure. Some researchers in the world have conducted researches on fracture reduction robots. Since 2005, the University of Tokyo and Osaka University have jointly developed a surgical robot for assisting the reduction of fractures of the femur and femoral neck (Warisawa et al. 2004). Until now, the prototype of the surgical robot has been built; however, since the system can only achieve the reduction through an indirect way, it has not been widely recognized in the clinical setting. The University of Rosenberg and Brunswick Engineering University have been using the 6-degrees-of-freedom (DOF) manipulator for the development of a direct fracture reduction robot since year 2006 (Füchtmeier et al. 2004). The master–slave remote manipulation is adopted, and a large 6-DOF manipulator with a high payload is used to provide the large reduction force. However, the manipulator structure results in the system body to be too large for clinical applications. In 2012, the University of West England launched a study on fracture reduction robots. They used a self-contained robot with a series-parallel hybrid structure to achieve fracture reduction inside the joint. And recently, the team used a somatosensory sensor device (Leap Motion) to realize noncontact robot control, and the results were presented at the 2017 ICRA meeting (Dagnino et al. 2015; Dagnino et al. 2017).

In China, the Harbin Institute of Technology also carried out a research on fracture reduction and developed a prototype of the fracture reduction robot based on the parallel robot structure. In addition, utilizing the advantages of static stiffness, positioning accuracy, payload/weight ratio, and stability of parallel robots, the Beijing Jishuitan Hospital and TINAVI (TINAVI Medical Technologies CO., Ltd., Beijing, China) have developed a 6-DOF parallel manipulator robot (PMR) for the reduction of long bone fractures. The system uses a 6-DOF joystick as the master end and the PMR as the slave end of the master–slave robot and manipulates the parallel reduction robot to perform the reduction operation by mapping method (Wang et al. 2013). Hung in Taiwan proposed a prototype system for the reduction robot of the operating bed type, which initially possesses automatic operation functions such as knee bending, thigh traction, and foot rotation (Hung and Lee 2010). Tang from the People's Liberation Army General Hospital developed a reduction system of the parallel robot based on preoperative CT and completed the specimen experiment (Tang et al. 2012).

The researches of screw navigation robot for traumatic orthopedics are slightly less than that for the joint and spinal surgery, which is mainly used for internal fixation or implant locking of the fractured end after reduction. The PinTrace orthopedic surgical robot system developed by Medical Robotics in Sweden can be used for navigation of femoral neck cannulated screw surgery (Lindequist 1992). The system uses a 6-DOF serial robotic arm to perform surgical navigation and uses a touchscreen for human–computer interaction. It was proven in clinical surgery that the system can improve the quality of surgery and reduce the cumulative radiation time during surgery. At present, the system has been marketed, but the market response is not satisfactory because the system is relatively simple in function, large in size, and expensive in price. The CRIGOS orthopedic surgical robot system (Brandt et al. 1999), jointly developed by Germany and France, is used to perform X-ray-guided orthopedic positioning. The system is based on intraoperative 2D X-ray images for surgical positioning and uses a miniaturized parallel robot for surgical navigation, which can assist the surgeon to complete the femoral neck cannulated screw surgeries and other operations. Currently, the system is in the principle prototype phase and has not been used in clinical practice. The Hebrew University of Jerusalem in Israel developed the MARS robotic system (Shoham et al. 2003) for assisting the distal locking of long intramedullary nails. The system adopts a small parallel robotic structure that is equivalent to SpineAssist (Sukovich et al. 2006) which can be attached to the intramedullary nail by means of a connection device. Then several X-ray films can be used to calculate the drilling path, and this small parallel robot is used to finally adjust the trajectory and complete the surgical navigation.

In China, Beijing University of Aeronautics and Astronautics (BUAA) took the lead in researching orthopedic robots, cooperating with Beijing Jishuitan Hospital and others to develop the first Chinese orthopedic navigation robot (Fig. 19.1) and carried out clinical application research of the system in different indications of orthopedic minimally invasive surgery (Wang et al. 2004; Yu et al. 2005).

In addition, Harbin Institute of Technology was among the earliest to carry out research on orthopedic robots and developed a teleoperation-assisted orthopedic robot system (Fu et al. 2004). The system uses Motorman's SV3 robot for surgical navigation and positioning and a 6-DOF parallel robot to perform traction and reduction of the affected limb and combines with the self-developed 7-DOF operating bed and automatic C-arm to assist the surgeon in completing the intramedullary nail procedure. The system integrates a variety of automated equipment, with a relatively complete surgical support function. However, it has not been able to be applied clinically due to its complexity and size.

In 2004, the Chinese University of Hong Kong developed a passive orthopedic robot to work out the instability of surgical operations under photoelectric navigation (Fig. 19.2) and successfully carried out a clinical application in trauma ortho-

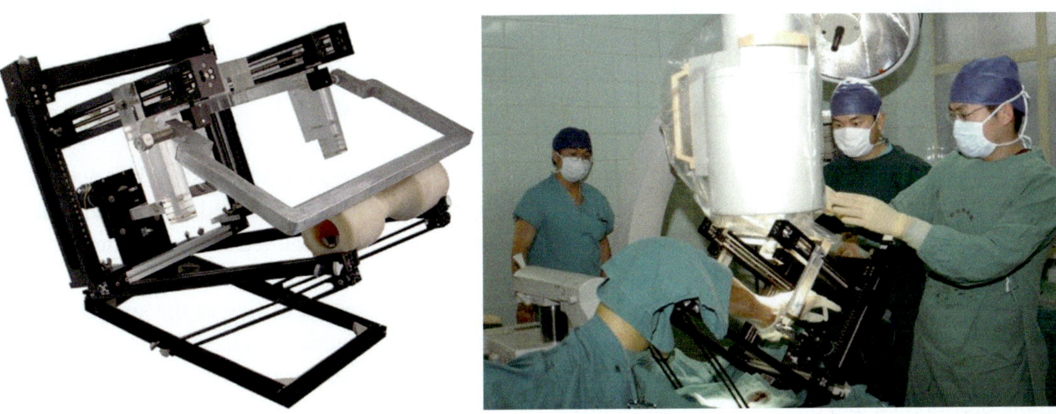

Fig. 19.1 Orthopedic navigation robot of BUAA

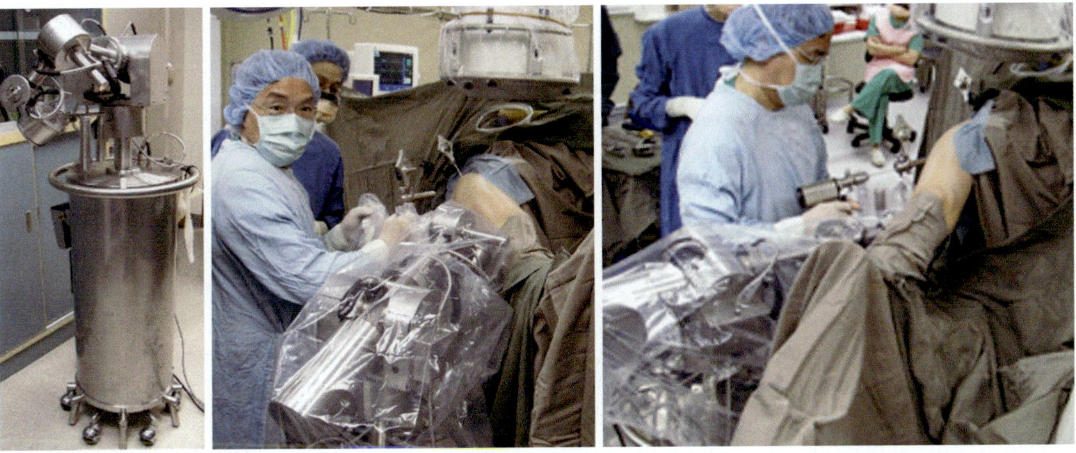

Fig. 19.2 Orthopedic robot at the Chinese University of Hong Kong

pedics (Kuang et al. 2012). The robot has a 6-DOF serial structure that uses an electromagnetic clutch for joint locking. In orthopedic surgery, the installation of a photoelectric tracer at the end of the robot enables the surgeon to operate the robot to the correct drilling position under the guidance of the photoelectric tracker and then lock the robot to stably hold the sleeve, ensuring that the path is not changed in the drilling process. So far, the system has completed over 20 clinical trials at the Prince of Wales Hospital of the Chinese University of Hong Kong and has achieved good results in improving the accuracy of surgery.

2 Overview of the Application of Navigation-Assisted Robot in Traumatic Orthopedics at Beijing Jishuitan Hospital

Beijing Jishuitan Hospital, Beijing University of Aeronautics and Astronautics, and TINAVI started the earliest research on orthopedic surgery robots in China for 15 years since 2002. They have succeeded in carrying out the first domestic case of robot-assisted orthopedic surgery, the world's first robot-assisted remote orthopedic surgery, and obtained the CFDA product registration certificate for the only orthopedic surgical robot in China. So far, three generations of orthopedic surgery robot products have been developed, and three CFDA product registrations for orthopedic surgery robots have been obtained. The third-generation product TiRobot® orthopedic surgery robot is currently the only orthopedic robotic system in the world that can perform full-spine, pelvic, and limb fracture surgery of international advanced level.

2.1 Robot Component

Orthopedic surgery robot, TiRobot® (TINAVI), consists of a robot arm, an optical tracking device, a surgical planning and controlling workstation, and surgical instruments.

The robot arm is an actuator for trajectory positioning in this system with 6 degrees-of-freedom (DOF). The optical tracking device is a binocular camera based on infrared light, where positioning error is smaller than 0.3 mm. The robot tracker and the patient tracker with reflection ballas are fixed, respectively. The optical tracking device locates the spatial position of the robot arm and the patient through the robot tracker and patient tracker correspondingly. The calibrator is used for acquiring mapping relation between the imaging space and the surgical space through fluoroscopic images matching coordinates in the calibrator images. The planning and controlling workstation are used for image processing, trajectory planning, coordinate calculating, data saving, and controlling robot arm movements.

2.2 Robot-Assisted Operation Principles

The robot-assisted surgical system has two major designs: (1) spatial guidance to obtain the spatial coordinates of the planned surgical trajectory and (2) trajectory positioning to control the movement of the robot according to the spatial coordinates of the planned trajectory and move the cannula system to the surgical position.

The system collects two fluoroscopic images using C-arm in different directions during the surgery for screw trajectory planning and spatial positioning. The imaging principle of C-arm conforms to the imaging principle of a pinhole camera, to acquire the spatial location of the surgical trajectory through a biplane localization algorithm. In controlling the movement of each joint of the robot arm, the sleeve fixed at the distal end of the robot arm will move exactly in reference to the planned trajectory. Firmly holding the sleeve, the operator can place guide wires along the sleeve, after which the cannulated screws can be inserted (Fig. 19.3).

The Department of Traumatic Orthopedics of Beijing Jishuitan Hospital used the TiRobot® orthopedic robot to perform minimally invasive surgery for pelvic acetabular fractures, percutaneous screw internal fixation for femoral

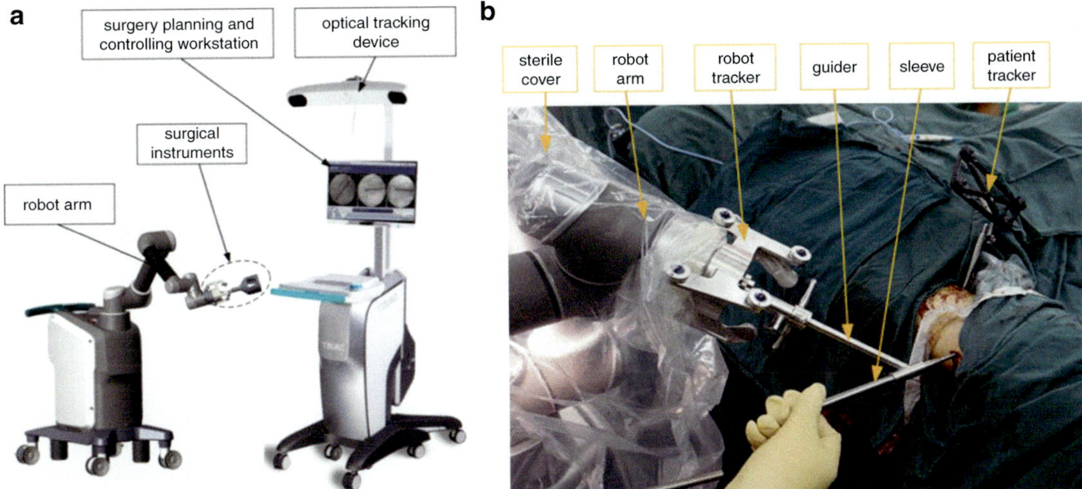

Fig. 19.3 (**a**) Main components of TiRobot®: a robot arm, an optical tracking device, a surgical planning and controlling workstation, and some surgical instruments. (**b**) Surgical instruments: robot arm is isolated by the sterile cover; robot tracker and patient tracker are fixed, respectively, at the distal end of the robot arm and on the patient; guider attaches to the robot arm and firmly holds the sleeve; sleeve can slide along the guider and invade patient

neck fractures, and multiple traumatic minimally invasive surgery for complicated pelvic fractures. Robot-assisted orthopedic minimally invasive surgery is a minimally invasive surgery based on image navigation and precise positioning of the robotic arm, which uses the intelligent and precise operation characteristics of the surgical robot. It is very suitable for percutaneous screw fixation for the treatment of fractures under image navigation and has the advantages of minimal invasion and accuracy and can reduce the time of intraoperative fluoroscopy and operation.

References

Brandt G, Zimolong A, Carrat L, et al. CRIGOS: a compact robot for image-guided orthopedic surgery. IEEE Trans Inf Technol Biomed. 1999;3(4):252–60.

Dagnino G, Georgilas I, Tarassoli P, et al. Design and real-time control of a robotic system for fracture manipulation. In: 2015 37th Annual International Conference of the IEEE Engineering in Medicine and Biology Society (EMBC). Piscataway, New Jersey: IEEE; 2015. p. 4865–8.

Dagnino G, Georgilas I, Morad S, et al. RAFS: a computer-assisted robotic system for minimally invasive joint fracture surgery, based on pre-and intra-operative imaging. In: 2017 IEEE International Conference on Robotics and Automation (ICRA). Piscataway, New Jersey: IEEE; 2017. p. 1754–9.

Fu L, Du Z, Sun L. A novel robot-assisted bone setting system. In: 2004 IEEE/RSJ International Conference on Intelligent Robots and Systems (IROS)(IEEE Cat. No. 04CH37566), vol. 3. Piscataway, New Jersey: IEEE; 2004. p. 2247–52.

Füchtmeier B, Egersdoerfer S, Mai R, et al. Reduction of femoral shaft fractures in vitro by a new developed reduction robot system 'RepoRobo'. Injury. 2004;35:S-A113-9.

Hung SS, Lee MY. Functional assessment of a surgical robot for reduction of lower limb fractures. Int J Med Robot. 2010;6(4):413–21.

Kuang S, Leung K, Wang T, et al. A novel passive/active hybrid robot for orthopaedic trauma surgery[J]. Int J Med Robot. 2012;8(4):458–67.

Lindequist S. PINTRACE: a computer program for assessment of pin positions in routine radiographs of femoral neck fractures. Comput Methods Prog Biomed. 1992;37(2):117–25.

Shoham M, Burman M, Zehavi E, et al. Bone-mounted miniature robot for surgical procedures: concept and clinical applications. IEEE Trans Robot Autom. 2003;19(5):893–901.

Sukovich W, Brink-Danan S, Hardenbrook M. Miniature robotic guidance for pedicle screw placement in posterior spinal fusion: early clinical experience with the SpineAssist®. Int J Med Robot. 2006;2(2):114–22.

Tang P, Hu L, Du H, et al. Novel 3D hexapod computer-assisted orthopaedic surgery system for closed diaphyseal fracture reduction. Int J Med Robot. 2012;8(1):17–24.

Wang T, Liu W, Hu L. BPOR: a fluoroscopy-based robot navigating system for distal locking of intramedullary nails. In: 2004 IEEE/RSJ International Conference on Intelligent Robots and Systems (IROS)(IEEE Cat. No. 04CH37566), vol. 4. Piscataway, New Jersey: IEEE; 2004. p. 3321–6.

Wang J, Han W, Lin H. Femoral fracture reduction with a parallel manipulator robot on a traction table. Int J Med Robot. 2013;9(4):464–71.

Warisawa S, Ishizuka T, Mitsuishi M, et al. Development of a femur fracture reduction robot. In: IEEE International Conference on Robotics and Automation, 2004. Proceedings. ICRA'04. 2004 2004 Apr 26, vol. 4. Piscataway, New Jersey: IEEE; 2004. p. 3999–4004.

Yu W, Chao Y, Lei H. Development of a compact orthopedic robot for distal locking of intramedullary nails. In: Proceedings of the 1st International Conference on Complex Medical Engineering, Japan 2005. Piscataway, New Jersey: IEEE; 2005. p. 183–7.

Research Study of Robotic-Assisted Pelvic Fracture Reduction

20

Xinbao Wu, Yu Wang, Gang Zhu, Junqiang Wang, Chunpeng Zhao, and Wei Tian

Abstract

This chapter reported some research works on reduction robot done by the Beijing Jishuitan Hospital. The main works include the designing for the structure of a reduction robot, the study on robot-assisted traction, the registration and tracking algorithm, and the master–slave operation method of the robot. This chapter will also mention the problems and disputes of robotic-assisted fracture reduction, which are the balance of the flexibility and the payload for a reduction robot, the lack of clinical reduction parameter, and the lack of a simulation system for robot testing before clinical application. Due to these problems, the fracture reduction robot will not be accepted by the orthopedist. We believe that the development of reduction robot in the future will be based on the answers to those questions.

X. Wu · J. Wang · C. Zhao
Trauma Orthopedic, Beijing Jishuitan Hospital, Fourth Clinical Hospital of Peking University, Beijing, China
e-mail: wuxinbao@jst-hosp.com.cn

Y. Wang · G. Zhu
School of Biological Science and Medical Engineering, Beihang University, Beijing, China
e-mail: wangyu@buaa.edu.cn

W. Tian (✉)
Department of Spine Surgery, Beijing Jishuitan Hospital, Fourth Clinical Hospital of Peking University, Beijing, China
e-mail: tianweijst@vip.163.com

Keywords

Pelvic fracture · Reduction robot · Research progress · Questions and disagreements Robot-assisted traction

1 Problems and Disputes of Robotic-Assisted Pelvic Fracture Reduction

Although many universities and research institutions have invested huge manpower, material resources, and financial resources to study fracture reduction robots, no product has entered the phase of large-scale clinical application until now.

This is due to the huge difference in the need for robot-assisted reduction surgery and robot-assisted positioning surgery. It is generally believed that since the bone is a rigid body structure, its geometry can be used as a basis for robotic operation planning during surgery. However, the fracture reduction is not just a simple spatial geometric movement, however a mechanical equilibrium process under the common constraints of many soft tissues. This is especially true for the pelvis. There are more than 20 important muscle ligaments attached on the pelvic ring. The pelvic fracture reduction process mainly needs to overcome the constraint force of soft tissues such as muscle ligaments. Therefore, in the robot-assisted pelvic reduction study, the reduc-

W. Tian (ed.), *Navigation Assisted Robotics in Spine and Trauma Surgery*,
https://doi.org/10.1007/978-981-15-1846-1_20

tion force and the operating space are a set of mutual trade-offs. Analysis of the existing problems of various fracture reduction robots has found that the following aspects need to be resolved:

The existing fracture reduction robot system cannot balance the operational flexibility and large load performance required for reduction. At present, the main configuration of the fracture reduction robot includes serial, parallel, and serial–parallel hybrid. Each arm of the serial robot is connected in series to perform the action, which has the characteristics of large operation space, high flexibility, and good maneuverability. However, some disadvantages exist in the fracture reduction robot with serial structures, such as small load–weight ratio, low positioning accuracy (caused by accumulated errors of each arm), and oversize. At present, some serial reduction robots are based on the development of a six-degree-of-freedom (DOF) industrial robot arm, having safety problems and being unable to be applied to the operating room environment. The parallel robot has the characteristics of large static stiffness, high positioning accuracy, large load–weight ratio, and good state maintenance, but it lacks operational flexibility. For the shortcomings of serial and parallel reduction robots, some researchers have proposed a serial–parallel hybrid configuration, hoping to effectively balance the operational flexibility and large load, but the control of the serial–parallel hybrid robot is more complicated. At present, there are no products that meet clinical requirements. Compared with the long bones such as the femur, the pelvic structure is complex, and the surrounding muscle and soft tissue are more abundant, the flexibility required for pelvic fracture reduction will be higher, and the reduction force will be greater. Therefore, the primary solution to be solved for the development of the pelvic fracture reduction robot system is how to ensure a flexible operation while providing a large reduction force.

1.1 Determination of the Mechanical Parameters of the Reduction Robot

Due to the bone-binding effect of the soft muscles and ligaments attached to the bone, it is necessary to provide a large restoring force during the fracture reduction to counteract the resistance of the soft tissues of the muscles and others. When the femoral shaft fracture is reduction, the required axial traction often reaches 250 N. However, due to the complex structure of the pelvis and the numerous muscles around the pelvis, the reduction force during the reduction of the pelvic fracture has not been reported yet, and this data is the key design parameter for the development of a pelvic fracture reduction robot that can be applied in clinical practice. How to obtain the mechanical parameters during the reduction of pelvic fractures is also an urgent problem to solve.

The current experimental research on fracture reduction robots is mostly carried out on the free bone. Considering the soft tissue of muscles, ligaments, and other soft tissues, there are few studies on the bone restraint. In order to simulate the actual operating environment more realistically, it is also important to construct a pelvic fracture reduction experimental platform containing soft tissues such as muscles and ligaments.

2 Structure and Procedure of Pelvic Fracture Reduction Robot System

Considering the complexity of pelvic fractures, parallel robots are difficult to meet the range of motion required for surgery. Therefore, we believe that the reasonable configuration of the pelvic fracture reduction robot is still a 6-DOF serial manipulator structure. At the same time, in order to solve the problem of insufficient reduction force of the robot, we introduced a robot-assisted traction device to resist the huge constraint force of muscles and soft tissues and reduce the required mechanical load of the mechanical arm to its rated load. The pelvic fracture reduction robot, TiRobot® orthopedic robot system, on its original basis, is equipped with a six-axis force-torque sensor (ATI mini45, USA) for real-time detection of forces and moments during reduction. The other end of the sensor is fitted with a fixed gripping kit, which is stably fixed by two handles on the iliac wing.

At present, sacroiliac screw internal fixation is a common treatment for sacroiliac (joint) fracture and dislocation. The surgical procedure can be described as: the doctor puts needle holders on the iliac wing and reduces the fractured pelvic with bare hands under the X-ray of the C-arm; then based on the surgeon's experience, under repeated X-ray fluoroscopy, 1–2 guide pins are inserted into the sacroiliac joint by bare hands. After reaming, the cannulated screw is inserted along the direction of the guide wire to the state of compression and fixation. And the guide wire should be taken out in the end. Such reduction process is time consuming and laborious, and the reduction effect is difficult to guarantee. The process is totally dependent on repeated X-rays and the personal experience of the surgeon. Moreover, repeated X-rays will cause radiation damage to both surgeons and patients. At the same time, the instability of the barehanded operation also increases the difficulty of surgery. In the experiment, we introduced traction equipment to balance the great constraint force of the muscles and ligaments around the pelvis. The positional correspondence between the preoperative computed tomography (CT) reconstructed three-dimensional (3D) model and the position of the intraoperative pelvis was established by registration. Under the guidance of the 3D model, the surgeon controls and operates the movement of machine through master–slave interaction, thus to achieve a closed fracture reduction. The application of the robotic system to assist the above fracture reduction process can significantly reduce the radiation damage to surgeons and patients from X-rays and reduce the errors caused by barehanded operation.

2.1 Experimental Study on Traction of Robot-Assisted Pelvic Fracture

The main significance of robot-assisted pelvic fracture traction is to balance the constraint force of muscle ligaments, and it generally uses the electric and pneumatic structures to realize the traction of one DOF of large load. In order to ensure the safety of traction, it is also necessary to implement a tracking system and a force sensor to implement double protection on force and position. In this study, an electric lower limb elastic traction platform was built using a gear-down motor, a roller linear guide, a 1D force sensor, etc.; see figure below at the right side. The system is fixed to the bed, the traction bow is elastically connected to the traction device by springs and ropes, and the 1D force sensor is used to measure the traction force on the elastic traction device (Fig. 20.1).

In this chapter, springs with different k values simulate the main muscle constraint forces near the pelvis. According to the study by Elabjer et al., 10 groups of muscles with great influence on pelvic displacement were selected in this study. And in accordance with the muscle properties reported in the literature, springs of different specifications were selected, and springs of different specifications were fixed by screws to the left side of the pelvis (affected side), thus simulating the restraining effect of surrounding muscles during pelvic reduction (see the upper left image). The radial muscles such as the gluteus medius and the gluteal muscle are simulated by a plurality of springs distributed in a certain area. The model consists of 10 groups, totaling 22 springs. The affected sacroiliac joint was separated to simulate the fracture of the dislocation that is common in clinical practice. When the fracture is caused, the affected pelvis undergoes a significant upward displacement under the force of the spring and the rotation of the book opening direction, which is consistent with the common clinical situation.

According to Bishop et al., this chapter selects the clinically commonly used path of iliac spine to iliac wing (channel 1) and the anterior inferior iliac spine to the greater sciatic notch (channel 2); then a screw holder 1 and the screw holder 2 of 5 mm diameter on the affected side is used for holding during reduction operation (Fig. 20.2). Two screw holders were inserted into the contralateral anatomical position for the fixation of the contralateral pelvis. The pelvic stabilization is achieved by the passive arm of multi-degree of freedom, so that the pelvis maintains the supine position commonly used in surgery.

In order to measure and record the reduction force during reduction, the experiment will install the reduction force-measuring device as shown in Fig. 20.3 to the screw holder. It is directly fixed to the screw holder by the quick connect device and will not change the physicians' operation habit of reduction. The reduction force measuring device mainly includes a

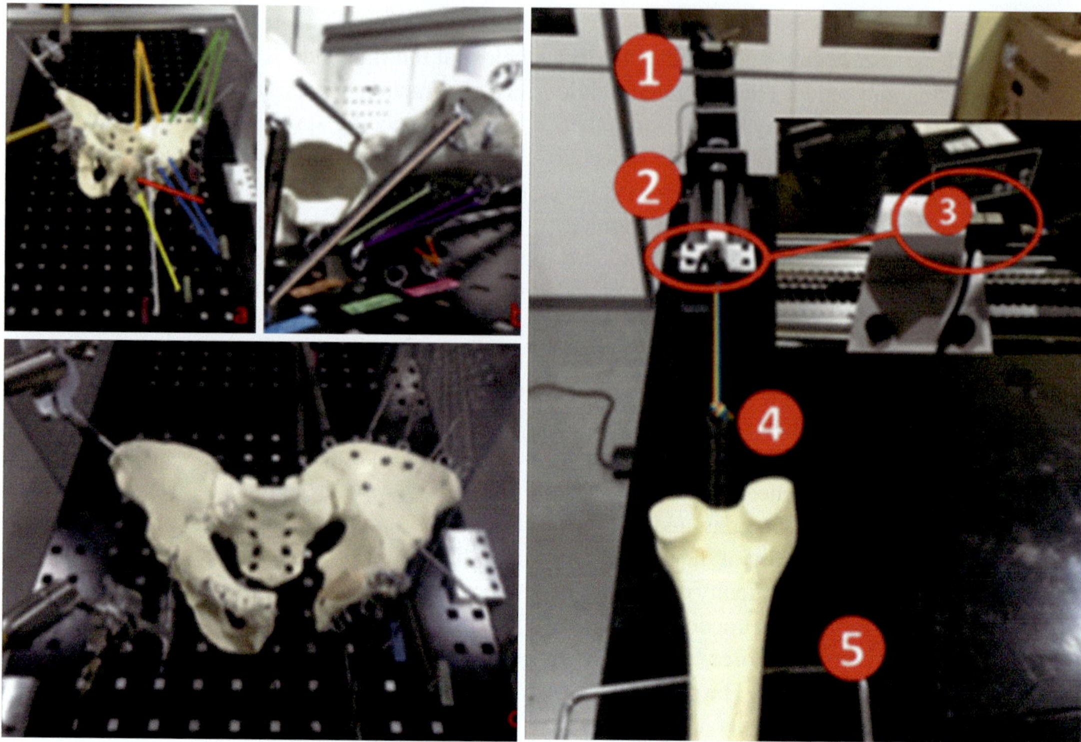

Fig. 20.1 Learning curve and reduction accuracy

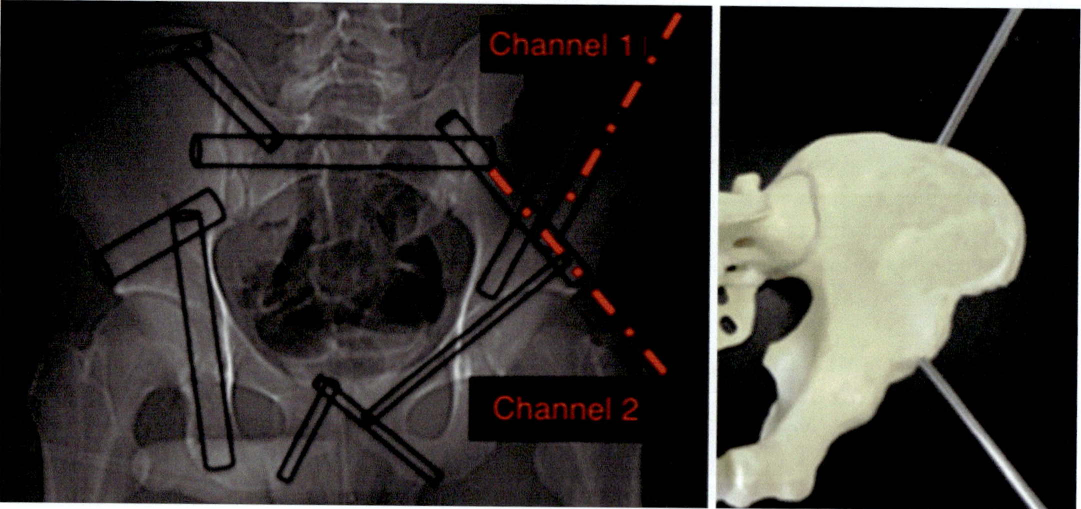

Fig. 20.2 Simulated reduction experimental platform and robot-assisted traction device for muscle pelvic fracture

quick connect device, an ATI 6D force sensor, and an operating handle. The ATI 6D force sensor and its associated acquisition software are used to measure and collect the reduction force, and the force in all directions during the reduction process is recorded in real time.

Repeated experiments were performed on the muscle constraint force simulation platform of the pelvic fracture reduction process. The tester held the two fixed needles at the same time to perform the reduction operation. When the pelvis returned to the anatomical position, it was

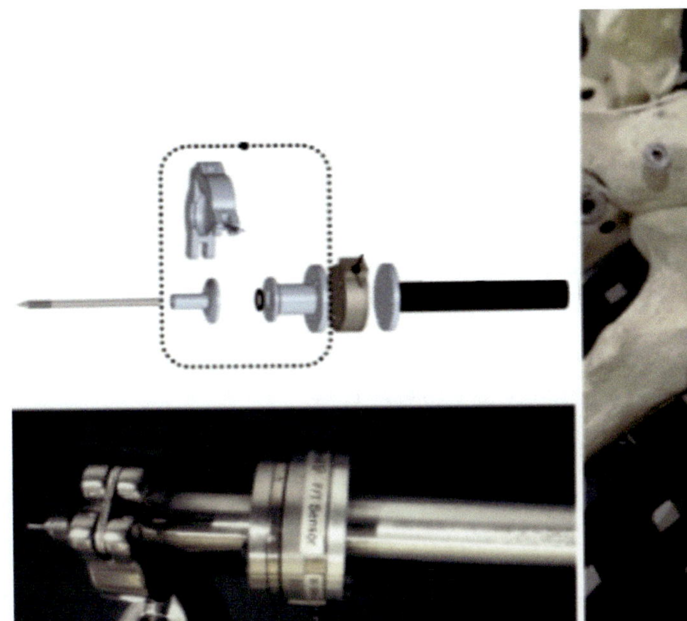

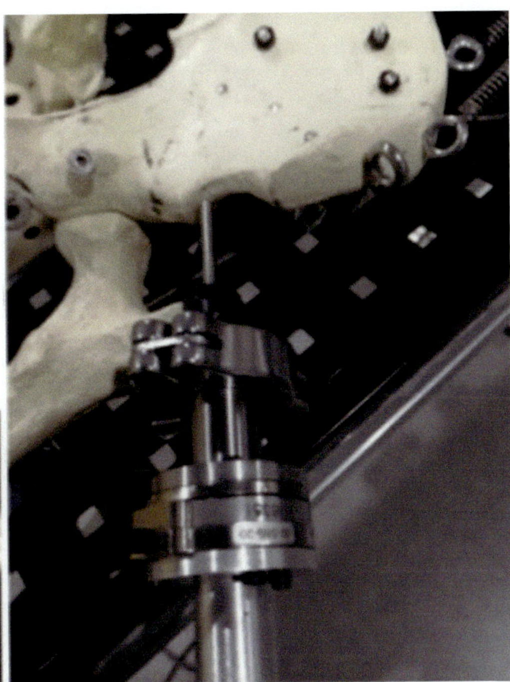

Fig. 20.3 Channel choosing of iliac spine

regarded as the completion of the reduction and the completion of an experiment when the correct reduction position was held for 10 s. Experiments were carried out under 0 kg, 5 kg, and 10 kg of lower limb tractive force, and each group of experiments were repeated five times. The reduction force data of 2 holding screws were measured, respectively, and the mechanical data of different lower limb traction forces were compared to analyze the effect of the lower limb elastic traction force on reduction force.

Experimental results show that the robot-assisted traction technology can reduce the reduction force required for the subsequent reduction operation to the rated working load (50 N) of the serial arm, thus becoming a limitation for solving the problem of insufficient reduction force of the robot (Fig. 20.4).

2.2 Registration Tracking Algorithm

In the experiment, the registration algorithm based on intraoperative fluoroscopy images is used to determine the spatial coordinates of several bone landmarks on the bone, and then match the corresponding bone markers on the preoperative CT.

Space positioning uses a special calibrator sleeve with an ATI force and torque sensor attached to the end and connected to the robot. Each point on the tool coordinate system can be converted to the robot end coordinate system by a known coordinate transformation matrix. During the X-ray filming phase, the sleeve is inserted between the X-ray digital plate and the see-through portion to obtain two positive side X-ray images (Fig. 20.5).

Since the image distortion of the flat C-arm is small, the imaging principle at any point P_i^{world} in the world coordinate system can be approximated by the pinhole model. At any shooting angle, there is

$$M \times P_i^{\text{world}} = \begin{bmatrix} m_{11} & m_{12} & m_{13} & m_{14} \\ m_{21} & m_{22} & m_{23} & m_{24} \\ m_{31} & m_{32} & m_{33} & m_{34} \end{bmatrix} \begin{bmatrix} x_i^{\text{world}} \\ y_i^{\text{world}} \\ z_i^{\text{world}} \\ 1 \end{bmatrix} = t \begin{bmatrix} u_i \\ v_i \\ 1 \end{bmatrix}$$

where the u_i, v_i is P_i of the image coordinates are obtained on the image by Hough transform, t is the normalization constant, and M is an affine

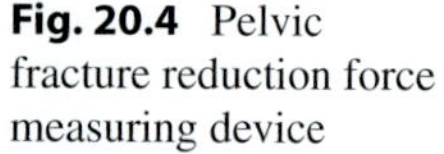

Fig. 20.4 Pelvic fracture reduction force measuring device

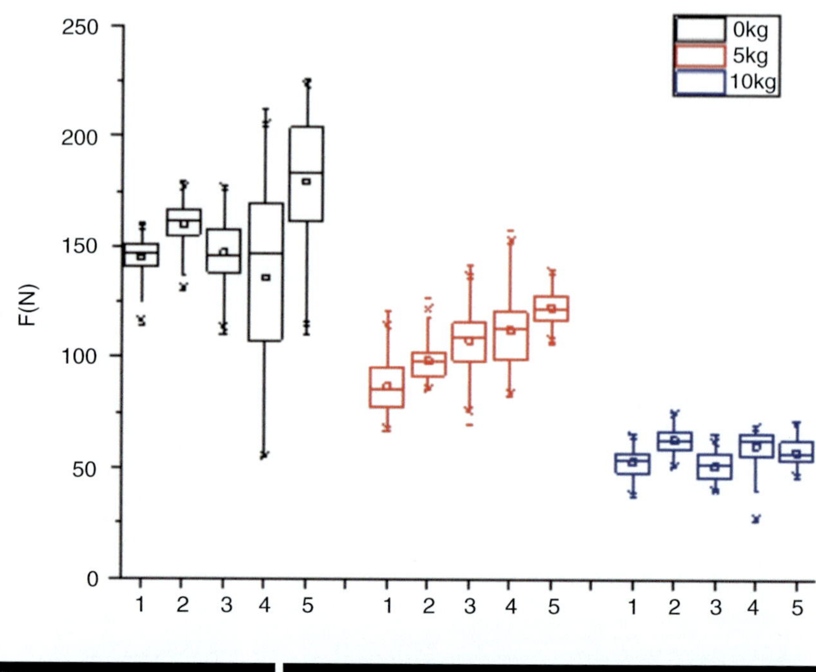

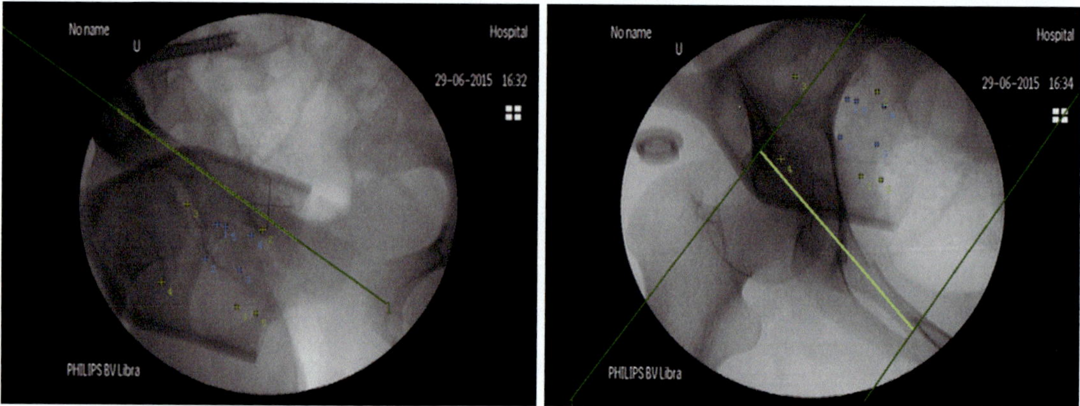

Fig. 20.5 Reducing force under traction assist is significantly reduced

transformation matrix. The M matrix has 12 unknowns; hence, with the space coordinates and image coordinates of more than six known points (in order to reduce the error, eight points are selected in this experiment), the M matrix can be obtained by the least square method.

The small steel ball on the calibrator can appear as a known point in the image because the scale tool is inserted between the C-arm launch and the patient during shooting. The spatial positions of these small steel balls are determined by the terminal pose of the connected robot. The position parameters (x, y, z, θ, φ, ϕ) relative to the NDI world coordinate system can be obtained by the NDI tracker fixed on the scale sleeve. The following coordinate transformation matrix exists, where

$$\begin{cases} r_{11} = \cos\psi \times \cos\varphi \\ r_{12} = \cos\psi \times \sin\varphi \times \sin\theta - \sin\psi \times \cos\theta \\ r_{13} = \cos\psi \times \sin\varphi \times \cos\theta + \sin\psi \times \sin\theta \\ r_{21} = \sin\psi \times \cos\varphi \\ r_{22} = \sin\psi \times \sin\varphi \times \sin\theta + \cos\psi \times \cos\theta \\ r_{23} = \sin\psi \times \sin\varphi \times \cos\theta - \cos\psi \times \sin\theta \\ r_{31} = -\sin\varphi \\ r_{32} = \cos\varphi \times \sin\theta \\ r_{33} = \cos\varphi \times \cos\theta \end{cases}$$

Therefore, there is a conversion relationship between the steel balls P_i on the calibrator and the tool hole A and tool hole B.

Based on the binocular vision principle, two different transformation matrices M_1, M_2 can be obtained at two different angles, and the marker points $P_{wi}(x_{wi}, y_{wi}, z_{wi})$ on the pelvis can be obtained. For any target points (u_{target}, v_{target}) on the image, there is an equation set:

$$\begin{cases} (u_{target}m_{31} - m_{11})X + (u_{target}m_{32} - m_{12})Y + (u_{target}m_{33} - m_{13})Z = m_{14} - u_{target}m_{34} \\ (v_{target}m_{31} - m_{21})X + (v_{target}m_{32} - m_{22})Y + (v_{target}m_{33} - m_{23})Z = m_{24} - v_{target}m_{34} \end{cases}$$

The solution of the equation is the spatial line connecting the optical center and the target point in space. The two spatial lines obtained at different shooting angles intersect at the target point. Considering the calculation error, the two straight lines may not intersect. Therefore, the spatial position P_{wi} of the target point relative to the robot base coordinate system is obtained by using the focus of the two straight lines of the vertical line as the target calculation result. In some open surgery, when more than three markers of the pelvis are exposed, the spatial location P_{wi} of the marker points can be obtained by clicking on the NDI probe.

The real-time tracking section is designed to combine the preoperative CT model with intraoperative NDI tracking device data so that doctors can see the entire bone without cutting the affected area. Before the operation, the CT image was established with Mimics. The pelvic reduction was taken as an example. The STL model was established for the left and right humerus, and the coordinates $P_{mi}(x_{mi}, y_{mi}, z_{mi})$ of the marker points for registration were obtained in the model coordinate system. When the passive control robot and the six-degree-of-freedom robot are, respectively, fixed to the left and right tibia, the NDI tracking targets are, respectively, installed at the ends of the passive arm and the active arm. In order to establish an optical tracking target (tracker) relationship with the model, a spatial positioning process is first required.

After positioning, the coordinates $P_{wi}(x_{wi}, y_{wi}, z_{wi})$, i = 1, 2, 3 of the feature points on the pelvis in the world coordinate system of the optical tracking device are obtained. At the same time, the optical tracking device transmits the coordinate transformation T_t^w between the optical tracking target and the tracking device world coordinate system. Thus,

$$P_{ti} = T_t^w \times P_{wi}$$

Create three coordinate points on the left and right ilium to establish a coordinate system:

$$\begin{cases} T = \left[\overset{\vee}{a}^T \ (\overset{\vee}{a} \times \overset{\vee}{b})^T \ (\overset{\vee}{a} \times \overset{\vee}{b} \times \overset{\vee}{a})^T \ P_{t1} \right] \\ \overset{\vee}{a} = P_{t1} - P_{t2} \\ \overset{\vee}{b} = P_{t2} - P_{t3} \end{cases}$$

With the same reason, it can obtain the following equation:

$$\begin{cases} T_b^m = \left[\overset{\vee}{a}^T \ (\overset{\vee}{a} \times \overset{\vee}{b})^T \ (\overset{\vee}{a} \times \overset{\vee}{b} \times \overset{\vee}{a})^T \ P_{m1} \right] \\ \overset{\vee}{a} = P_{m1} - P_{m2} \\ \overset{\vee}{b} = P_{m2} - P_{m3} \end{cases}$$

Make the optical tracking device world coordinate system coincide with the 3D environmental coordinate system. For any point $P(x, y, z)$ on the pelvis, there is a relationship:

$$T_m^c \times T_b^m \times P = T_t^w \times T_b^t \times P, \ T_m^c = T_t^w \times T_b^t \times \left(T_b^m\right)^{-1}$$

Since the optical tracking device can provide position information T_t^w at a high frequency, with the above formula, the relative position of the bone block can be continuously updated in the 3D model display environment, thereby realizing 3D implementation tracking (Fig. 20.6).

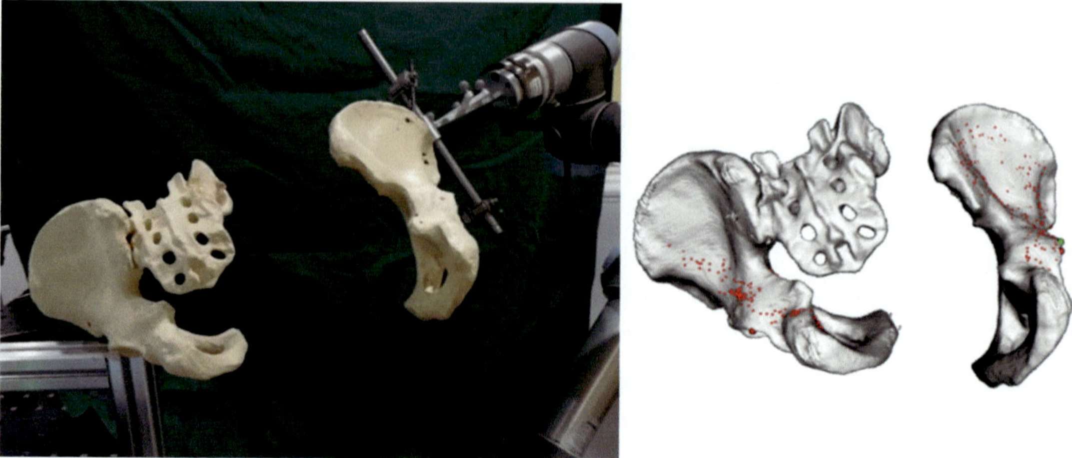

Fig. 20.6 Intraoperative X-ray image-based positioning

2.3 Study on Master–Slave Operation of Pelvic Fracture Reduction Robot

For complex pelvic fracture reduction requirements, it is still necessary to rely on doctors' experience to achieve the reduction operation, that is, in the real-time tracking of the bone block, the master–slave operation mode in which the robot controls the robot to gradually reduction. Based on the sterility of the operating room and the need for sensing force during reduction, this book provides two master–slave modes of operation in the laboratory phase.

One is a reduction control mode based on somatosensory interaction. This is a noncontact master–slave control mode that uses a somatosensory interactive camera (Kinect V2, USA) to track human bones, recognize the movements of the human body, and achieve master–slave control of the robot. Considering the complexity of the pelvic structure and the uncertainty of the reduction task, we collect the position information of the one-handed gesture and the palm of the human hand as a control signal in real time. Gestures are divided into hands, fists, and pointing movements (the index and middle fingers are straight and close together, and the other refers to the fist; this position is called lasso). Due to the lack of precision of the somatosensory camera and the stability of the human hand, it is difficult for us to master the pelvic robot reduction with master–slave control that is completely consistent with the gesture. Here, we use the gesture signal as a switch to control the robot to translate or rotate in a certain direction at a constant speed and stop at a suitable position. The speed of movement can be adjusted by two pointing actions. The control command in the coordinate system of the somatosensory camera is converted to the motion in the robot coordinate system, and the coordinate conversion relationship of the motion direction is:

$$\overset{\vee}{V}_{\text{robot}} = R_{\text{tool}}^{\text{base}} \times R_{\text{NDI}}^{\text{tool}} \times R_{\text{moving}}^{\text{NDI}} \times \overset{\vee}{V}_{\text{moving}}$$

$$\overset{\vee}{W}_{\text{robot}} = R_{\text{tool}}^{\text{base}} \times R_{\text{NDI}}^{\text{tool}} \times R_{\text{moving}}^{\text{NDI}} \times \overset{\vee}{W}_{\text{moving}}$$

The relevant control methods are as follows: (1) Define the control hand and mode hand: In this study, due to the left pelvic fracture, we define the left hand as the control hand and the right hand as the mode hand; (2) control the hand information acquisition: in order to prevent misoperation, the robot only receives motion information while controlling a fist. When controlling the hand fist, the system records the spatial position of the control hand as the initial position until the control hand state becomes the hand, and the initial position is cleared; (3) the mode hand information acquisition: the mode hand state information is used to control the motion mode. When the mode hand state is the hand, the corresponding motion is the translation; when the mode hand is the fist, the corresponding is the rotation; when the mode hand is the pointing, the corresponding is the increase or decrease of the speed; (4) the movement direction is determined: the somatosensory camera continuously collects and controls the palm of the hand. The position information is compared with the initial position, and the direction in which the motion is maximum is considered to be the desired direction of motion, thereby completing the decoupling of the motion direction. As shown in (Fig. 20.7), (5) during the operation, the force signal of the robot is detected in real time. As a safety factor, the control robot stops protecting the soft tissue and nerve in time.

The ergonomic experiments of senior clinicians show that this control method has a learning time period, the reduction accuracy meets the clinical needs, and has the natural noncontact anti-infective advantage and is expected to be applied to the robot reduction control in the future clinical.

In addition, the reduction robot in this chapter can also be controlled in real time using force feedback devices (Omega 7, Switzerland). This control method eliminates the sterility advantage of noncontact control and increases equipment cost but has the advantage of allowing the end mechanical signal to be fed back to the operator in real time, which is of significant value in dangerous surgery involving sacral nerves exposure due to sacral foramina fracture. As shown in the figure, the force feedback device has 7-DOF and the advantages of high rigidity and good stability. It can be used as an operating lever to control the movement of the robot and can also feedback the force received by the end sensor of the robot to make the operator feel human. The force feedback device is a parallel mechanism close to the base part, providing three degrees of freedom of position. The rear end series mechanism provides 3-DOF of posture, and the end of the device is a holding position with a holding degree of freedom. Due to the parallel structure limitation of the force feedback device, the device has a small moving space; thus, we use the seventh clamping degree of freedom as the switching quantity of the motion. When the degree of freedom is the clamping state, the force feedback device moves synchronously with the robot. When the DOF is released, the force feedback device movement does not affect the robot pose (Fig. 20.8).

In general, the robot master–slave reduction time of the pelvic model bone is about 3–6 min, and 3D image navigation is used throughout. Since only X-ray images are needed during the

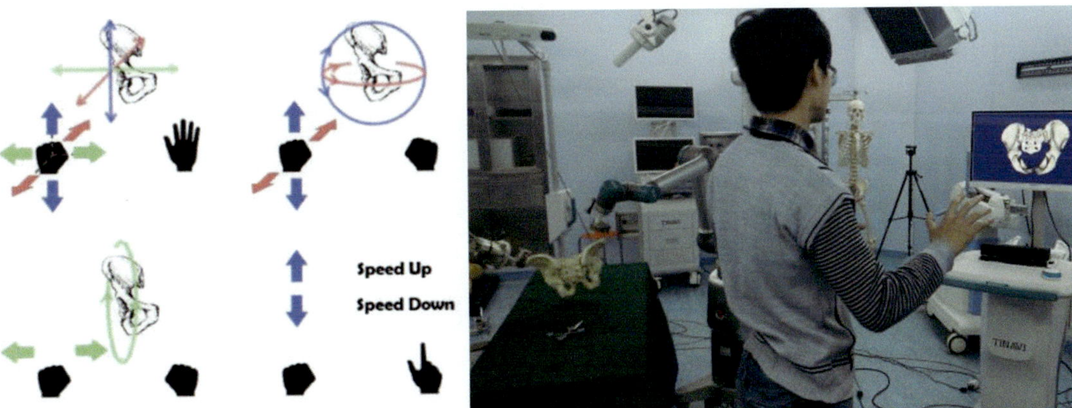

Fig. 20.7 Real-time tracking of reduction robot and bone block

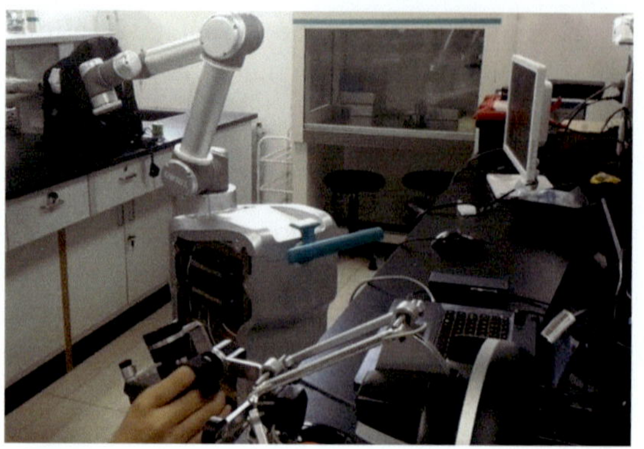

Fig. 20.8 Somatosensory interaction control method and scene

registration process, the operation time can be reduced, and the amount of surgical radiation can be reduced. Considering the possible errors in registration, the model bone test error of general robot-assisted pelvic fracture surgery is 5 mm, which is in line with clinical application requirements. With the development of registration and control technology, it is expected to achieve more accurate anatomical reduction (Fig. 20.9).

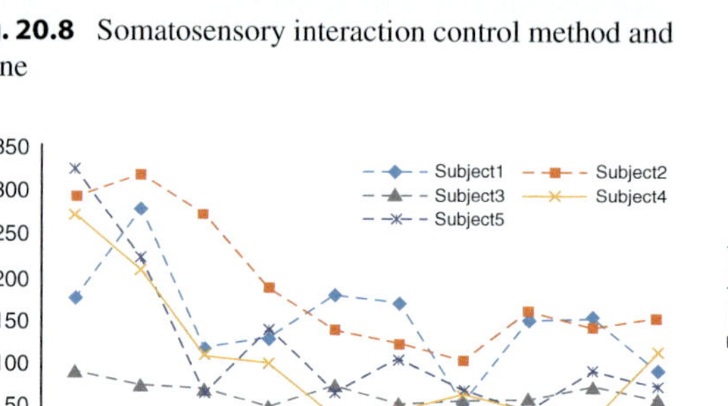

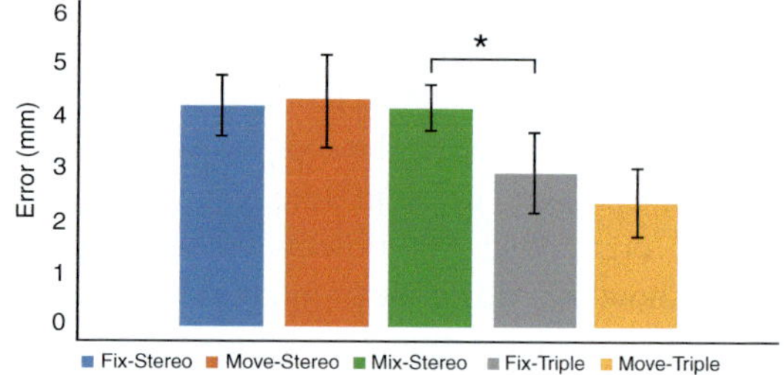

Fig. 20.9 Master–slave control based on force feedback

21 Application of Navigation-Assisted Robot in Internal Fixation of Fracture

Junqiang Wang, Xinbao Wu, Chunpeng Zhao, Wei Han, Teng Zhang, Meng He, Li Zhou, Yonggang Su, and Wei Tian

Abstract

This chapter mainly describes the application of navigation-assisted robot in internal fixation of fracture. There are many deficiencies in the traditional surgical treatment of pelvic acetabular fracture and femoral neck fracture. The appearance of robot solves these problems and provides a precise treatment scheme for the fracture. Taking TiRobot orthopedic surgery robot as an example, this chapter describes in detail the standardized operation procedure of the percutaneous cannulated screw internal fixation for femoral neck fracture and pelvic acetabular fracture, including sacroiliac joint, acetabular column, and symphysis of the pubis. The practical results of clinical cases were given. The advantages of robot-assisted orthopedic surgery are summarized, and the shortcomings and future development of the robot are pointed out.

Keywords

Navigation-assisted robot · Application Pelvic acetabular fracture · Femoral neck fracture · Percutaneous cannulated screw fixation

1 Robot-Assisted Pelvic Acetabular Fracture Percutaneous Fixation

1.1 Background

Pelvic acetabular injuries are mostly caused by high-energy injuries, accounting for about 3% of all orthopedic fractures, while the mortality rate is as high as 13.4%, and more than half of patients accompanied with other injuries (Wong et al. 2015). Pelvic acetabular fractures are generally considered to be a complex problem in orthopedics because pelvic fractures are mostly unstable, and damage to the pelvis and loss of stability can also cause damage to surrounding soft tissues and other bone injuries. As well as complications, especially in the early stages of such fractures, complications such as hemorrhagic shock are easily caused, which can easily threaten the life of the patient. Therefore, if the treatment of pelvic fracture type injury is not appropriate, it is easy to cause poor recovery and disability.

J. Wang · X. Wu · C. Zhao · W. Han · T. Zhang
M. He · L. Zhou · Y. Su
Trauma Orthopedic, Beijing Jishuitan Hospital, Fourth Clinical Hospital of Peking University, Beijing, China
e-mail: wuxinbao@jst-hosp.com.cn; suyonggang@pku.org.cn

W. Tian (✉)
Department of Spine Surgery, Beijing Jishuitan Hospital, Fourth Clinical Hospital of Peking University, Beijing, China
e-mail: tianweijst@vip.163.com

W. Tian (ed.), *Navigation Assisted Robotics in Spine and Trauma Surgery*,
https://doi.org/10.1007/978-981-15-1846-1_21

The reduction technique of pelvic and acetabular fractures usually adopts open reduction and internal fixation, but such traditional reduction method has large incision, large amount of bleeding, and great physical damage to the patient, and traditional open reduction and internal fixation surgery are likely to cause intraoperative blood vessels or neurological injuries, with prominent postoperative infections and other complications.

With the development of computer and navigation technology, minimally invasive orthopedics has gradually developed into a new trend in the treatment of acetabular pelvic injuries. For minimally invasive surgery for pelvic and acetabular fractures, percutaneous screw placement is typically performed by fluoroscopic guidance or fluoroscopy-based computer navigation guidance. Compared with the operation of conventional fluoroscopy, the navigation-assisted sacroiliac joint screw internal fixation has obvious advantages in the fluoroscopy time: the fluoroscopy time of the sacroiliac screw placement under navigation guidance is about 0.14–2.10 min, and the intraoperative fluoroscopy time of the freehand operation is about 1.40–4.40 min; in the accuracy of screw placement, the accuracy of the navigation-guided sputum screw can reach more than 95%, and the hand is free. The accuracy of the operation is about 76–95% (Eastman and Routt Jr 2015). However, the structure of the pelvis is complicated, the fracture position is deep, and the bony passage is relatively narrow. Compared with the traditional surgery mainly relying on the doctors' personal experience, the navigation-based treatment can increase the accuracy of screw placement and reduce the accuracy. X-ray radiation can cause damage, but it is more suitable for patients with small fracture displacement and closed reduction (Von Keudell et al. 2015). Moreover, even if the navigation tool can accurately locate and guide the surgical tool to reach the target position, it is limited by the instability of the manual operation and the pelvic region and its strict surgical positioning requirements, and the ideal fracture fixation effect is still more difficult to achieve in real surgical operations. With recent advancement of surgical robot technology, orthopedic surgery robots have also begun to enter the field of orthopedic applications, such as robotic positioning system for femoral neck fractures, assisted femoral neck fractures, cannulated screw internal fixation, and robotic positioning system for pelvic fractures. Assisted sacroiliac joint screw fixation, orthopedic robots can improve the operation accuracy of traditional surgical operations, improve the surgical treatment effect, and reduce the damage of fluoroscopy radiation to the surgeon and the patient (Li et al. 2014).

The robotic-assisted acetabular pelvic fracture internal fixation technique is to use the screw fixation technique to minimally invasively fix the fractures of various parts of the acetabulum and pelvis. For any positional screws designed by the doctors for fixed fractures, if the only design plan can be determined by preoperative or intraoperative images, it can be considered a clinical indication for robotic-assisted internal fixation. In addition, in order to facilitate clinical application, we divided the surgical indications into two parts: the acetabulum and the pelvis according to clinical needs. The acetabular fractures can be divided into acetabular anterior column screws, acetabular posterior column screws, and acetabular roof screws. The pelvic fracture is divided into the pubic symphysis screw of the anterior pelvic ring and the pubic screw, and the sacroiliac joint screw of the posterior ring.

The use of the acetabular anterior column screw is suitable for all types of acetabular fractures that require fixation of the acetabular anterior column. As shown in Fig. 21.1, the screws are generally placed in antegrade placement from the acetabular anterior column along the acetabular anterior column.

The acetabular posterior column screw is suitable for all types of acetabular fractures that require fixation of the posterior column of the acetabulum. It is divided into an anterior posterior column screw and a retrograde posterior column screw. The anterior posterior column screw is 1–2 cm from the inner side of the less pelvic margin, and 2 cm in front of the area about the sacroiliac joint is inserted into the bone-rich site along the posterior column according to the fixation requirement of fracture (Fig. 21.2). The retrograde posterior column screw is opposite to the antegrade posterior column screw. The ischial

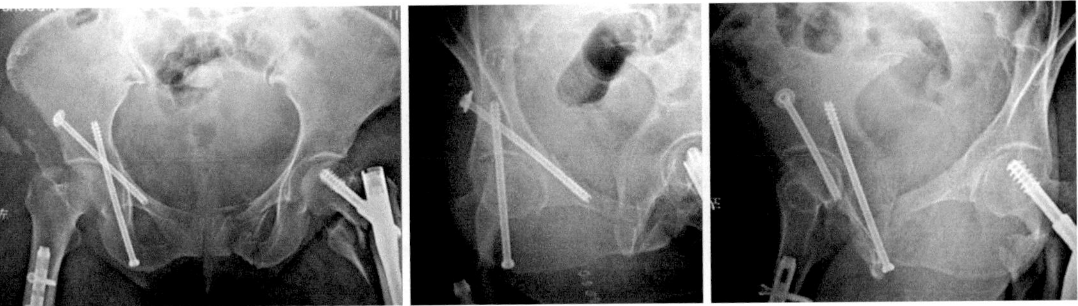

Fig. 21.1 Anterior acetabular screw and retrograde acetabular posterior column screw

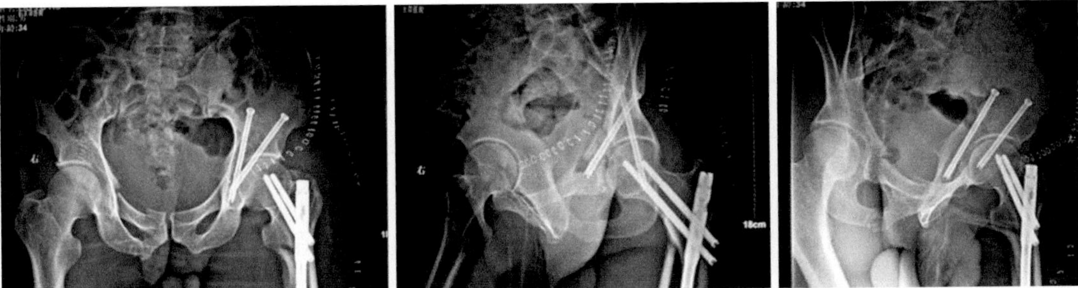

Fig. 21.2 Anterior acetabular screw and acetabular posterior anterior screw

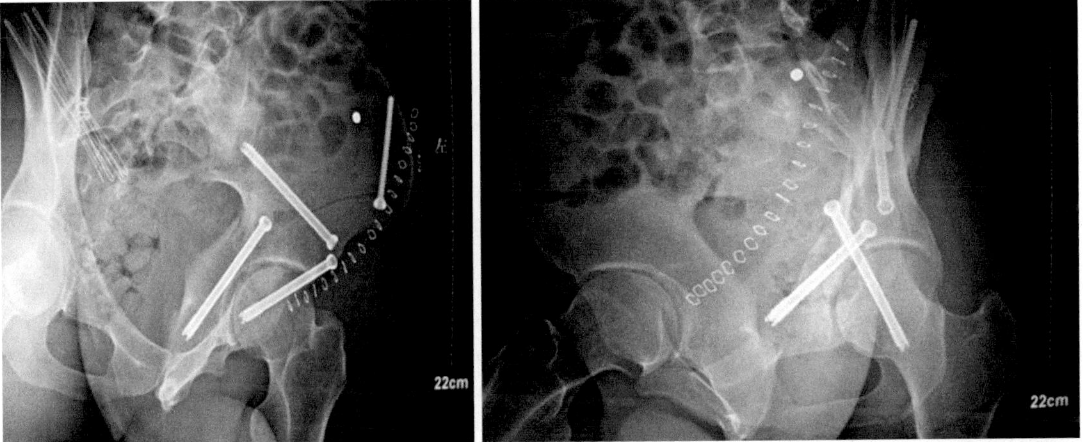

Fig. 21.3 The acetabular apex, the acetabular posterior anterior screw, and the acetabular anterior column screw

tuberosity is used as the incision point. The proximal end of the screw is inserted into the acetabular posterior column, which is generally used to fix the lower acetabular posterior column fracture line, as shown in Fig. 21.1.

The acetabular roof screw is used to fixate the acetabular anterior or posterior column fracture above the acetabular apex. It is usually inserted from the anterior and posterior iliac spine in the direction of the sacroiliac joint. It can fixate the high acetabular posterior column fracture in the downward direction and the low fracture of the humeral wing in the horizontal direction, as shown in Fig. 21.3.

The pubic symphysis screw of the anterior pelvic ring is suitable for the pelvic symphysis separation injury. It is usually inserted into the other side of the pubic symphysis to fixate the pubic symphysis, as shown in Fig. 21.4.

The anterior bronchial pedicle screw is used to fixate the anterior ring pubic symphysis fracture. Generally, the high pubic bronchus fracture is treated with an antegrade pubic screw (e.g., the acetabular anterior column screw), while the low pubic bronchus fracture is treated with an anterior pubic screw from the top of the acetabular bone, as shown in Fig. 21.5.

Sacroiliac joint screws are used to treat sacroiliac joint injuries and sacrum fractures, the most important treatment for posterior pelvic ring injury. The screw enters the iliac crest 1 or 2 vertebral body through the patella outer plate through the sacroiliac joint and the iliac wing safety zone, as shown in Fig. 21.6.

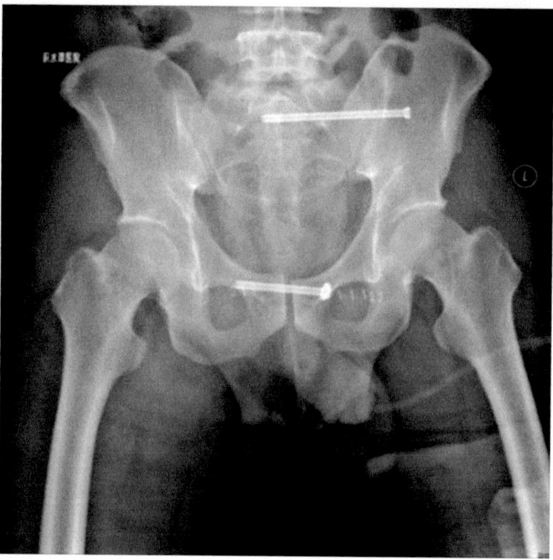

Fig. 21.4 Pubic symphysis screw and sacroiliac joint screw

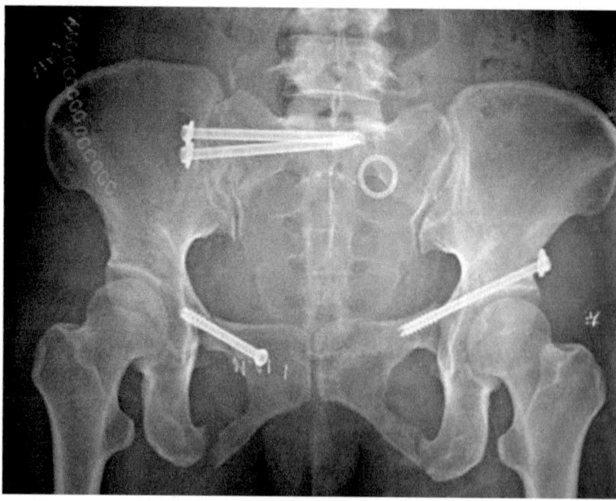

Fig. 21.5 The pubis branch antegrade, retrograde screw

1.2 Robot-Assisted Sacroiliac Joint Screws Internal Fixation

Percutaneous sacroiliac screw fixation under fluoroscopic guidance for unstable pelvic ring fractures is becoming increasingly popular worldwide. It was first described by Routt and has steadily gained popularity, with advantages of minimal invasion to compromised soft tissue, limited blood loss, and decreased infection rates, compared with conventional open techniques (Schweitzer et al. 2008; Routt Jr. et al. 2000; Routt Jr. et al. 1997). However, it requires detailed knowledge and experience to accurately correlate the sacral osseous landmarks with their corresponding fluoroscopic images and find a secure screw corridor using rotating inlet, outlet and lateral fluoroscopic views (Giannoudis et al. 2007), because incorrect placement of SI screws may result in implant-related and neurovascular complications (Altman et al. 1999; Stephen 1997; Stöckle et al. 2001). Statistically, the rates for malposition of the screw under fluoroscopic guidance have been reported to range from 2% to 15% (Hinsche et al. 2002; Templeman et al. 1996), with an incidence of neurologic injury between 0.5% and 7.7% (Templeman et al. 1996). Given this, fluoroscopy and computer-assisted techniques have been widely used to achieve an accurate screw placement. Currently, the conventional freehand fluoroscopy technique is very common for intraoperative visualization realized via image intensifier, which is possible in only one plane at a time, meanwhile requiring complex hand–eye coordination (Salari et al. 2015; Bastian et al. 2015; Zwingmann et al. 2009). As such, it is a highly demanding and challenging operative technique. Recently, computer-assisted orthopedic surgery, that potentially increases the accuracy and efficiency of percutaneous targeting, has utilized image navigation systems and purpose-built robots. The 2D- or 3D-fluoroscopy-based naviga-

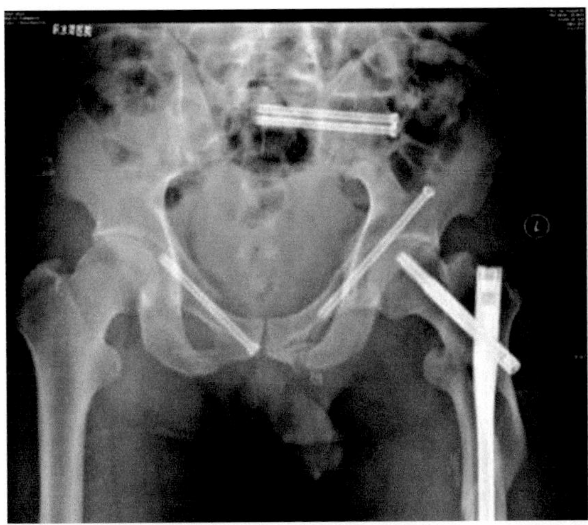
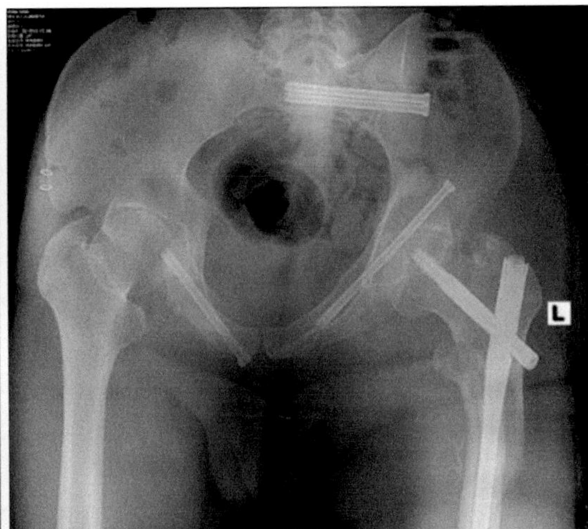

Fig. 21.6 Sacroiliac joint screws and antegrade, retrograde pubic screw

tion system makes it possible for simultaneous representation in up to four planes, which means a substantial improvement for the operator (Wang et al. 2011; Wu et al. 2015). Moreover, this advantage reduces the time of repeated C-arm movements during surgery and optimizes precise and simultaneous visualization of the surgical instruments in relation to the patient's anatomy in the all desired image planes. However, navigation does not solve the problem of precise manipulation of guide wire insertion and calculate the screw trajectory, which can be expediently alternated with a robot application. Robot-assisted orthopedic surgery is believed to potentially improve the precision of implant placement and decrease radiation and operative time. Several manufacturers research and produce hardware and software products for orthopedic surgery (Lang et al. 2011). Notably, TiRobot® is an orthopedic surgery robot which can be used for implantation of SI screws, especially useful in SI screw fixation for unstable pelvic injury. The method, studied in cadaver and cohort studies, has shown a high accuracy.

1.3 Robot-Assisted Sacroiliac Joint Screws Internal Fixation

Possessing the only registered license from the Food–Drug Administration in China, TiRobot® has been certified for use in orthopedic surgery, including SI screw implantation. At the beginning of the surgical procedure, the patient was prepared through positioning, sterilizing, and draping. The patient tracker was fixed on the contralateral anterior superior iliac spine of the surgical side, and a C-arm was placed on the same side of the patient. All parts of the robot were placed on the distal side of the patient, while the robot tracker and calibrator were assembled at the distal end of the robot arm. After the calibrator was fixed, pelvic inlet, outlet, and lateral intraoperative fluoroscopic images were taken. The fluoroscopic images were automatically imported into the planning and controlling workstation. Based on these fluoroscopic images, the surgeon planned the surgical trajectory for SI screw insertion and generated spatial positioning orders for the robot arm. The arm was moved automatically according to orders from the surgical planning and controlling workstation and completed the surgical trajectory positioning.

During the positioning process, the surgeon controlled accuracy through adjusting the screw trajectory on the fluoroscopic image, as necessary. When the positioning accuracy was smaller than 1.00 mm, the guide wire was placed into the sleeve. The instrumentation was then concluded through implantation and fixation of the SI screw over the guide wire without the assistance of the robot. Following the implantation, the surgeon verified accuracy through a comparison between the inserted screw's position and the intraoperative planned screw's position through fluoroscopy.

1.3.1 Illustrative Clinical Case 1

A 33-year-old male patient sustained pelvic fractures in a car accident. The preoperative X-ray film and computed tomography (CT) scan showed a C3-type injury involving sacral fractures combined with separation of the sacroiliac joint (Fig. 21.7). The patient was treated with SI screw fixation using TiRobot® (Fig. 21.8). Different from conventional freehand technique, the workstation of the robot can plan and calculate the surgical trajectory of the SI screw. To verify the accuracy of robotic planning intraoperatively, fluoroscopy verification for guide wire insertion was necessary (Fig. 21.9). Postoperative images showed that the positioning of the S1 and S2 screws had been excellent according to evaluation criterion (Fig. 21.10).

1.3.2 Illustrative Clinical Case 2

A 24-year-old female patient was admitted for surgery 4 days after a car accident injury. According to the preoperative examination, there

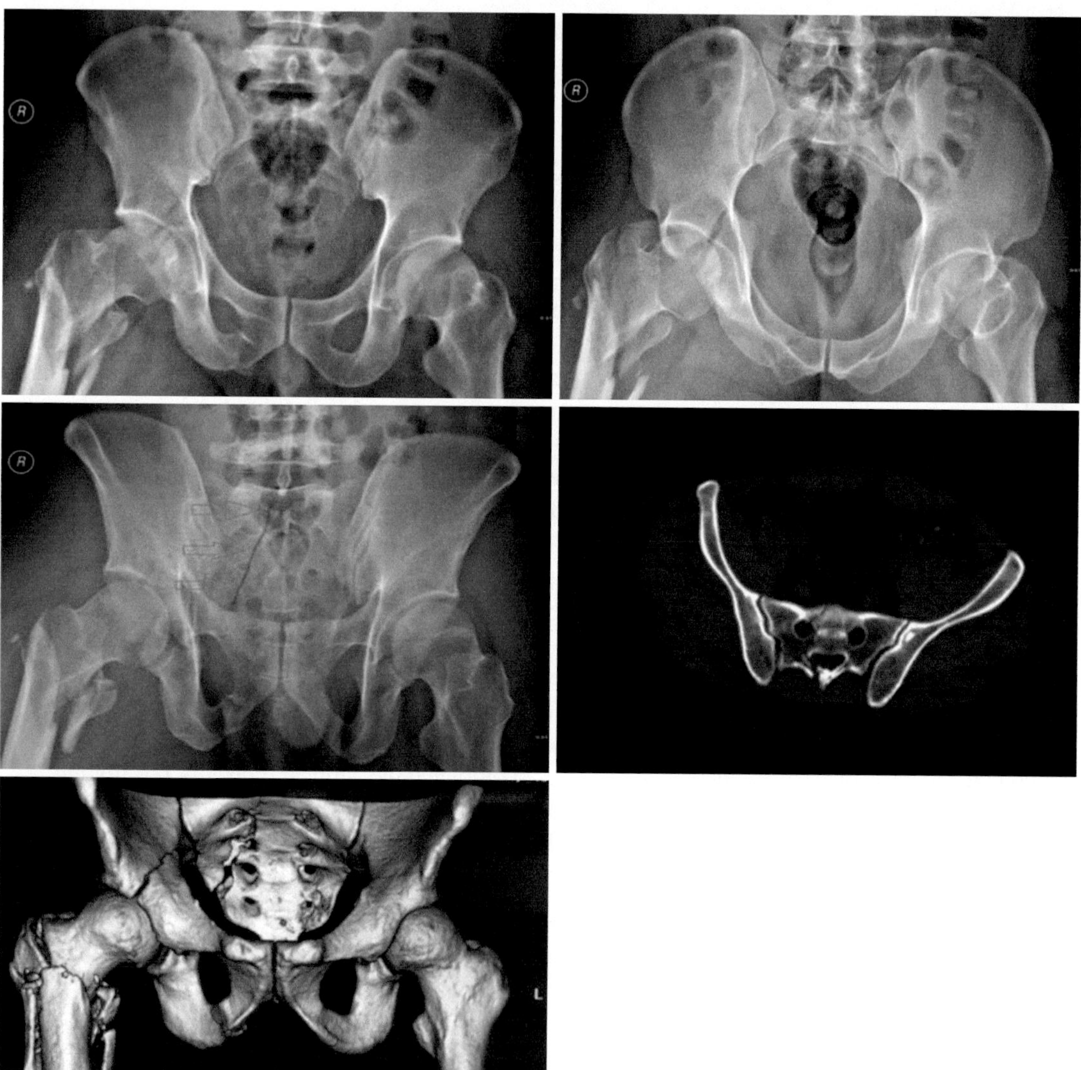

Fig. 21.7 Patient was examined preoperatively by X-ray and CT scan; the result was sacral fractures combined with separation of the sacroiliac joint

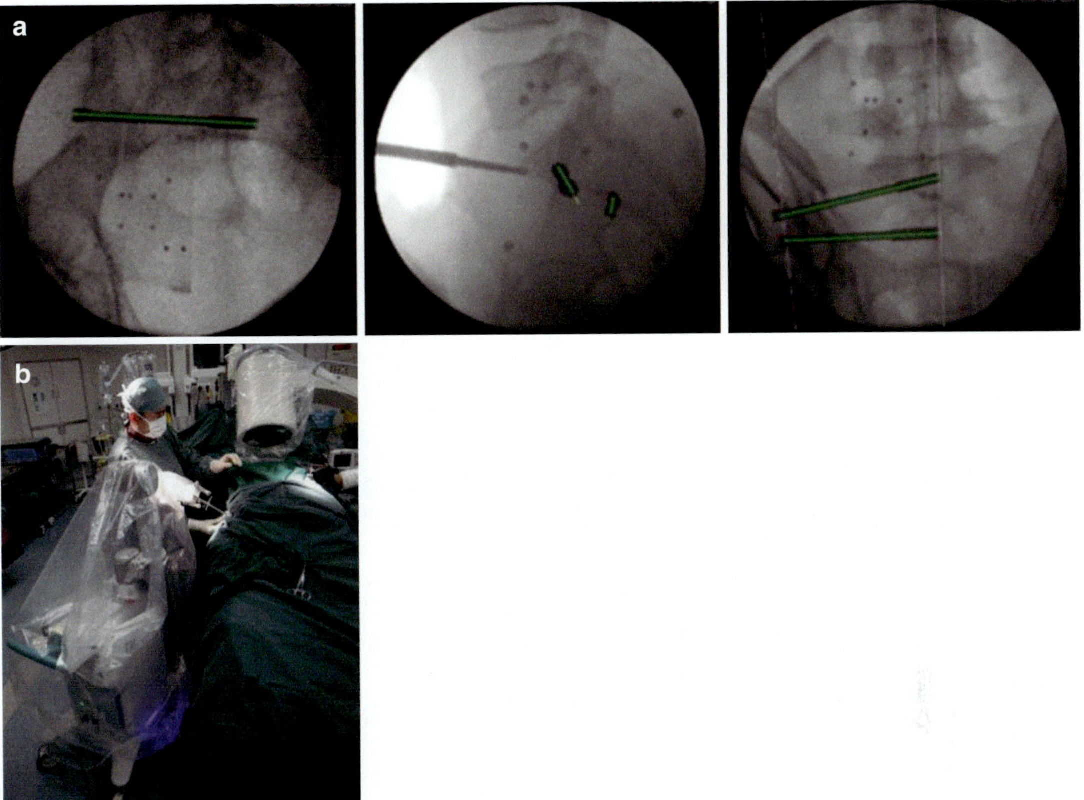

Fig. 21.8 (**a**) Planning image of the sacroiliac screw on the pelvis inlet, outlet, and lateral side. (**b**) Implantation of sacroiliac screws with the robot

were sacral fractures combined with separation of the sacroiliac joint. The operator implanted screws using the freehand technique, but the S1 screw passed IN–OUT–IN between the sacrum and the ilium, which was found in the postoperative X-ray image and CT scan (Fig. 21.11). However, there were no postoperative complications including nerve palsy and revision.

1.4 Robot-Assisted Anterior Column and Pubis Combined Screw Internal Fixation

1.4.1 Acetabular Anterior Column Fracture

Background

Simple acetabular anterior column fractures are not common, accounting for about 6% of acetabular fracture (Letournel and Judet 1993; Matta 1996). The anterior column of the acetabulum starts from the iliac crest, accounting for about 2/3 of the tibia, including the anterior half of the acetabulum, distal to the pubic symphysis. All fractures involving this part are called anterior column fractures. According to anatomy, the anterior column can be divided into the iliac segment, the acetabular segment, and the pubis segment. According to the fracture site, the fracture of the distal anterior iliac spine is a low anterior column fracture; the fracture line involves sputum, which is a high fracture (Wang et al. 2016). For low anterior column fractures, especially those distal to the anterior column acetabular segment, sometimes considered part of a pelvic fracture, minimally invasive fixation can be performed using the acetabular anterior column screw. For high acetabular anterior column fractures involving the ankle, it can lead

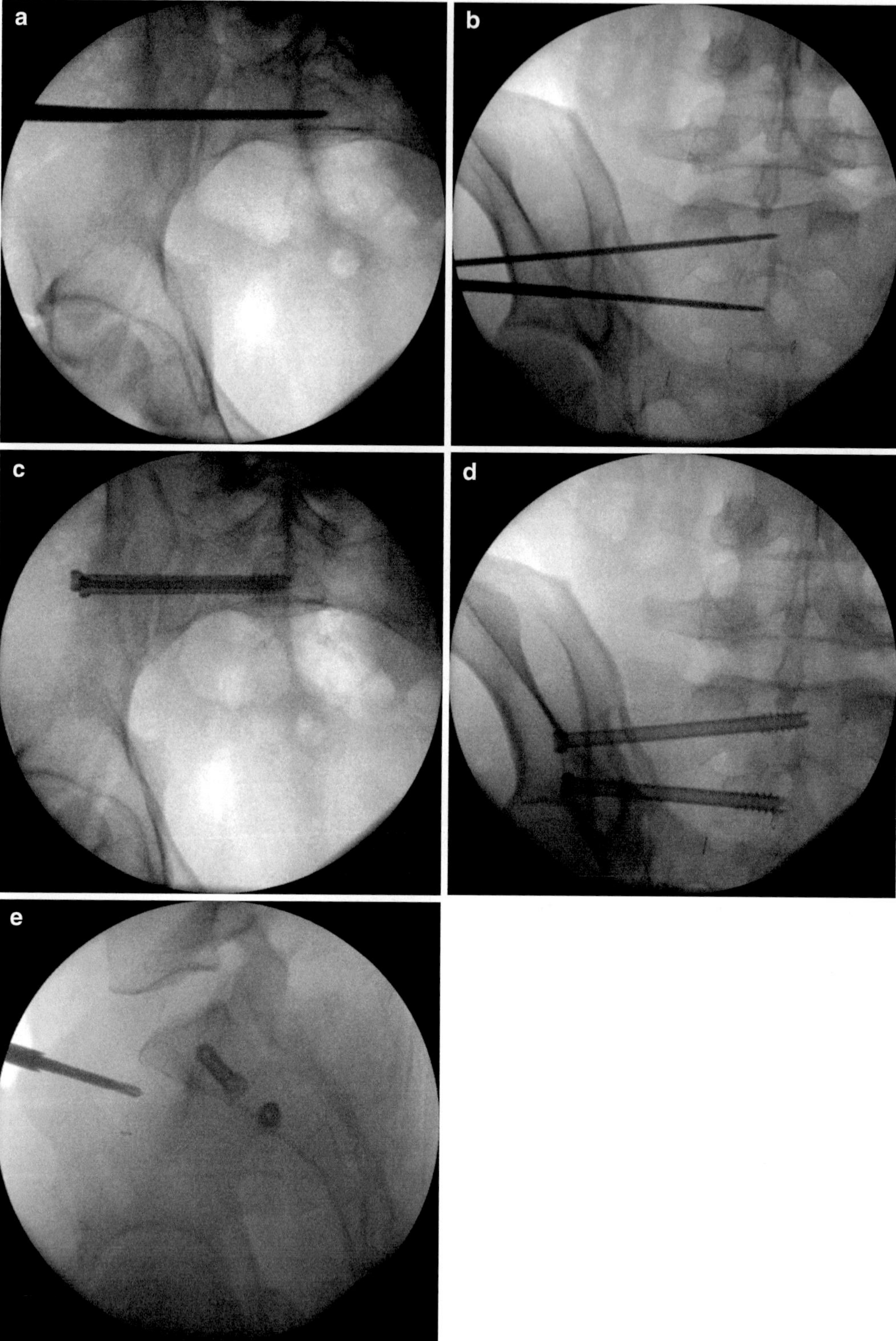

Fig. 21.9 Verifying location of guide wires and sacroiliac screws intraoperatively. (**a**) Inlet view of guide wires' location, (**b**) outlet view of guide wires' location, (**c**) inlet view of SI screws' location, (**d**) outlet view of SI screws' location, (**e**) lateral view of SI screws' location

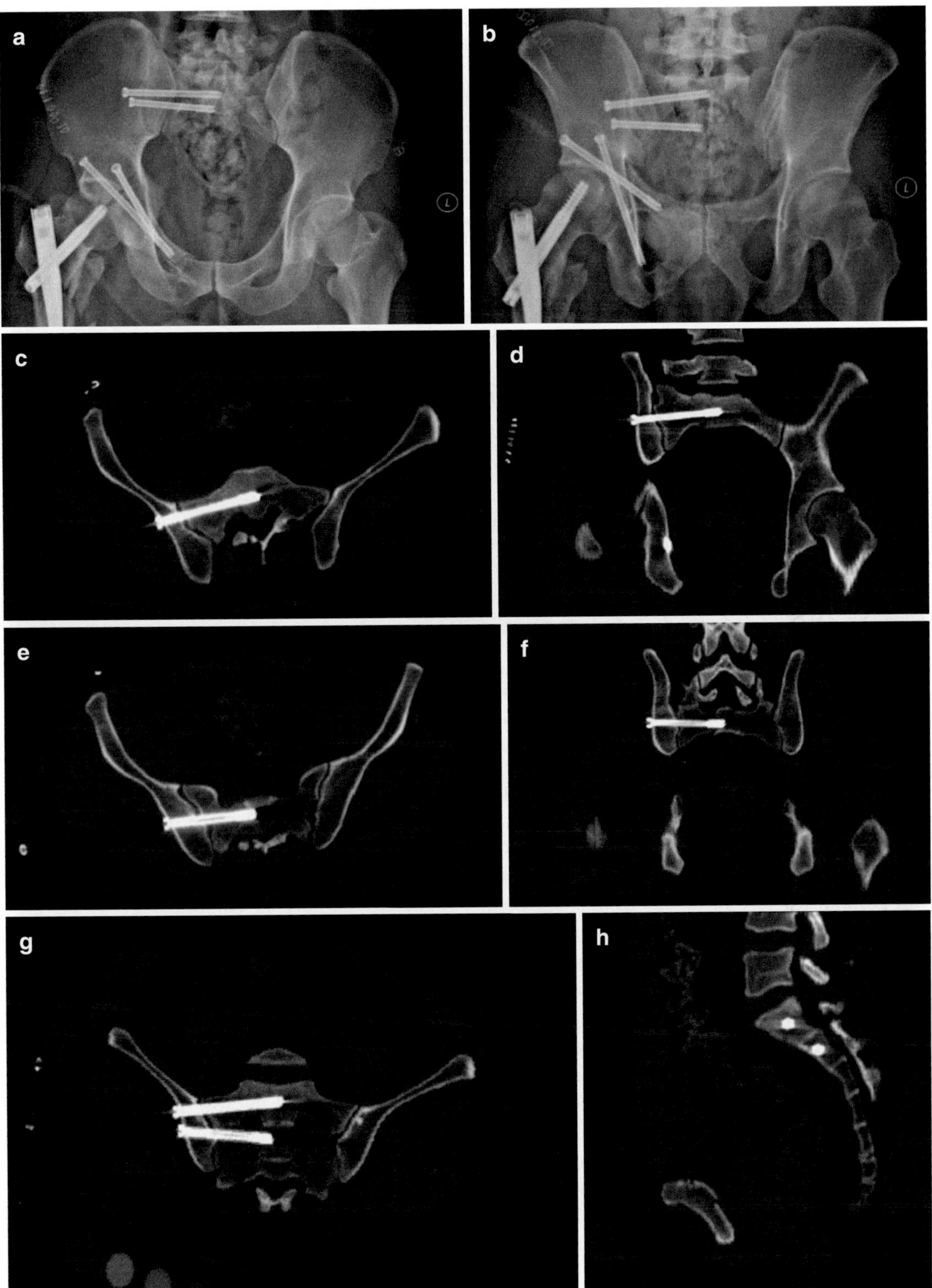

Fig. 21.10 The patient was examined by X-ray and CT scan postoperatively. (**a**) Inlet view, (**b**) outlet view, (**c**) S1 axial CT scan, (**d**) S1 coronal CT scan, (**e**) S2 axial CT scan, (**f**) S2 coronal CT scan, (**g**) angled sacral coronal CT scan, (**h**) sacral sagittal CT scan

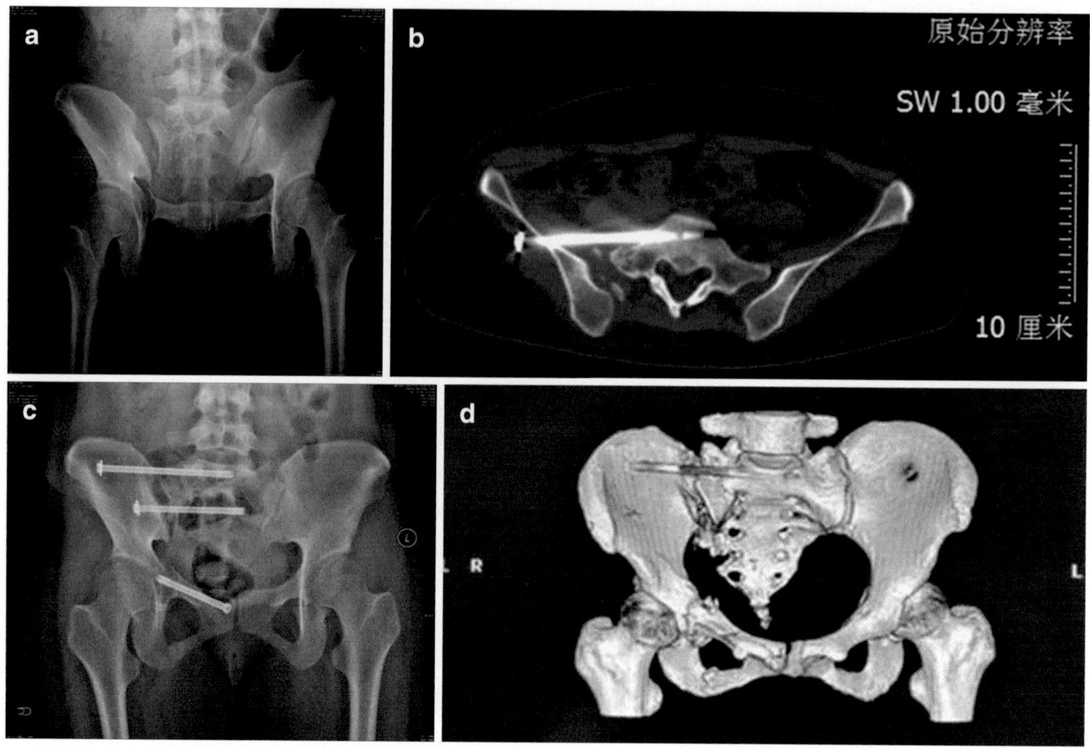

Fig. 21.11 By contrast, between preoperative and postoperative images, the S1 screw passed IN–OUT–IN between the sacrum and the ilium was found. (**a**) Preoperative outlet view, (**b**) postoperative CT image, (**c**) postoperative outlet view, (**d**) postoperative reconstruction CT image

to damage in the weight-bearing area, which can be fixed with acetabular screws (Zhao et al. 2017). This section describes the use of acetabular anterior column screws to fix the anterior column fracture of the acetabular segment. Although simple acetabular anterior column fractures are not common, many types of acetabular fractures combined with anterior column fractures require surgical fixation. Therefore, it is common to use the screw technique to fix the acetabular anterior column fracture during the treatment of acetabular fractures. In general, the anterior approach should be used in the traditional acetabular anterior column fracture, and the sacral approach and the Stoppa approach + the armpit approach (joint approach) can reveal all anterior columns. The exposure and internal fixation of the fracture can be performed in both surgical approaches. However, no matter which kind of incision is made, it involves the exposure and protection of important blood vessels, including the femoral blood vessels of the inguinal hernia, the extra-orbital vessels of the Stoppa approach, and the traffic branches of the nostrils. Therefore, the traditional open reduction surgery is complicated, which may cause complications such as vascular injury and hemorrhage.

The use of robotic technology can avoid a wide range of surgical exposure and reduce the side damage caused by surgery. Because the anterior column of the acetabulum is relatively anatomically fixed, the use of screws to fix the anterior column can achieve good position maintenance and compression of the fracture end (Zhao et al. 2011).

Robot-Assisted Screw Fixation for Acetabular Anterior Column Fracture

The surgical procedure for surgical robot-assisted acetabular anterior column screw internal fixation is as follows:

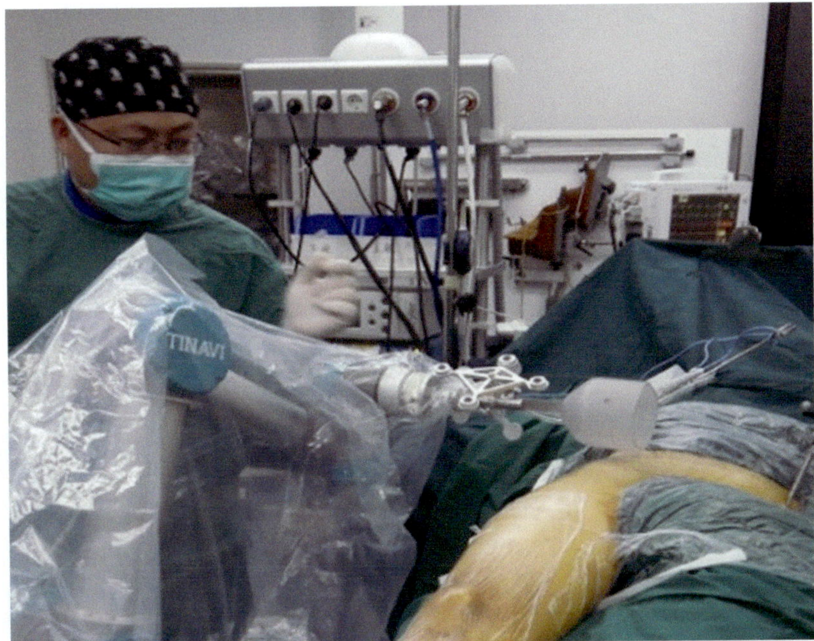

Fig. 21.12 Installing the robot end tracker and calibrator

1. The use of a fully transparent surgical bed facilitates the acquisition of images during surgery to prevent occlusion of metal objects during image acquisition. The patient is in a supine position, completing the closed reduction of the fracture and maintaining the fracture position
2. Place the robot on the sterile sleeve and install the robot end tracker and calibrator (Fig. 21.12). Move and fix it to the appropriate position next to the operating bed to ensure that the robotic arm working space is up to the operative region. The optical tracking camera is placed on the patients' foot, and the mobile C-arm is placed on the opposite side of the surgeon. Place the patient tracker on the healthy side or the affected side of the anterior superior iliac spine (Fig. 21.13). Use the C-arm to obtain the fluoroscopic image of the exit oblique position and inlet position of the affected acetabular obturator with the robot positioning marker (Fig. 21.14) and transmit it to the master station. Based on the typical marker points and the bony landmark structure, the surgeon performs surgical screw path planning on the master control system planning software (Fig. 21.15).

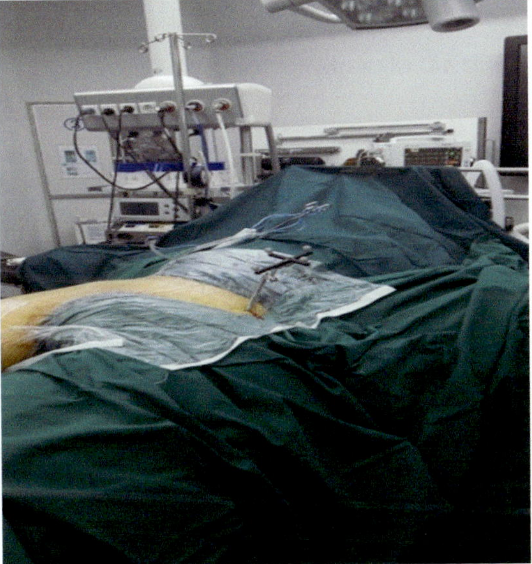

Fig. 21.13 Installing the patient tracker

3. Robot-assisted nailing: The operation posture of the robot arm is simulated by using the robot arm posture simulation module in the planning software. The control software of the main control system controls and monitors the robot arm to move along the planned path to the target position after con-

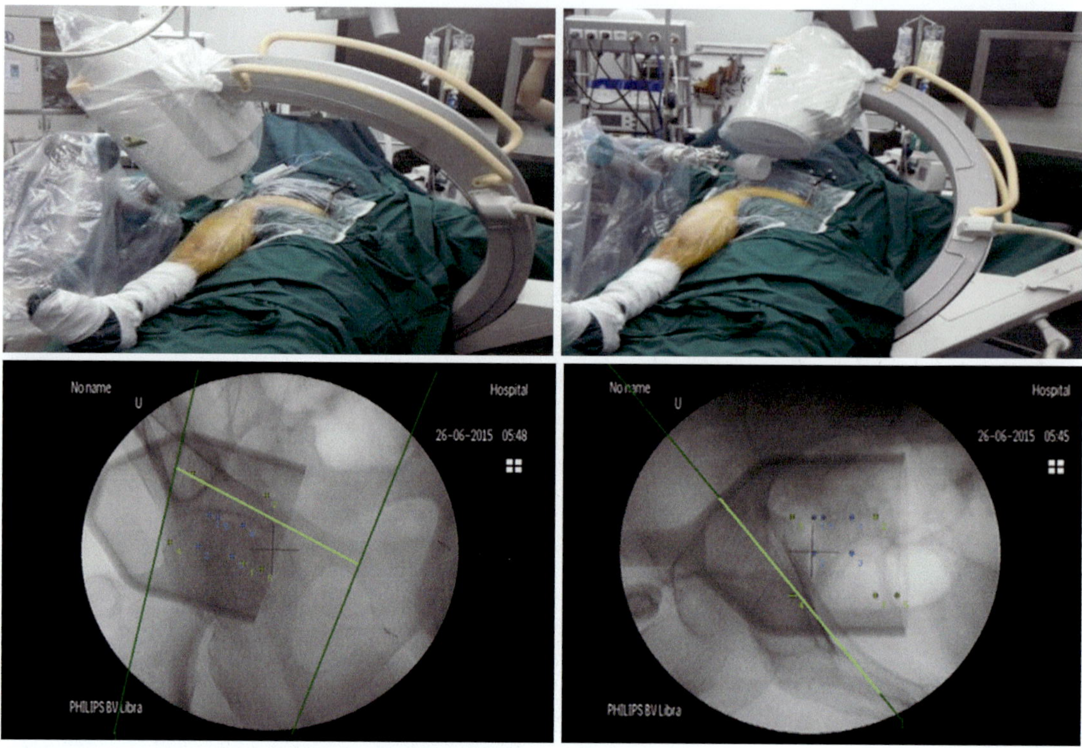

Fig. 21.14 Obtain the fluoroscopic image

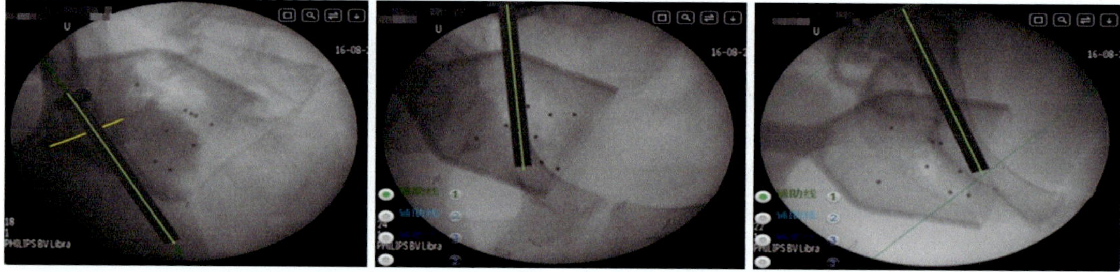

Fig. 21.15 Acquire the images at obturator exit oblique position and inlet position image and plan on the software

firming the posture of the robot arm is suitable for subsequent operation. Install a guide sleeve at the end of the arm, make a 2 cm small incision at the entry point, bluntly separate the subcutaneous tissue, and bring the tip of the sleeve to the cortical bone of the nail. Check whether the nail point and virtual probe direction are in the planning software. In line with the plan, if the software shows that it has a large deviation from the planned path, the robot can fine-tune the path. After the path is confirmed accurately, the guide wire is drilled into the bony channel through the sleeve under the perspective monitoring (Fig. 21.16).

4. Perspective verification path: After confirming the position of the guide wire, insert the cannulated screw (Fig. 21.17), and finally confirm that the position of the cannulated screw is good, and then withdraw the guide wire, simply by flushing the incision and suturing it.

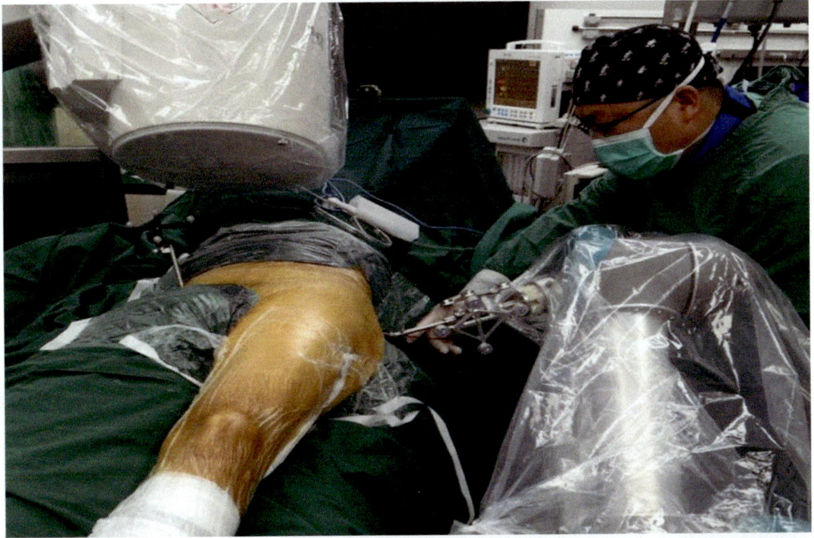

Fig. 21.16 Insert the front post screw guide wire according to the robot travel path

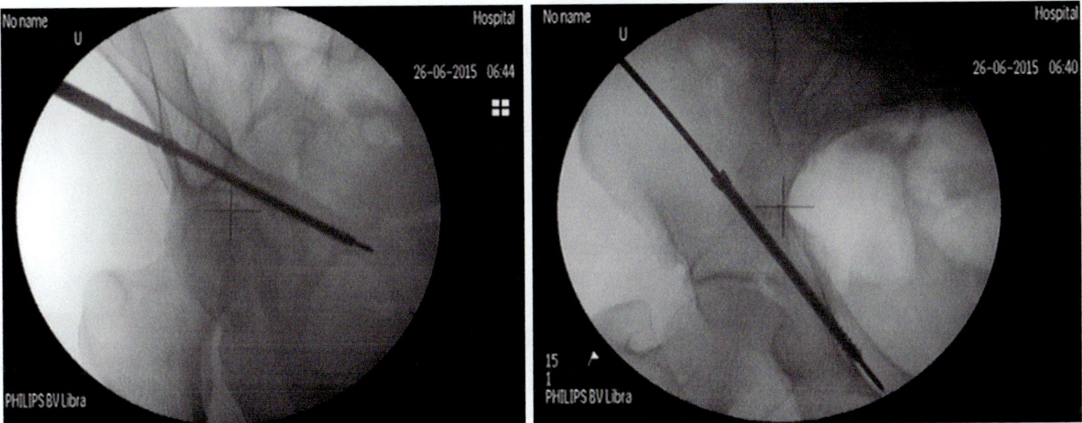

Fig. 21.17 Insert the front post screws and verify the screw position

1.4.2 Symphysis Pubis Screw

Background

The pubic symphysis separation injury, that is, the B1-type pelvic fracture, is generally fixed with plate screws (Tile et al. 2003), but the placement of the plate requires an anterior incision to reveal the pubic symphysis. For cases requiring closed reduction, minimally invasive internal fixation is also a treatment option for percutaneous screw fixation. Perspective guidance, computer navigation, and robotics can assist in the internal fixation of the pubic symphysis screw.

Robot-Assisted Internal Fixation of the Pubis Symphysis Screw

As with the acetabular anterior column screws, the surgical procedure for robot-assisted placement of the pubic symphysis screws is identical, except that the required fluoroscopic images are different. The patient is lying on his back in the orthopedic operating table. First, a closed reduction was performed for the fracture. In general, we use the external fixation bracket to close the pubic symphysis separation injury (Fig. 21.18), and then the robot is placed, and the calibrator and the tracker are installed. The pubic symphysis screw insertion requires the collection of the

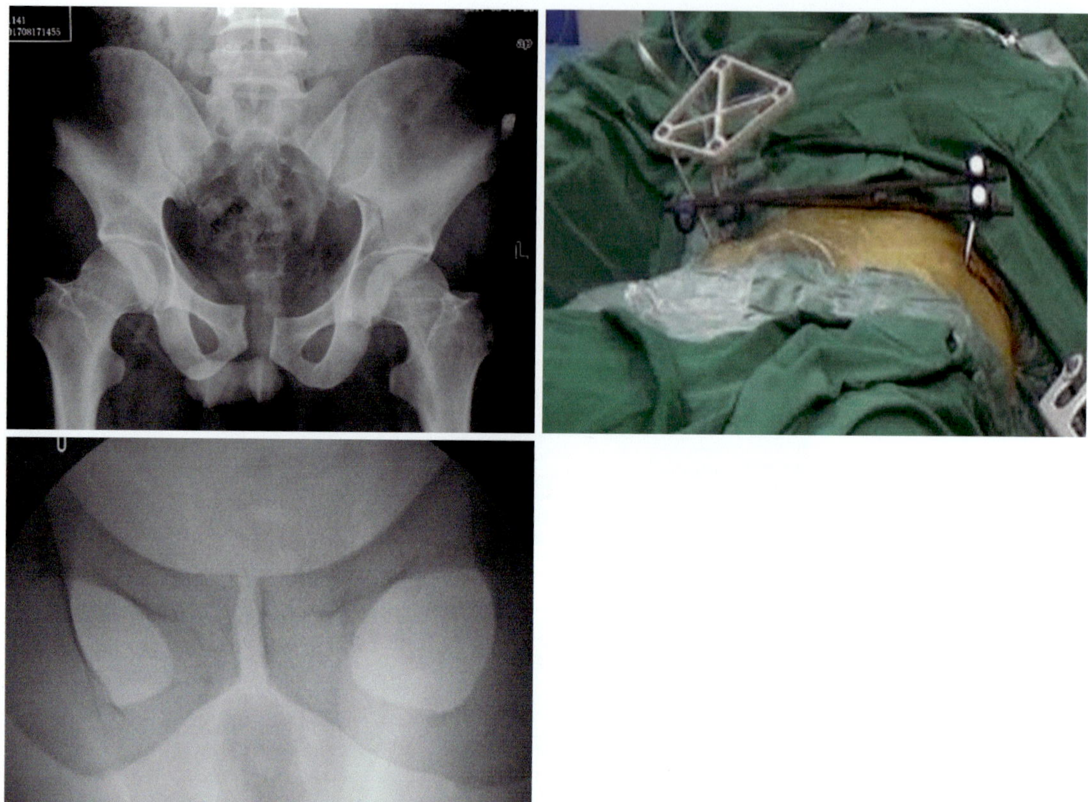

Fig. 21.18 Using the external fixator to restore the pubic symphysis separation injury

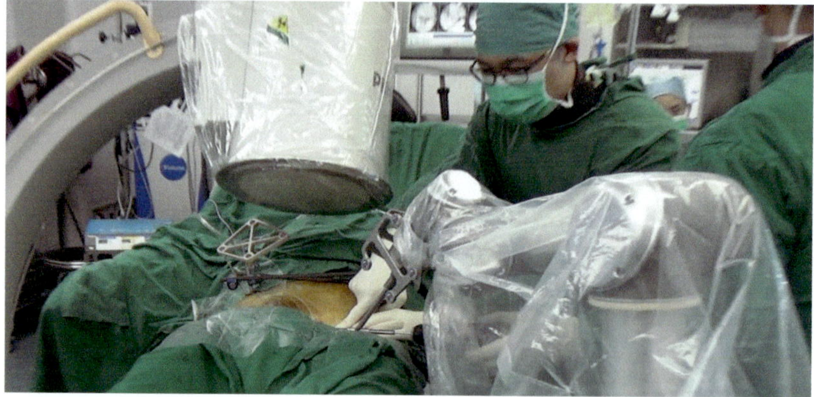

Fig. 21.19 Using the robot to plan the pubic symphysis screw channel, insert the screw guide wire

exit and entrance points of the pubic symphysis. After the image is acquired, the robotic arm is moved to the planned position after the software master control system is completed (Fig. 21.19) and inserted through the guide sleeve at the end of the arm. The guide wire for the screw can be placed into the pubic symphysis screw after fluoroscopy (Fig. 21.20).

1.5 Robot-Assisted Posterior Column Screw Internal Fixation

1.5.1 Background

Simple posterior column fractures account for only 3–5% of acetabular fractures (Letournel and Judet 1993). More posterior column fractures are

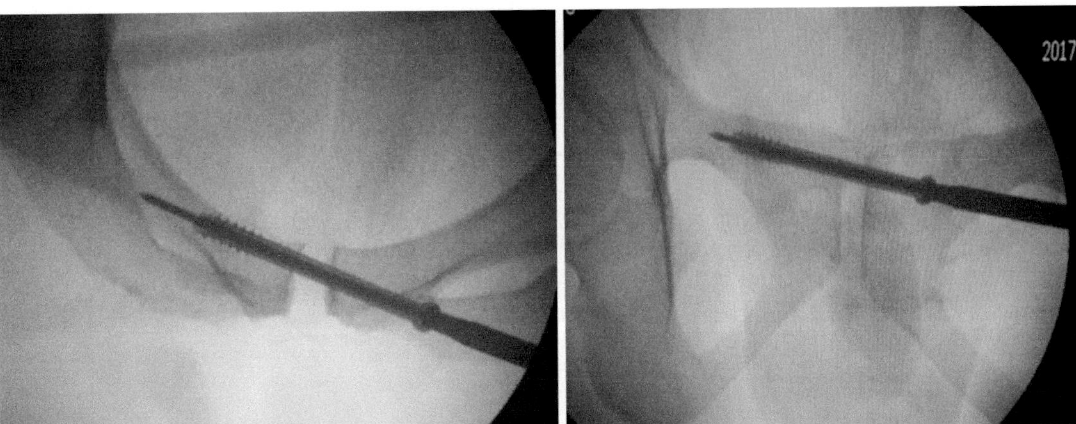

Fig. 21.20 Verify the pubic symphysis exit entry and check the position of the pubic symphysis screw

found in acetabular transverse fractures, T-shaped fractures, and double-column fractures. Imaging is characterized by fractures and discontinuities in the squat line. The goal of the posterior column fracture is to restore the anatomical alignment of the acetabulum and effectively fix it. For a slightly displaced (<2 mm) posterior column fracture, antegrade or retrograde percutaneous screw fixation can be used to reduce surgical trauma. For fractures requiring open reduction, especially acetabular transverse fractures, T-shaped fractures, and double-column fractures, in many cases, the anterior and posterior column fractures can be restored through the anterior approach, and the screws are used to advance from the iliac fossa. The posterior column is fixed so that the posterior approach can be avoided to reduce surgical trauma and complications (Shiramizu et al. 2003; Stockle et al. 2000). In order to accurately insert the posterior column screw, there are studies to measure the anatomy of the posterior column. The maximum length of the screw that can be used is 74.7–122.4 mm, the narrowest part of the channel is 13.4–26.9 mm, and the distance from the hip joint is 3.1–6.9 mm (Puchwein et al. 2012). When the screw is inserted antegrade, the "safe area" of the entry point is a triangular area, the center of which is about 32.5 mm from the leading edge of the sacroiliac joint. The posterior column channel is wider, allowing multiple screws to be placed (Jung et al. 2017). In some cases, a percutaneous retrograde posterior column screw can be used, and the patient should be placed in the lateral or prone position. Under the intraoperative imaging monitoring, selecting the appropriate entry point does not increase the risk of sciatic nerve injury (Mouhsine et al. 2005; Azzam et al. 2014). Moreover, with the aid of computer-assisted technology, the accuracy of screw placement is greatly improved under the aid of navigational 2D or 3D images (Ochs et al. 2010). In clinical practice, the usual antegrade placement method has the following drawbacks: (1) If the position of the fracture line of the posterior column is too low, it will cause the screw to be inserted difficult to cross the fracture line; (2) sometimes the fracture block at the posterior column is long and narrow. If the position of the screw is poor or repeated, it is easy to cause the bone to break. (3) If the screw is not deep enough, the holding force is weak, and it is prone to failure. (4) Surgery depends on repeated fluoroscopy during surgery. The damage is large. (5) The surgeon has insufficient experience, and the insertion is wrong or even impossible to put in (Fig. 21.21). Therefore, the use of navigation robot-assisted technology can help doctors reduce the learning curve of the operation.

1.5.2 Robot-Assisted Posterior Column Screw Fixing Method

The surgical procedure for orthopedic surgery robot-assisted posterior column screw fixation is as follows:

1. The use of an all-transparent surgical table facilitates the acquisition of images during surgery to prevent occlusion of metal objects

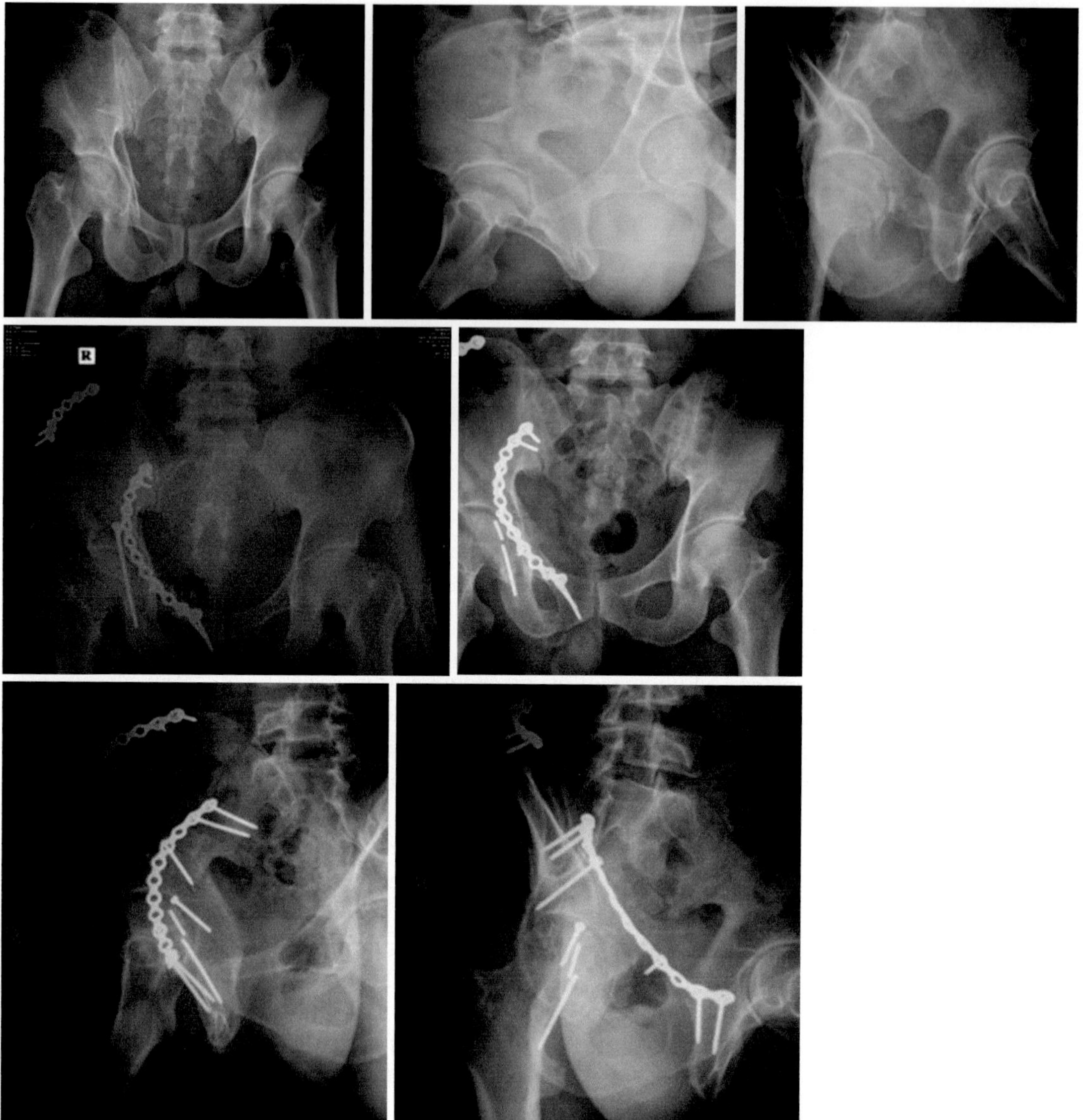

Fig. 21.21 Patients with double-column fractures, with a single anterior approach for anterior column fracture open reduction and internal fixation, free antegrade posterior column screw fixation, no screw placement deviation into the hip and femoral head during surgery, postoperative review the screw breaks into three parts

during image acquisition. The screw was in an anterograde placement, and the patient was placed in a supine position; the screw was in a retrograde placement, and the patient was placed in a prone position to complete the closure or open reduction of the fracture and the maintenance of the fracture position.

Place the robot on the sterile sleeve and install the robot end tracker and calibrator. Move and fix it to the appropriate position next to the operating bed to ensure that the robotic arm working space is up to the operative region. The optical tracking camera was placed on the foot side of the patient, and the C-arm was put on the opposite side of the surgeon. Place the patient tracker on the healthy side or the affected side of the anterior superior iliac spine (prone position in the posterior superior

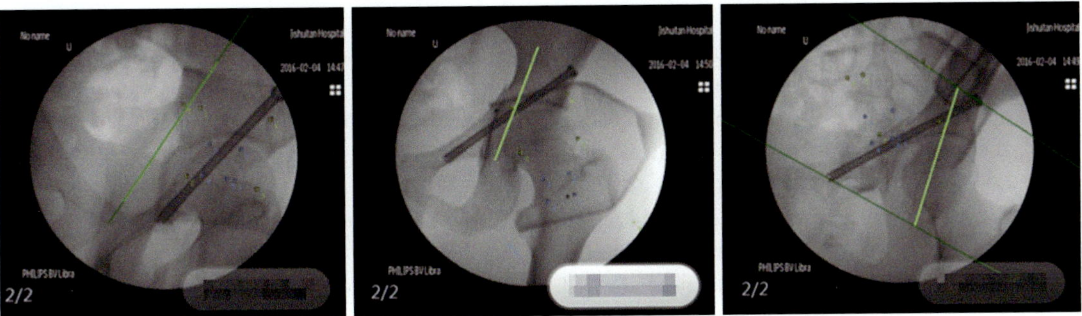

Fig. 21.22 Patients with acetabular fractures have been treated with anterior column screws, and the posterior column screw orientation (line) is performed at the sacral, ortho, and obturator exits

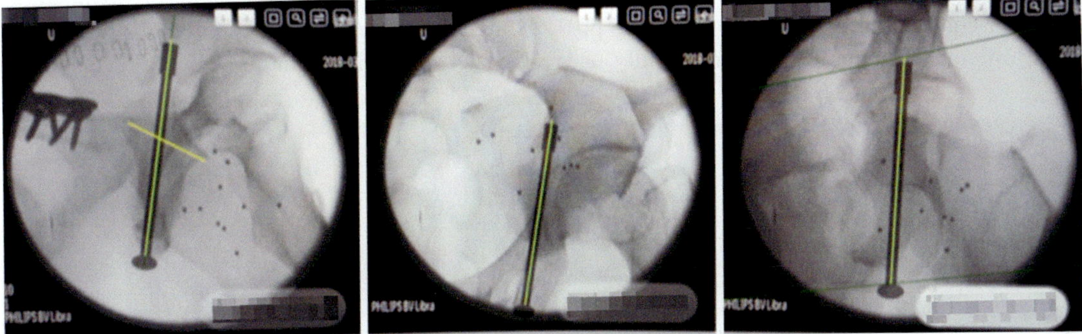

Fig. 21.23 Retrograde screw placement planning for posterior column fractures

iliac spine). Use the C-arm to obtain the fluoroscopic image of the affected acetabular sac, the obturator oblique position, and the pelvic anterior containing the robotic locating points and transmitted to the master workstation. Based on the typical marker points and the bony landmark structure, the surgeon performs surgical screw path planning on the master control system planning software (Fig. 21.22).

2. Robot-assisted nailing: The operation posture of the robot arm is simulated by using the robot arm posture simulation module in the planning software. The control software of the main control system controls and monitors the robot arm to move along the planned path to the target position after confirming the posture of the robot arm is suitable for subsequent operation. Install the guide sleeve at the end of the arm. Note that the direction of the guide wire will pass through the abdominal cavity. Therefore, make a small incision at the lateral humeral ridge of the insertion point and separate it along iliac intraosseous plate to avoid damage to the organ. To the cortical bone of the nail point, confirm whether the direction of the nail point and the virtual probe is in accordance with the planning in the planning software. If the software shows that it has a large deviation from the planned path, the robot can fine-tune the path. After the path is confirmed accurately, under the perspective monitoring, a guide wire is drilled into the bony channel through the sleeve. If retrograde placement is used in the prone position, only a small incision is required to detach the soft tissue to the bone surface (Fig. 21.23).
3. Perspective verification path: After confirming the position of the guide wire in perspective, screw in the cannulated screw, and finally confirm that the position of the cannulated screw is good, and then withdraw the guide wire and flush the incision.

1.5.3 Clinical Applications

In most cases, acetabular fractures are high-energy injuries. Patients can have pelvic fractures and other limb fractures. Using navigation robot-assisted surgery can reduce the "secondary damage" and minimize surgical trauma (Fig. 21.24).

If the acetabular fracture needs open reduction, a single incision can be used. First, the anterior and posterior columns are cut and repositioned. The anterior column is fixated with a steel plate, and then the point is inserted from the iliac fossa, and a posterior column screw is placed under the guidance of the navigation robot (Fig. 21.25).

In special cases, the percutaneous retrograde posterior column screw is used to fixate the posterior column fracture. The patient usually uses the prone position. Pay attention to the blunt dissection of the soft tissue to the bone surface. Place the guide wire and screw under the sleeve protection to avoid wrap around the tissue and the sciatic nerve (Fig. 21.26).

1.5.4 Summary

The acetabular posterior column channel is a bone channel between the fossa iliac and the ischial tuberosity. The channel is long and has a large diameter. It is used to fix the posterior column fracture. It is often used to avoid posterior open reduction. There is no important structure nearby, and the screw should be avoided. It should not enter the hip joint. Navigation robot-assisted posterior column screws are placed in

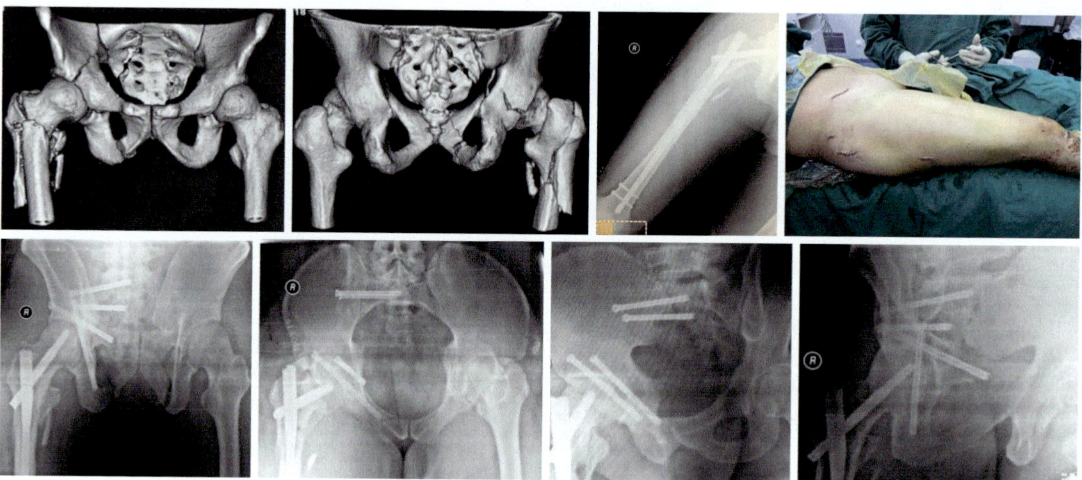

Fig. 21.24 Middle-aged male, car accident leading to pelvic fracture, acetabular fracture, fracture below femur thick grand, using supine position, navigation robot-assisted descending sacroiliac joint screw, anterior column and posterior column screw fixation, femoral bone fixation. Postoperative photos showed that the internal fixation was percutaneous minimally invasive fixation

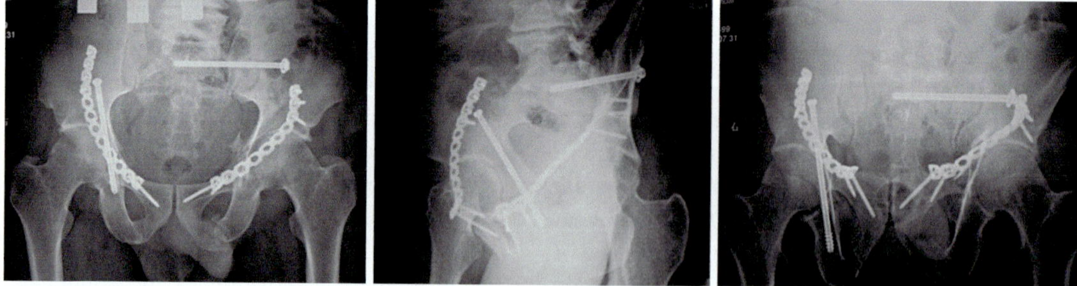

Fig. 21.25 After the front column steel plate is fixated, the posterior column fracture is fixated with long screws in the posterior column channel

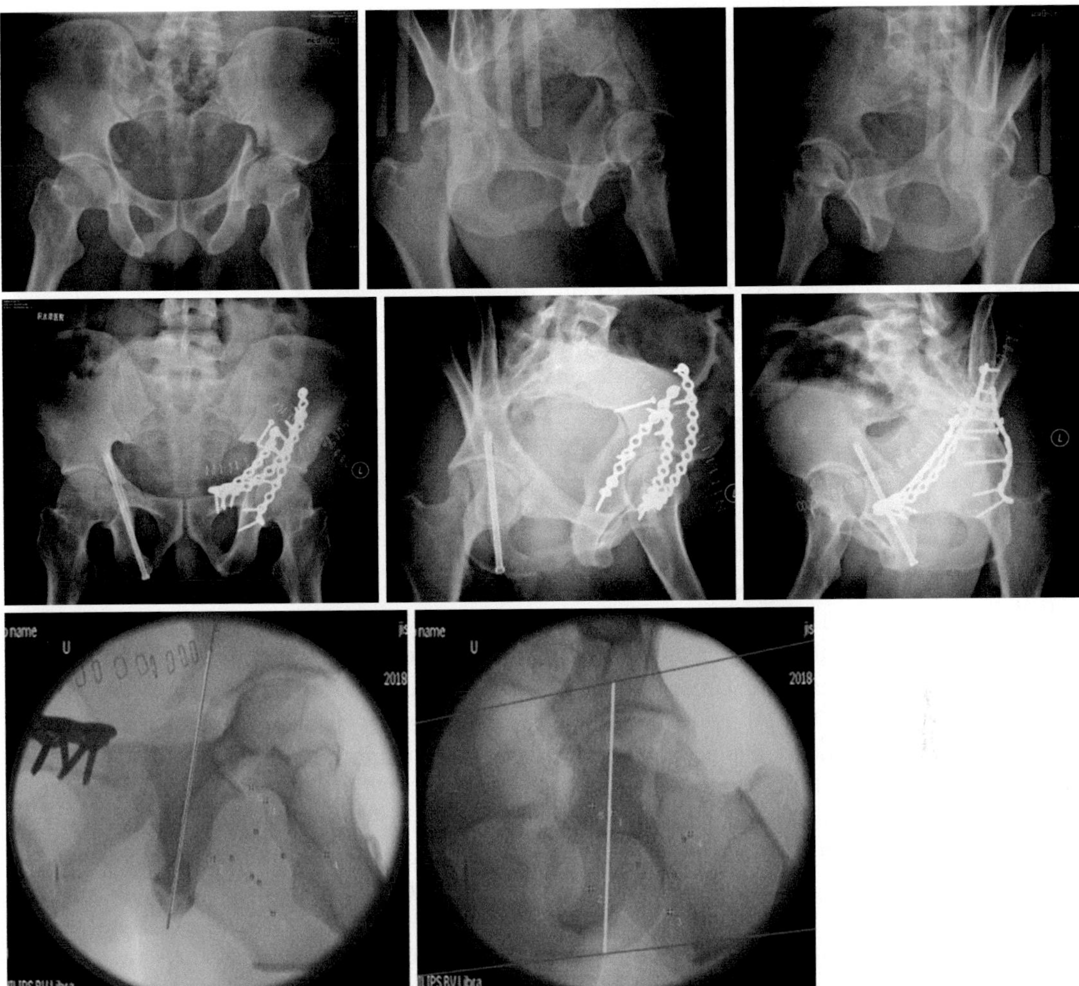

Fig. 21.26 The patients' left acetabular double-column fracture. A single anterior approach cannot be used to reduce the fracture; hence, the anterior and posterior combined approach for open reduction and plate fixation. The simple posterior column fracture on the right side was slightly displaced; hence, the prone position navigation robot-assisted percutaneous retrograde posterior column screw was used

three ways: percutaneously placed in the antegrade direction. Note that it cannot be cut along the distal end of the arm of the arm. It needs to be cut laterally along the humeral ridge and separated along the iliac intraosseous plate to avoid injury and the organ; after the reduction of the fracture through the anterior incision, the screw is implanted antegrade, because it is relatively safe to be exposed under direct vision; when the prone position is inserted through the retrograde screw, attention should be paid to the blunt dissection to avoid injury to the sciatic nerve. Robots can reduce the learning curve, but they are not a substitute for the doctors' theoretical knowledge; hence, it is still necessary to be familiar with the anatomy of the site.

1.6 Robot-Assisted Acetabular Screw Internal Fixation

1.6.1 Background

The upper acetabular channel is a bone channel between the anterior iliac spine and the posterior superior iliac spine. The channel is long, and the bone mass is large. It is often used as a fixed position for the external fixation of the pelvis. For iliac crescent fractures, lateral compression fractures (lateral compression type II/LC2), and acetabular anterior column fractures, in many cases doctors choose to use the anterior or posterior approach. Open reduction plate screws internal fixation (Judet et al. 1964). However, as early as more than 20 years ago, Starr et al. introduced a technique for percutaneous placement of screws in the acetabulum (LC2 screw) (Crowl and Kahler 2002), which protects bone blood and reduces soft tissue scars, reducing the amount of surgical bleeding and reducing the infection rate (Routt Jr. et al. 1995). Therefore, percutaneous minimally invasive techniques have greatly reduced surgical complications and obtained good clinical results (Vigdorchik et al. 2012). Another application of the acetabular screw is the iliac screw, which is used to hold the tibia to maintain stability throughout the fixation system. The INFIX screw of the anterior pelvic ring can be used to fix the anterior pelvic ring fracture, which reduces extensive incision. The internal fixation of the wound avoids the inconvenience caused by the external fixation frame and provides enough biomechanical stability (Santos et al. 2011). In the posterior pelvic ring, the iliac screw system can be used to fix unstable sacral fracture, spinal surgery, and pelvic tumor resection. Accurate placement of the appropriate length and diameter of the tibial nail can be provided biomechanically, suggesting very good stability (Puchwein et al. 2012). However, it is still quite difficult and challenging to insert the screws by hand in the upper acetabulum. Although there are no important structures adjacent to each other, the incorrectly inserted screws lose their function (Fig. 21.27). In order to accurately insert the screw into the acetabulum, it has been studied to measure the channel. The maximum length of the channel is 127.2–163.9 mm, the narrowest part is 9.9–23.6 mm, and the distance from the hip is 14.8–25.1 mm (Ochs et al. 2010). And with the aid of computer-assisted technology, the accuracy of screw placement is greatly improved under the aid of navigation of 2D or 3D images during surgery.

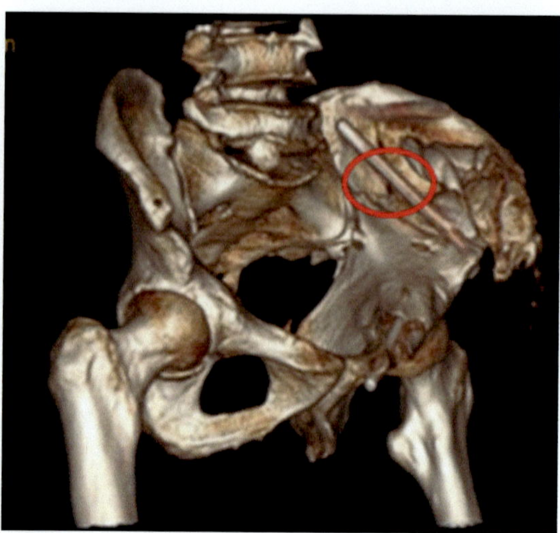

Fig. 21.27 The screw inserted by freehand pierced the iliac cortex and lost its fixation

1.6.2 Robot-Assisted Acetabular Screw Fixation Method

The surgical procedure for orthopedic surgery robot-assisted acetabular screw fixation is as follows:

1. The use of an all-transparent surgical table facilitates the acquisition of images during surgery to prevent occlusion of metal objects during image acquisition. The screws were in a retrograde placement (front to back), and the patient was placed in a supine position; the screws were in an anterograde placement (from the posterior to the front), and the patient was placed in a prone position to complete the closure or open reduction of the fracture and the maintenance of the fracture site.
2. Place the robot on the sterile sleeve and install the robot end tracker and calibrator. Move and fix it to the appropriate position next to the operating bed to ensure that the robotic arm working space is up to the operative region. The optical tracking camera is placed on the patients' foot, and the mobile C-arm is placed on the opposite side of the surgeon. Place the patient tracker on the healthy side or the affected side of the anterior superior iliac spine (prone position in the posterior superior iliac spine). Use the C-arm to obtain the fluo-

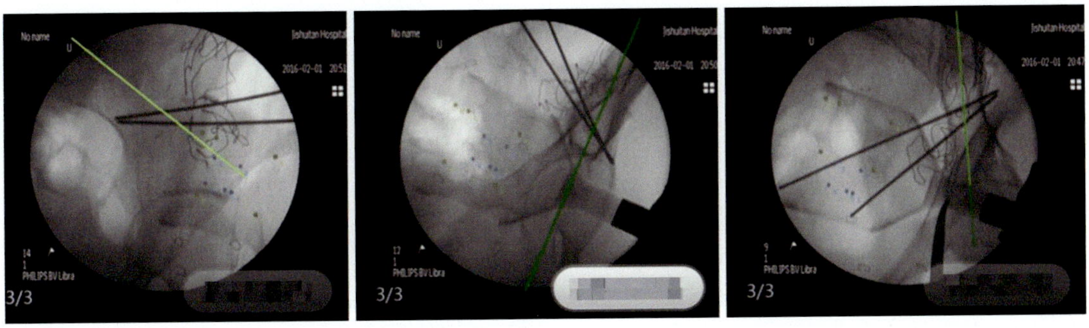

Fig. 21.28 After the tibiofibular fracture is cut open and the Kirschner wire is temporarily fixed, the screw position is planned from the left to the right in the oblique position of acetabular iliac bone and obturator outlet oblique position and the closed orifice oblique position

roscopic image of oblique position of acetabular iliac bone and obturator outlet oblique position (tear drop position), the closed orifice oblique position with the robot's locating point and transmitted to the master workstation. Based on the typical marker points and the bony landmark structure, the surgeon performs surgical screw path planning on the master control system planning software (Fig. 21.28).

3. Robot-assisted nailing: The operation posture of the robot arm is simulated by using the robot arm posture simulation module in the planning software. The control software of the main control system controls and monitors the robot arm to move along the planned path to the target position after confirming the posture of the robot arm is suitable for subsequent operation. Install a guide sleeve at the end of the arm, make a 2 cm small incision at the entry point, bluntly separate the subcutaneous tissue, and bring the tip of the sleeve to the cortical bone of the nail. Check whether the nail point and virtual probe direction are in the plan software. In line with the plan, if the software shows that it has a large deviation from the planned path, the robot can fine-tune the path. After the path is confirmed accurately, the guide wire is drilled into the bony channel through the sleeve under the perspective monitoring.
4. Perspective verification path: After confirming the position of the guide wire in perspective, screw in the cannulated screw, and finally confirm that the position of the cannulated screw is good, and then withdraw the guide wire and flush the incision.

1.6.3 Clinical Applications

Clinically, when the screw is inserted to fixate the fracture, it is not necessarily along the posterior aspect of the iliac spine to the anterior and posterior iliac spine. According to the different forms of the humeral fracture, the insertion direction of the screw on the acetabulum can be adjusted to make the screw and the fracture line. Pressurization of the fracture end is formed vertically (Fig. 21.29).

For crescent-shaped fractures, the prone position can be used to fix the fracture from the posterior and forward screws (Fig. 21.30).

When the iliac screw is placed in the upper area of the acetabulum, the anterior annulus is fixed between the anterior and posterior iliac spine and placed along the upper acetabular sac (Fig. 21.31). For posterior ring fixation or lumbosacral fixation, the humeral nailing point is located in the anterior superior iliac spine, and the target direction is the anterior superior iliac spine or the upper acetabular rim (Fig. 21.32).

1.6.4 Summary

The upper acetabular channel is anatomically wide, and the placement of the screw is relatively safe. The advantage of the robot-assisted insertion screw is that when the fracture is fixed by the compression screw, the optimal position can be placed according to the fracture shape to obtain a

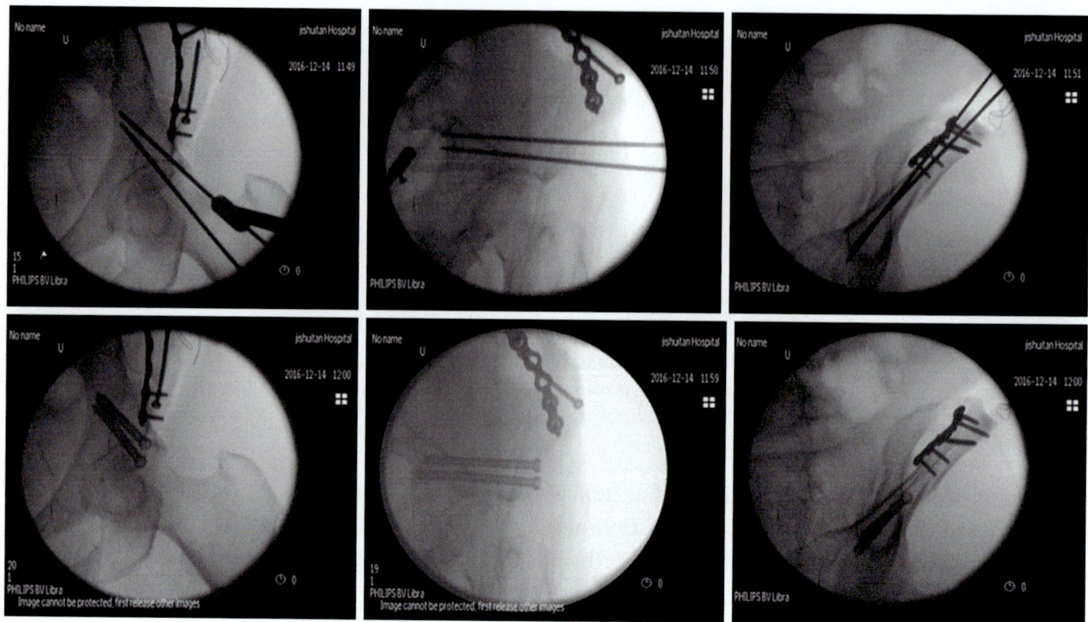

Fig. 21.29 After the reduction of the iliac fracture, according to the fracture morphology, the cannulated screw guide wire was placed percutaneously, and two screws were placed to make the screw perpendicular to the fracture line

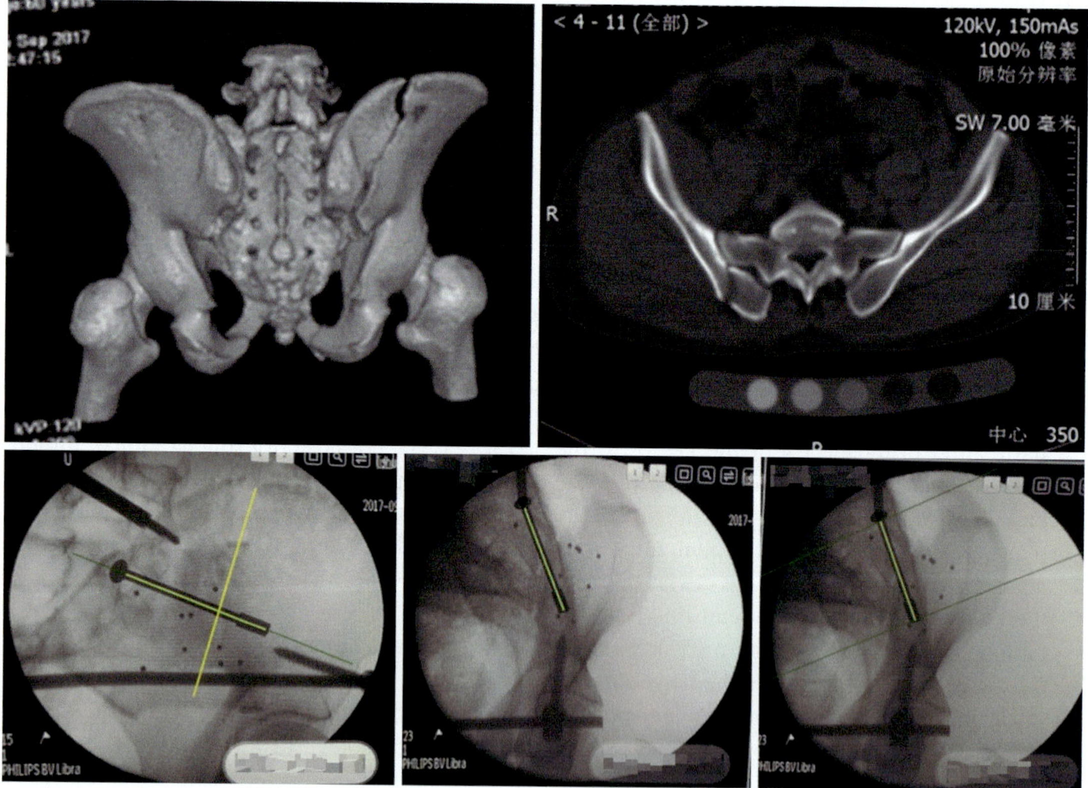

Fig. 21.30 Intraoperative planning of the crescent fracture and image after screw placement

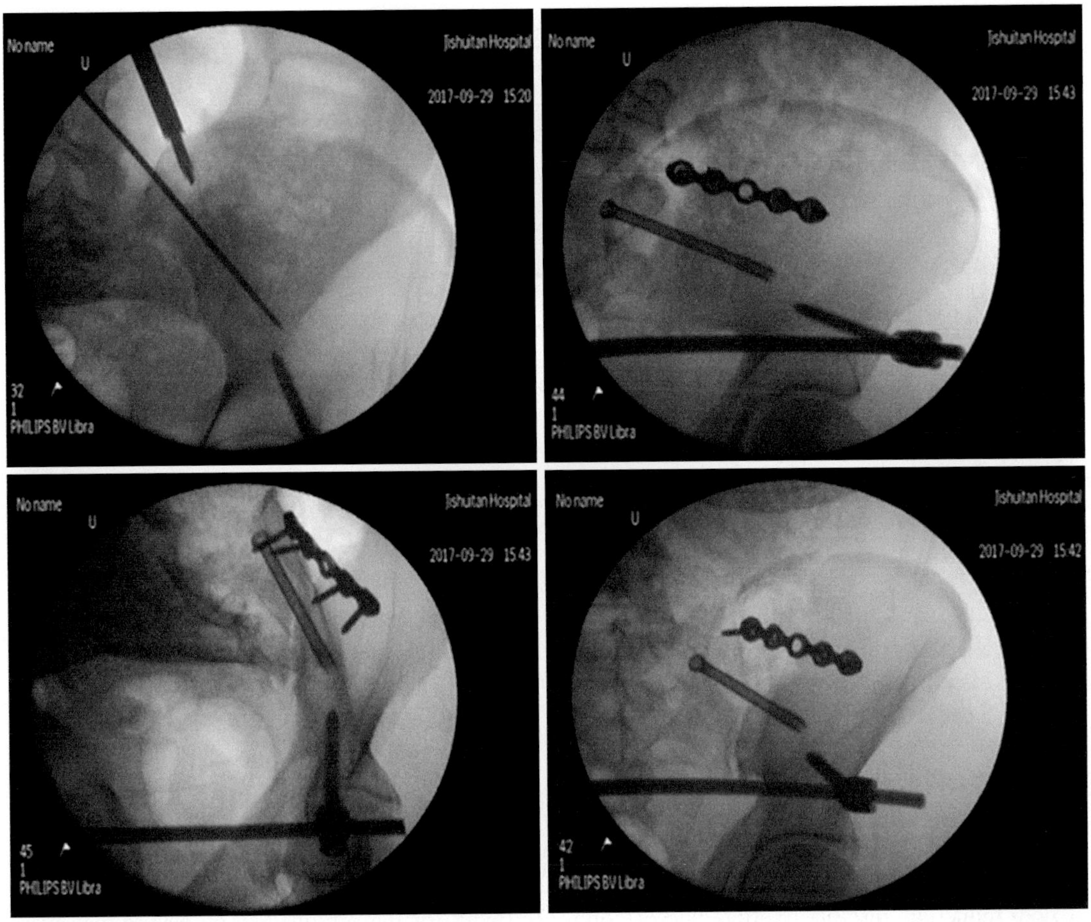

Fig. 21.30 (continued)

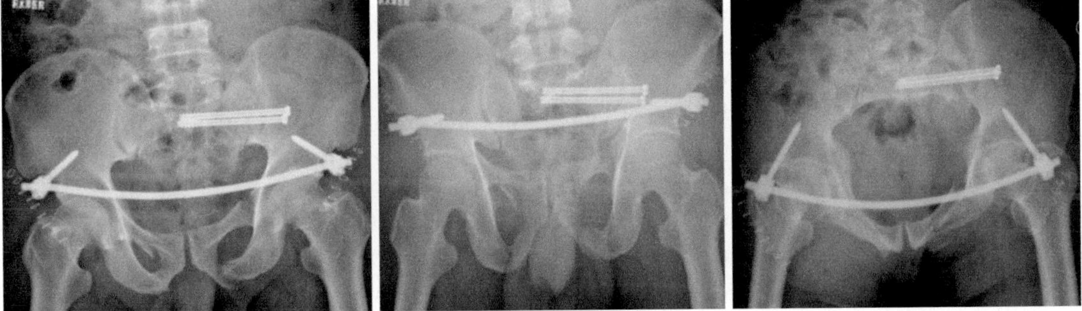

Fig. 21.31 The anterior annulus of the pelvic fracture was fixed with INFIX. The robot-assisted humeral nail was placed on the acetabular upper channel, and the posterior ring injury was fixated with a robot-assisted sacroiliac joint screw

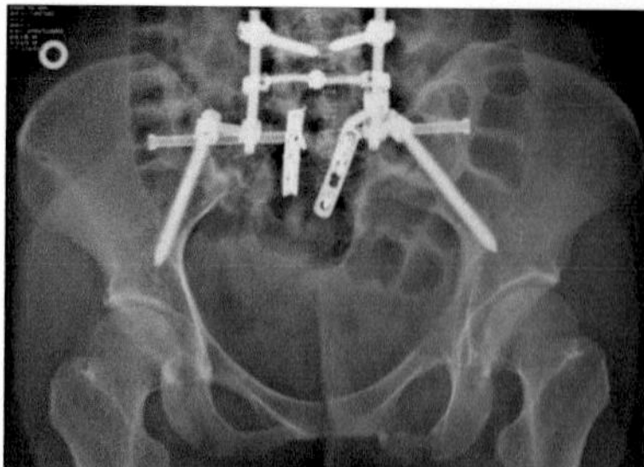
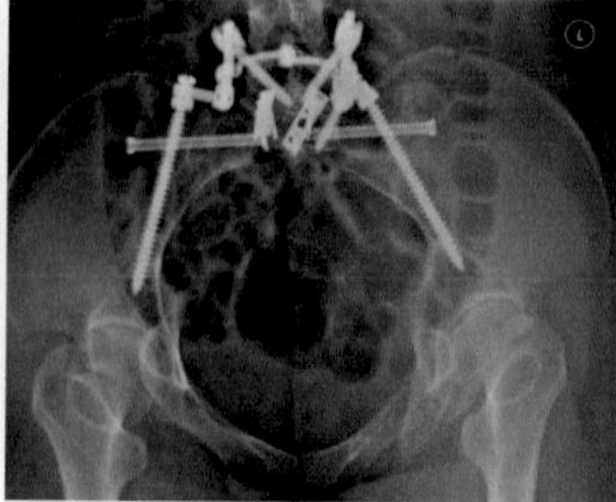
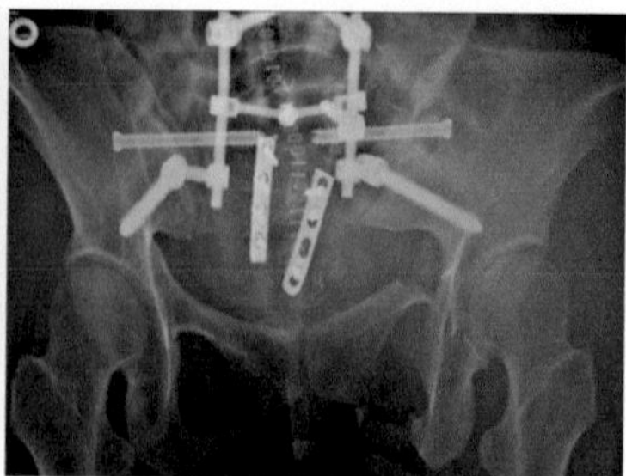

Fig. 21.32 In patients with pelvic fractures, the posterior ring injury is a humeral H-shaped fracture. The lumbosacral fixation and bilateral sacroiliac joint screw fixation are used. The tibial screw and the iliac screw are assisted by the navigation robot. The iliac nail is accurately placed to ensure that the direction is correct and enough length to obtain the control strength

stable fixation. Use long screws to increase stability when the iliac screw holds the pelvic ring in a stable position.

2 Robot-Assisted Femoral Neck Fracture Percutaneous Screw Internal Fixation

2.1 Background

Femoral neck fractures are the most common type of hip fracture, approximating 53%. Factors such as poor reduction, instable fixation, and osteoporosis can lead to many postoperative complications (Thiele et al. 2007). Slobogean GP showed that the incidence of avascular necrosis was 14.3% and nonunion was 9.3% after femoral neck fracture. In addition, the postoperative complications of femoral neck fracture are evident, of which varus shortening accounted for 7.1%, internal fixation failure accounted for 9.7%, and infection accounted for 5.1% (Slobogean et al. 2015). In the United States, annual problems associated with femoral neck fractures cost about $10 billion (Schmidt et al. 2005). Therefore, femoral neck fractures have higher requirements for treatment.

Minimally invasive reduction and internal fixation is an important method to treat displaced femoral neck fractures in recent years. Schep et al. found that the precise position and orientation of intraoperative fixation screws are closely related to the stability of the fracture and whether it is re-displaced and the healing of the fracture. Accurate screw placement ensures that the fixation of the fracture is more secure and can be effective to reduce the incidence of surgery-related complications (Schep et al. 2004). Ideal screw placement requires a good reduction of fracture in the anteroposterior and lateral fluoroscopy images, while reducing the number of adjustments of the pre-guide wire and the drill before the screw is placed, which can reduce the incidence of iatrogenic fractures induced by multiple insertions of the guide wire (Gurusamy et al. 2005). However, due to the instability of manual operation and the inability to perform real-time perspective during surgery, it is difficult for the orthopedists to ensure that every screw is in an ideal position. At the same time, doctors, patients, and related surgical personnel are exposed to radiation for a long time, causing greater damage to the bodies.

There are many treatments for the femoral neck, such as DCS, DHS, plate–screw fixation, and joint replacement. Although many studies have pointed out that the biomechanical stability of plate–screw fixation is the most stable (Aminian et al. 2007). Due to the large damage to patients, for the current treatment of young femoral neck fractures, most orthopedic surgeons still use cannulated screws to fix them. After the screw was placed, the head end of the cannulated screw was located within 5 mm below the cartilage of the femoral head. The cannulated screw was considered to have cortical support within 3 mm of the femoral neck from the cortical bone. However, there is so much difficulty to realize ideal screw placement by manual operation.

Computer-assisted orthopedic surgery refers to a new technique for improving intraoperative vision and improving operational accuracy through navigation systems and robotic devices while surgically operating. It has been considered a clinical advantage in the past few years (Nolte and Beutler 2004). In vitro simulated surgery using a cannulated screw to fix a femoral neck fracture demonstrated that the computer-assisted orthopedic surgery system significantly improved the parallelism and the dispersion of the screws in the femoral neck (Wang et al. 2011). Beijing Jishuitan Hospital has a wealth of experience in the use of biplanar navigation robots to assist the placement of femoral neck cannulated screws. The specific procedure of the procedure will be described below.

2.1.1 Preparation

Patient was placed on the traction bed after anesthesia. Attach the feet to the traction bed and pull the affected limb along the longitudinal axis of the body.

2.1.2 Reduction

Under fluoroscopy, closed or limited open reduction method can be used to restore anatomical structure of femoral neck. The tracker and the optical navigation camera were used to track the spatial variation of the surgical site in real time, and the accuracy is less than 0.3 mm.

2.1.3 Preparation of the Robot

When disinfection and drape was finished, move and fix the robot to the appropriate position next to the operating bed to ensure that the robotic arm working space is up to the operative region. The optical tracking camera, which was used to track the spatial variation between patient and robotic arm in real time, was placed on the foot side of the patient, and the C-arm was put on the opposite side of the surgeon.

2.1.4 Image Collection and Registration

A Schanz wire was placed in the anterior superior iliac spine of the affected side, and patient tracker was fixed on it. Cover the robot arm with sterile protective sleeve, and then assemble the robot tracker and tap ruler. The image including marking points was obtained and transmitted to the master workstation software for registration.

2.1.5 Surgical Path Planning

Master workstation planning software used the AP view and lateral view of femoral neck to confirm screw channel, based on typical identification points and bone marker structure. The surgical planning must consider the safety and the optimal mechanical distribution of screws. Screws should be between the upper and lower cortical boundaries of the femoral neck on Ap view image and between the anterior and posterior cortical boundaries of the femoral neck on lateral view image. Based on the premise of no penetration, disperse the screws as much as possible to provide better biomechanical stability. The length of the screws depend on the tip apex distance (TAD) (Fig. 21.33).

2.1.6 Mechanical Arm Operation

The operation posture of the robot arm is simulated by using the robot arm posture simulation module in the planning software. The control software of the main control system controls and monitors the robot arm to move along the planned path to the target position after confirming the posture of the robot arm is suitable for subsequent operation. Install the guide sleeve at the end of the robot arm, and the positioning principle of the guide sleeve is as follows: (a) Guide sleeve should always move in the clean area, leaving enough working space. (b) Leave room for the surgeon to implant the guide wire. (c) Ensure real-time tracking guide sleeve and patient tracer by optical tracker to facilitate real-time monitoring accuracy.

2.1.7 Guide Wire Placement

Make a small incision at the entry point, and then separate the subcutaneous tissue gently. Insert the sleeve until it touches the cortical bone. Verify that the entry point and direction of the virtual guide wire conform to the plan, and if not, the doctor can fine-tune the path through the robot. Through the perspective after the guide sleeve

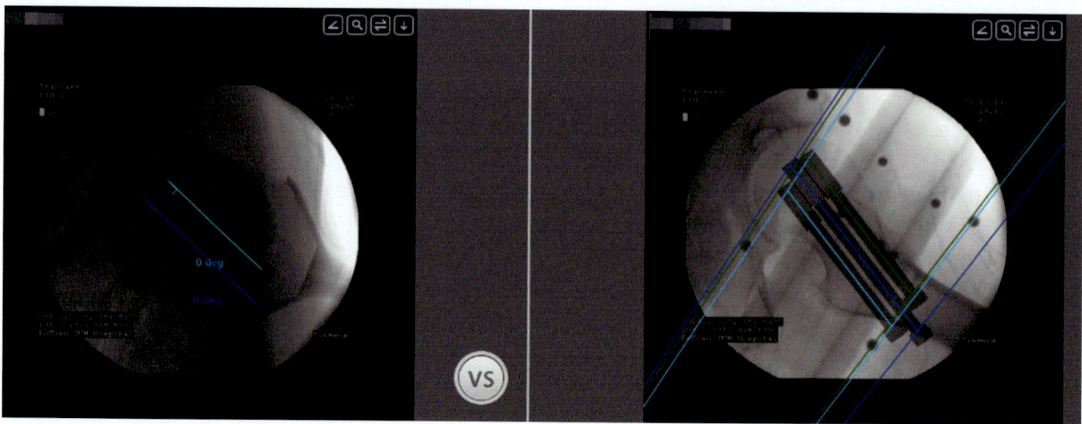

Fig. 21.33 Navigation robot operating platform shows planned screw placement, screw length, and parallelism between screws

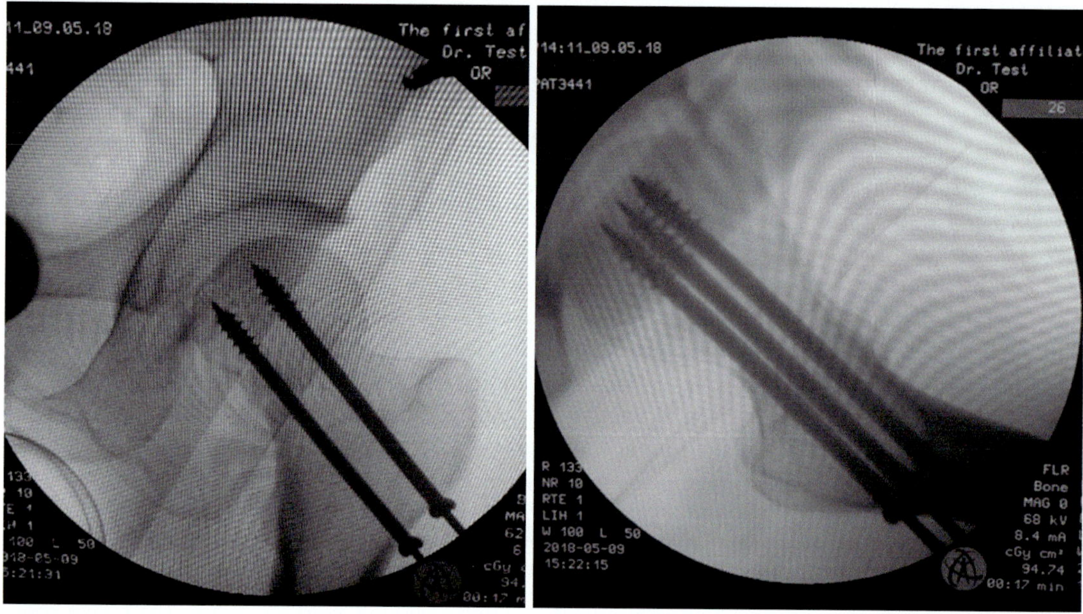

Fig. 21.34 Navigation robot-assisted placement of three inverted triangular cannulated screws intraoperative images

contacts the bone surface, the AP and lateral view images are verified to ensure that the implant path is consistent with the planned path. The guide wire is drilled into the bone channel through the sleeve under fluoroscopic monitoring after the path was confirmed correctly.

2.1.8 Screw Placement and Verification

Place the cannulated screws along the guide wires. Confirm the position of screws again (Fig. 21.34), and then pull out the guide wire. Flush and suture the wound.

The reduction and internal fixation techniques for the treatment of femoral neck fractures should be strict, and orthopedic surgeons should have good 3D anatomy and radiology concepts. It is difficult for surgeons to ensure that every screw is in an optimal position, due to the visual errors of human visual inspection and the instability of manual operation. At the same time, because of the limited size of the femoral neck space, frequently adjustment guide wire and screw in conventional surgery may cause local osteoporosis and even iatrogenic fractures. At present, the use of navigation technology allows the surgeon to see the position of the guide wire and the femoral neck more intuitively during surgery. The number of guide wire adjustments obtained by Müller et al. in 2012 using the 3D navigation system (the average adjustment of each guide wire is about three times) and average operation time is 38.0 min (Muller et al. 2012), but photoelectric navigation still has human instability. The use of a biplanar robot can perfectly provide the ideal planned path to the surgeon through the robotic arm. From January to April 2016 in Jishuitan Hospital, 30 cases were treated with biplanar navigation robot-assisted femoral neck cannulated screw placement, and a total of 90 screws were placed according to the statistical data, in which only one guide wire was adjusted, the average fluoroscopy time was 5.7 s, and the average screw placement time was 12.7 min, while the fluoroscopy time for conventional cannulated screw placement in the hospital was 28.3 s (Zhao et al. 2006). It can demonstrate that the use of the biplanar robot-assisted cannulated screw insertion can achieve accurate replacement, without multiple adjustments, and can reduce the fluoroscopy time.

There are also shortcomings in the biplanar navigation robot system: (1) Because the navigation robot system needs to collect preoperative images and connect with related instruments and equipment, the preoperative preparation time will be too long. (2) Because the iliac bone needs to be placed with an optical tracker, it will cause some damage to the patient. (3) The spatial error of the 2D navigation robot is 0.3 mm. However, during the actual operation, the mechanical arm may be too close to the patient, and the soft tissue may cause a certain blockage, which will cause a slight deviation that can be adjusted by the fine adjustment function again. (4) Because the channel provided by the mechanical arm is outside the body, when the guide wire passes through the cortical bone of femoral neck and femur moment, the small elastic deformation may cause the guide pin to deflect in the bone due to the harder bone barrier, resulting in deviations in the original planning direction, which require the surgeon to have aplenty surgical experience and adjust it in time throughout the operation. At present, the robot system is relatively expensive, and the operation cost is higher than that of the conventional surgery.

References

Altman DT, Jones CB, Routt ML Jr. Superior gluteal artery injury during iliosacral screw placement. J Orthop Trauma. 1999;13:220–7. https://doi.org/10.1097/00005131-199903000-00011.

Aminian A, Gao F, Fedoriw WW, Zhang LQ, Kalainov DM, Merk BR. Vertically oriented femoral neck fractures: mechanical analysis of four fixation techniques. J Orthop Trauma. 2007;21(8):544–8. https://doi.org/10.1097/BOT.0b013e31814b822e.

Azzam K, Siebler J, Bergmann K, Daccarett M, Mormino M. Percutaneous retrograde posterior column acetabular fixation: is the sciatic nerve safe? A cadaveric study. J Orthop Trauma. 2014;28(1):37–40. https://doi.org/10.1097/BOT.0b013e318299c8fb.

Bastian JD, Jost J, Cullmann JL, Aghayev E, Keel MJ, Benneker LM. Percutaneous screw fixation of the iliosacral joint: optimal screw pathways are frequently not completely intraosseous. Injury. 2015;46:2003–9. https://doi.org/10.1016/j.injury.2015.06.044.

Crowl AC, Kahler DM. Closed reduction and percutaneous fixation of anterior column acetabular fractures. Comput Aided Surg. 2002;7(3):169–78. https://doi.org/10.1002/igs.10040.

Eastman JG, Routt ML Jr. Correlating preoperative imaging with intraoperative fluoroscopy in iliosacral screw placement. J Orthop Traumatol. 2015;16(4):309–16. https://doi.org/10.1007/s10195-015-0363-x.

Giannoudis PV, Tzioupis CC, Pape HC, Roberts CS. Percutaneous fixation of the pelvic ring: an update. J Bone Joint Surg Br. 2007;89:145–54. https://doi.org/10.1302/0301-620X.89B2.18551.

Gurusamy K, Parker MJ, Rowlands TK. The complications of displaced intracapsular fractures of the hip: the effect of screw positioning and angulation on fracture healing. J Bone Joint Surg Br. 2005;87(5):632–4. https://doi.org/10.1302/0301-620X.87B5.15237.

Hinsche AF, Giannoudis PV, Smith RM. Fluoroscopy-based multiplanar image guidance for insertion of sacroiliac screws. Clin Orthop Relat Res. 2002;395:135–44. https://doi.org/10.1097/00003086-200202000-00014.

Judet R, Judet J, Letournel E. Fractures of the acetabulum: classification and surgical approaches for open reduction. Preliminary report. J Bone Joint Surg Am. 1964;46:1615–46.

Jung GH, Lee Y, Kim JW, Kim JW. Computational analysis of the safe zone for the antegrade lag screw in posterior column fixation with the anterior approach in acetabular fracture: a cadaveric study. Injury. 2017;48(3):608–14. https://doi.org/10.1016/j.injury.2017.01.028.

Lang JE, Mannava S, Floyd AJ, Goddard MS, Smith BP, Mofdi A, et al. Robotic systems in orthopaedic surgery. J Bone Joint Surg Br. 2011;93:1296–9. https://doi.org/10.1302/0301-620X.93B10.27418.

Letournel E, Judet R. Fractures of the acetabulum. Berlin: Springer-Verlag; 1993.

Li J, Wu T, Xu Z, Gu X. A pilot study of post-total knee replacement gait rehabilitation using lower limbs robot-assisted training system. Eur J Orthop Surg Traumatol. 2014;24(2):203–8. https://doi.org/10.1007/s00590-012-1159-9.

Matta JM. Fractures of the acetabulum: accuracy of reduction and clinical results in patients managed operatively within three weeks after the injury. J Bone Joint Surg Am. 1996;78(11):1632–45.

Mouhsine E, Garofalo R, Borens O, Wettstein M, Blanc CH, Fischer JF, et al. Percutaneous retrograde screwing for stabilisation of acetabular fractures. Injury. 2005;36(11):1330–6. https://doi.org/10.1016/j.injury.2004.09.016.

Muller MC, Belei P, Pennekamp PH, Kabir K, Wirtz DC, Burger C, et al. Three-dimensional computer-assisted navigation for the placement of cannulated hip screws. A pilot study. Int Orthop. 2012;36(7):1463–9. https://doi.org/10.1007/s00264-012-1496-7.

Nolte LP, Beutler T. Basic principles of CAOS. Injury. 2004;35(Suppl 1):S-A6–16. https://doi.org/10.1016/j.injury.2004.05.005.

Ochs BG, Gonser C, Shiozawa T, Badke A, Weise K, Rolauffs B, et al. Computer-assisted periacetabular screw placement: comparison of different fluoroscopy-based navigation procedures with conventional technique. Injury. 2010;41(12):1297–305. https://doi.org/10.1016/j.injury.2010.07.502.

Puchwein P, Enninghorst N, Sisak K, Ortner T, Schildhauer TA, Balogh ZJ, et al. Percutaneous fixation of acetabular fractures: computer-assisted determination of safe zones, angles and lengths for screw insertion. Arch Orthop Trauma Surg. 2012;132(6):805–11. https://doi.org/10.1007/s00402-012-1486-7.

Routt ML Jr, Kregor PJ, Simonian PT, Mayo KA. Early results of percutaneous iliosacral screws placed with the patient in the supine position. J Orthop Trauma. 1995;9(3):207–14.

Routt ML Jr, Simonian PT, Mills WJ. Iliosacral screw fixation: early complications of the percutaneous technique. J Orthop Trauma. 1997;11:584–9. https://doi.org/10.1097/00005131-199711000-00007.

Routt ML Jr, Nork SE, Mills WJ. Percutaneous fixation of pelvic ring disruptions. Clin Orthop Relat Res. 2000;375:15–29. https://doi.org/10.1097/00003086-200006000-00004.

Salari P, Moed BR, Bledsoe JG. Supplemental S1 fixation for type C pelvic ring injuries: biomechanical study of a long iliosacral versus a transsacral screw. J Orthop Traumatol. 2015;16:293–300. https://doi.org/10.1007/s10195-015-0357-8.

Santos ER, Sembrano JN, Mueller B, Polly DW. Optimizing iliac screw fixation: a biomechanical study on screw length, trajectory, and diameter. J Neurosurg Spine. 2011;14(2):219–25. https://doi.org/10.3171/2010.9.SPINE10254.

Schep NW, Heintjes RJ, Martens EP, van Dortmont LM, van Vugt AB. Retrospective analysis of factors influencing the operative result after percutaneous osteosynthesis of intracapsular femoral neck fractures. Injury. 2004;35(10):1003–9. https://doi.org/10.1016/j.injury.2003.07.001.

Schmidt AH, Asnis SE, Haidukewych GJ, Koval KJ, Thorngren KG. Femoral neck fractures. AAOS. Instr Course Lect. 2005;54:417–45.

Schweitzer D, Zylberberg A, Córdova M, Gonzalez J. Closed reduction and iliosacral percutaneous fixation of unstable pelvic ring fractures. Injury. 2008;39:869–74. https://doi.org/10.1016/j.injury.2008.03.024.

Shiramizu K, Naito M, Yatsunami M. Quantitative anatomic characterisation of the pelvic brim to facilitate internal fixation through an anterior approach. J Orthop Surg (Hong Kong). 2003;11(2):137–40. https://doi.org/10.1177/230949900301100206.

Slobogean GP, Sprague SA, Scott T, Bhandari M. Complications following young femoral neck fractures. Injury. 2015;46(3):484–91. https://doi.org/10.1016/j.injury.2014.10.010.

Stephen DJ. Pseudoaneurysm of the superior gluteal arterial system: an unusual cause of pain after a pelvic fracture. J Trauma. 1997;43:146–9. https://doi.org/10.1097/00005373-199707000-00037.

Stockle U, Hoffmann R, Nittinger M, Sudkamp NP, Haas NP. Screw fixation of acetabular fractures. Int Orthop. 2000;24(3):143–7.

Stöckle U, König B, Hofstetter R, Nolte LP, Haas NP. Navigation assisted by image conversion. An experimental study on pelvic screw fixation. Unfallchirurg. 2001;104:215–20. https://doi.org/10.1007/s001130050717.

Templeman D, Schmidt A, Freese J, Weisman I. Proximity of iliosacral screws to neurovascular structures after internal fixation. Clin Orthop Relat Res. 1996;329:194–8. https://doi.org/10.1097/00003086-199608000-00023.

Thiele OC, Eckhardt C, Linke B, Schneider E, Lill CA. Factors affecting the stability of screws in human cortical osteoporotic bone: a cadaver study. J Bone Joint Surg Br. 2007;89(5):701–5. https://doi.org/10.1302/0301-620X.89B5.18504.

Tile M, David H, et al. Fracture of the pelvic and acetabulum. Philadelphia: Lippincott Williams & Wilkins; 2003.

Vigdorchik JM, Esquivel AO, Jin X, Yang KH, Onwudiwe NA, Vaidya R. Biomechanical stability of a supra-acetabular pedicle screw internal fixation device (INFIX) vs external fixation and plates for vertically unstable pelvic fractures. J Orthop Surg Res. 2012;7:31. https://doi.org/10.1186/1749-799X-7-31.

Von Keudell A, Tobert D, Rodriguez EK. Percutaneous fixation in pelvic and Acetabular fractures: understanding evolving indications and contraindications. Oper Tech Orthop. 2015;25(4):248–55. https://doi.org/10.1053/j.oto.2015.08.007.

Wang JQ, Zhao CP, Su YG, Zhou L, Hu L, Wang TM, et al. Computer-assisted navigation systems for insertion of cannulated screws in femoral neck fractures: a comparison of bi-planar robot navigation with optoelectronic navigation in a Synbone hip model trial. Chin Med J. 2011;124:3906–11. https://doi.org/10.3760/cma.j.issn.0366-6999.2011.23.014.

Wang MY, Wu XB, et al. Fractures of the acetabulum(骨盆髋臼骨折). Beijing: Beijing Science and Technology Press(北京科学技术出版社); 2016. p. 131–3.

Wong JM, Bewsher S, Yew J, Bucknill A, de Steiger R. Fluoroscopically assisted computer navigation enables accurate percutaneous screw placement for pelvic and acetabular fracture fixation. Injury. 2015;46(6):1064–8. https://doi.org/10.1016/j.injury.2015.01.038.

Wu T, Chen W, Zhang Q, Zheng ZL, Lyu HZ, Cui YW, et al. Biomechanical comparison of two kinds of internal fixation in a type C zone II pelvic fracture model. Chin Med J. 2015;128:2312–7. https://doi.org/10.4103/0366-6999.163377.

Zhao CP, Wang JQ, Yu W, et al. Experimental study of biplane orthopedic robot system-assisted cannulated screw fixation for femoral neck fracture(双平面骨科机器人系统辅助股骨颈骨折空心螺钉内固定术的实验研究). Chin J Orthop Traumatol(中华创伤骨科杂志). 2006;8(1):50–5.

Zhao CP, Wang JQ, et al. Computer navigation assisted minimally invasive treatment of acetabular fracture(计算机导航辅助下髋臼骨折的微创治疗). Chin J Orthop Traumatol(中华创伤骨科杂志). 2011;13(12):1116–20.

Zhao CP, Wang JQ, et al. Robot assisted percutaneous screws in the treatment of acetabular and pelvic fractures(机器人辅助经皮螺钉治疗髋臼骨盆骨折). J. Peking Univ (北京大学学报). 2017;49(2):274–80.

Zwingmann J, Konrad G, Kotter E, Südkamp NP, Oberst M. Computer-navigated iliosacral screw insertion reduces malposition rate and radiation exposure. Clin Orthop Relat Res. 2009;467:1833–8. https://doi.org/10.1007/s11999-008-0632-6.

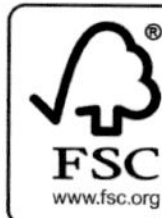

MIX
Papier aus verantwortungsvollen Quellen
Paper from responsible sources
FSC® C105338

If you have any concerns about our products,
you can contact us on
ProductSafety@springernature.com

In case Publisher is established outside the EU,
the EU authorized representative is:
Springer Nature Customer Service Center GmbH
Europaplatz 3, 69115 Heidelberg, Germany

Printed by Libri Plureos GmbH
in Hamburg, Germany